WORKING THE ROOTS

Over 400 Years of Traditional African American Healing

WORKING THE ROOTS

Over 400 Years of Traditional African American Healing

By Michele E. Lee

J. Douglas Allen-Taylor
Editor

WADASTICK PUBLISHERS
Oakland, California

TABLE OF CONTENTS

AUTHOR'S INTRODUCTION

African American traditional medicine, like jazz and the blues, is an American classic that emerged out of the necessity of its people to survive. It's a fusion of African, Native American, European and other healing traditions associated with the period of colonization and slavery in the United States. *African American* traditional healing is STRONG MEDICINE.

Working the Roots: Over 400 Years of Traditional African American Healing is a book that honors the ancestors who survived the Middle Passage and preserved the healing traditions. It also honors all who carry on those traditions today in its diverse and expanded forms.

Working the Roots is the culmination of a collection of first-hand interviews, conversations, and apprenticeships I experienced with over 20 traditional healers mainly in the southern region of the United States. It chronicles my sojourn to the land of my ancestors in search of their medicinal knowledge and their prescriptions for healthy living.

I gathered the majority of this information over the course of six years, from 1996-2002. Four of those six years I lived in rural North Carolina down a dirt road. It is here where I would experience the holistic foundation of Black American culture—the spiritual connected to the physical connected to the mental connected to the entire community.

I started this journey by interviewing the elders on both sides of my family from Louisiana and Mississippi. I used a tape recorder and a 35 mm camera to document, and learned how to ask open-ended questions so that the healer could talk freely while sharing the knowledge and experiences through the many stories. I was led to other healers by word of mouth, much like the discipline is passed down.

Working The Roots is presented in two parts: Part I: The Narratives and Part II: The Ailments and Medicines. Not all of the people I interviewed or worked with are represented in the collection of narratives in Part I. However, their healing knowledge is incorporated in the section following the narratives, Part II: The Ailments and Medicines.

I am eternally grateful to everyone I interviewed. This book could not have happened without their generosity and willingness to share.

Our ancestors had vast medical knowledge and spiritual strength that gave us the resilience to survive our predicament in slavery and colonization. *Working The Roots* is rich with herbal and naturopathic remedies that were used to treat and cure many ailments from the common cold, pneumonia, bronchitis and fevers to arthritis, measles, high blood pressure, cuts, wounds and more. It also contains routines for preventive health maintenance that are still applicable today. Many of these routines and philosophy of preventive healing were brought across the ocean from the African continent, and have been nurtured for half a millenium between the American shores.

Also included in the book are peoples' experience with that special blend of spirit-work and medicinal work that comes directly out of the African religious tradition and is known by various names on the American continent: rootworking, conjuring, hoodoo, vodoún, voodoo, Santería, and so forth.

The healing narratives in Part I are presented in the following six chapters: 1) The Southeast; 2) The Mississippi Valley And West; 3) Strong Medicine (includes Native American healing traditions by themselves along with the rich blending of African American and Native American traditions, bloodlines and shared history); 4) Spirit Work (conjurin, hoodoo, juju, voodoo and goofering narratives); and 5) Coming Full Circle (three people who have rekindled the healing tradition of their ancestors after two to three generations of its absence in their families). Images accompany each narrative.

The various medicines, remedies, disease preventions, health maintenance regimens, and conjure and hoodoo remedies in Part II are presented as an historical and educational reference for several hundred specific treatments, many with images and detailed instructions for what people did to prevent illness, cure illness when it occurred, and maintain good physical and spirit health. The portion of the book contains all of the information gathered from the interviews in Part I and organizes it in an easily-accessible index form. Part II also contains a Guide to Cultural Terms and a Glossary of Medical Terms.

Working The Roots can be read in three distinctly different ways.

You can follow the narratives in the order they appear in the book, as you would any story. It was written as a journey, following the slave trade from Africa across the Atlantic, crossing the American continent from the southeastern sea coast to the Pacific shores, and concluding with the wisdom of those who reached back in time to recapture and preserve the original teachings.

Alternatively, you can use the book as a guide to learn about a particular medicinal or spirit-practice that was used, learn the properties of the medicines, where to find them, and how they were best prepared. Also, you can follow the interesting stories of those who have the knowledge and did or still do the practices.

Or finally, you can experience *Working The Roots* at random, opening the book to whatever particular person or practice might interest you at any given time.

However you choose to experience *Working The Roots*, I truly thank you for reading this book. I hope you can hear your elders and ancestors talking to you. They knew what they were doing and their knowledge can help us live holistic and healthy lives today.

Michele Elizabeth Lee

ACKNOWLEDGEMENTS

I thought it would take me four or five years to write *Working the Roots*. Now, some 20 years later, I finally have a story, a slice of history, a body of work that I hope makes a peoples' history (those people being African Americans) a little more complete. And now that the work is completed, I want to thank the many, many people who have supported me through this process.

Two decades have passed since I started *Working the Roots* in 1996. The world is so different and few are living who have real-time memory of those horrific eras long gone—slavery and Jim Crow—and what the African American had to do to stay healthy and survive. First and foremost, I thank the elders and traditional healers who agreed to share their wisdom and stories with me. Many of them have crossed over by now. Had I started this book today, it would not have rendered the same information. Their names, as well as the names of all I interviewed, are listed in Part II of this book.

My family has been my biggest support, morally and financially. There is a running joke that we have about how long it has taken me to complete this project. Many in my family think I have two books written or that it is a never-ending project. Those people in my family who I wish to thank for my support are: my children and my ex-husband, Leon Dockery, Milon Lee-Dockery and Nora Irene-Elizabeth Dockery; my mother and father, Beverly E. Lee and the deceased Edward Oliver "Pete" Lee; my aunt and uncle, Dr. Jem Hing Lee and Frankie Hutchins-Lee; my sister-cousin Yacine Bell, aka Earlene Anne Perry (and her daughters); my brothers Eric and Keith Lee and sister-in-love, Kimberly Bankston-Lee; my favorite cuttys of all time, Lonnie Paul Poindexter, James Allen Gordon, III, and Robert Ware; and my "other mother" Mary Lovelace O'Neal.

Next I'd like to thank my first editors, readers and researchers: Jacqueline Luckett, Asual Aswad, Brian Bers, Roxie Mason, ToReadah Mikell, Itta Aswad, Asha Ransom, and Lauren Westerschulte. To the numerous friends and other relations who have been cheering this effort to completion for many years I am eternally grateful.

My Editor, Jesse Douglas Allen-Taylor, has been invaluable. I am eternally grateful to him for his selfless commitment over the past five years to see this project to completion. He gets the importance of this. His particular-ness about things (which he bluntly calls being anal) has made *Working the Roots* the best it could be. To my impatience he once answered, "the Cubans have a saying: 'we go slow because we are in a hurry.'" It eased many impetuous feelings that threatened to overcome me. This book is as much his as it is mine, and we turn it over to everyone.

Finally and of supreme importance, eternal gratitude for the Divine Creator, the Mistress and Master of the laws of the universe, the God and Goddess, the Great Father and Mother spirit who planted the idea for this book in my head 20-something years ago. Through the peaks and valleys, I have persevered!

For our ancestors, our elders elders, and the generations that carried
this holistic science through and beyond the Middle Passage.

PREFACE

Working the Roots: Over 400 Years of Traditional African American Healing represents a small window into the immense knowledge, perseverance and ingenuity that came into being when two great cultures came together on the continent of North America beginning in the seventeeth century and continuing down through this day. This book contains a small portion of the medical expertise that enslaved Africans brought from their homeland and blended with the knowledge of the healing arts they found already present among the indigenous people of America. The two cultures were compatible on many levels and eventually their bloodlines mixed, resulting in a people blended at the edges and creating a more powerful combined healing discipline.

This intermixed pool of Black and Red healing practices was enriched by the addition of folk medicine knowledge and practices adopted from the European colonizers.

For African Americans especially, these self-care practices were essential for survival during colonization, slavery and Jim Crow. But Blacks, the Indians, and Whites all used traditional healing not only because it was cheaper and they were excluded from mainstream health care, but because IT WORKED! It was something they could trust.

Traditional healers are as varied in their methods to healing as doctors are today. Their common thread is that they respect the spirit-mind-body connection and embody a holistic approach to their healing discipline. Many of their natural healing remedies include using roots, herbs, bark, animal by-products, natural oils, minerals, and other resources in a creative and diverse array of forms and combinations. Laying hands on a person to massage and move energy in addition to prayers and affirmation was also a part of the healing regimen and could be used independently or with the medicine traditional healers prescribed.

Hexing, juju, conjuring, goofering, or putting roots or a spell on someone for good or bad is also a practice used by many rootworkers. Those who use these particular practices are the alchemists of the African American healing traditions and use the spirit world, unseen natural forces, elements and root and herb combinations to work their magic.

Most families relied on one person as their primary consultant amongst the recognized community of great healers or rootworkers in their vicinity. This community of experts sometimes shared remedies, asked advice and consulted with each other. No one owned the knowledge or the medicine. These traditional healers knew the curative properties of the medicines they used, and understood that one remedy may work for one person but not the next. Using the wrong plant, remedy combination or dosage could do some serious damage. Keeping the community healthy was of prime importance.

African American traditional healing was a science that was passed down by word of mouth in families over the course of generations. Folks who practiced this medicine had a preventive philosophy "to be as strong and healthy as you can be so you won't get sick."

Unfortunately, many folks abandoned this philosophy and the use of traditional healing during the Great Migration[1] to the northern states. They often shed their "old timey" ways for what they felt was sophistication and modernization. "My children moved up North and aren't interested in this old medicine," is a phrase you hear often among the traditional healers who remained in the South. Thus, the chain was broken.

And many of the ones who stayed in the South weren't interested either. Tragically, the practice was not passed down for two, three, even four generations in some families. "When you die, you take that knowledge with you." These are the wise words of Ms. Sally McCloud, and many of the elders I interviewed echoed the same sentiment. They all wished they had asked more questions growing up but, "We didn't ask questions back then." Often folks I interviewed would say, "All of the people who really knew the roots are gone."

In my own family, two generations passed before traditional healing was rekindled again by me. By

---

[1]   The Great Migration was the movement of over one million African Americans out of the rural southern United States from 1914 to 1950. African Americans moved to escape the problems of racism in the South and to seek out better jobs and an overall better life in the North.

the time I realized how valuable those healing practices were, my great-grandmother, Fortuna Pijeaux had crossed-over at the age of 94, taking most of her knowledge with her.

Unfortunately, much of the knowledge of my great-grandmother and other traditional healers was not recorded. We will never know how much we lost as a people, but we certainly can begin recording what is left, asking questions and sharing the information with each other that we were either fortunate or foresighted enough to retain.

It's been over one hundred years since African Americans began the Great Migration out of southern fields to northern cities, and nearing two hundred years since the forced migration of Native American tribes out of the Southeast to what was called the "Indian Country" of Oklahoma (an atrocity known as the Trail of Tears). Sadly, many people in the Black and Native American communities all across the nation now suffer from chronic health problems like high blood pressure, diabetes, heart disease, alcoholism and obesity. These are killers! All of the healers I interviewed admitted that these chronic illnesses did not plague their communities when they were growing up in the South. One healer commented that diabetes and heart disease was something you read about in a book.

This critical health crisis is largely attributed to the continuing legacy of colonization and slavery and the consequences of living in an urban environment, an inequitable society, unhealthy diets and lack of exercise. Also, abandoning the "ol' timey" preventive health maintenance routines that kept immunity up and the body strong has been greatly underestimated and has also compromised peoples' health. One of the purported benefits of taking regular doses of cod liver oil is that it supports and strengthens the immune system. Many abandoned this practice after leaving the South. Could it be that taking those regular doses of cod liver oil helped keep colds, flu and other illnesses at bay?

Even though the traditional healing practices of African Americans are not as prevalent as they were in the past, they are by no means disappearing. Some folks did bring the tradition up North (both healing and root working) and blended and expanded it with knowledge from other cultures. Today, more and more people are taking control of their health and searching for safe and holistic alternatives to Western medicine or for traditional health practices that can complement Western medicine. Many are going back to their roots, remembering what their parents and grandparents did and considering whether they should be doing some of the same things today for their health.

A healthy diet, exercise, seasonal tonics, colon cleansings, and that daily dose of cod liver oil are just a few preventive and health maintenance routines people are incorporating into their lives today. These routines were also a staple in African American healing traditions. Cod liver oil (fish oil) is rich with Omega 3's and is similar to the flaxseed oil used in many traditional and doctor-based medicines and healing regimens. Taking seasonal doses of castor oil, senna tea or eating chalk or clay has similar effects as colon cleansings. Yellow root, the wonder herb that boosts your immunity, "cleans yo blood out" and "sets your body right," is the same as goldenseal.[2]

Traditional African American healing is an integral and important part of American history, much like the Revolutionary War, Emancipation Proclamation, Blues, Bluegrass, Powwows, Jazz, Suffrage, and Civil Rights. This discipline kept Blacks, Native Americans, and Whites healthy and strong during the tenuous development of our country.

For example, 18th century historical accounts of the introduction of the practice of smallpox innoculation in America state that it was an enslaved African named Onesimus who showed his "master," the Reverend Cotton Mather, how to innoculate against the disease. This eventually led to a successful vaccine that saved millions of lives. Before a vaccine, smallpox killed close to half a million people each year in Europe in the 1700's. And Boston's worst smallpox epidemic, 1721-1722, infected over half of the 10,700 population and killed 844. Africans had used this ancient practice well before the Europeans came during the slave trade. Smallpox came to North America on the many ships that brought the colonists to New England in the 1700's. The Native Americans of the Western Continents, already fighting for their land and against colonization also had to contend with this foreign disease which decimated many tribes. Tragically, the majority of people died from this disease, either from coming in contact with someone already infected or from the smallpox infected blankets given to them

---

[2] Flaxseed oil, colon cleansings, and goldenseal are all a staple of modern medicine, both as practiced by holistic healers and Western doctors.

by the U.S. Army as a part of their genocidal germ warfare strategy.

The African saying, "It takes a whole village to raise a child," is also appropriate for, "It takes a whole village to heal a community." In this spirit, *Working the Roots: Over 400 Years of Traditional African American Healing* is dedicated to remembering the healing traditions of our ancestors and to everyone who is on the path to healthy living.

May we continue to preserve and share our ancient knowledge to heal humanity and all life on Mother Earth. Remember that our ancestors speak to and through us.

PART I: HEALING NARRATIVES

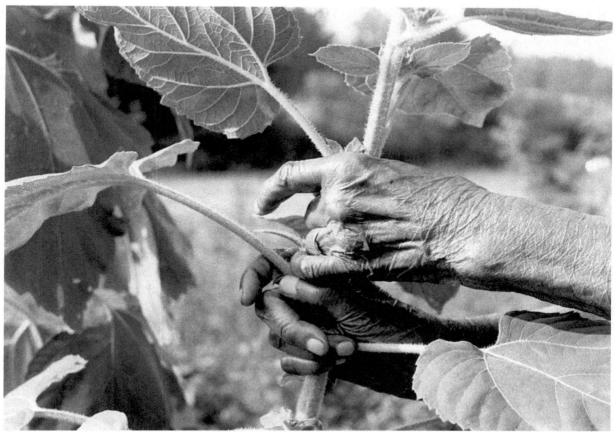

Hands of Ms. Sally McCloud
Image I-1

"Yeah, they kep that kettle on in the winter time. Kep it made up, strained out. And when one of us gets a cough, maybe once or twice, they go in that icebox and get that medicin. They say 'come on.' Don' care how bitter it was or how sweet it was, you had to drink it. And they didn't carry us to no doctor neither. Didn' have to. Didn' have no money to pay no doctor. We had to try to keep groceries here, pay bills. No, we didn' have no money to throw away like that. Thank God we made it."
Ms. Sally McCloud, Sand Hills region, Laurel Hill, North Carolina

1

Chapter 1 - Reclaiming Our Natural Healing Tradition

Introduction

The Southern region of the United States is hurricane country. Periodically, these massive monsters of water and wind come howling out of the depths of the Atlantic to pounce upon the fragile coastline of these states and to batter, break, and subdue the land beyond.

The great African American novelist and anthropologist Zora Neale Hurston, a child of Eatonville near Florida's eastern coast, best described a hurricane's effects in her 1937 novel *Their Eyes Were Watching God*:

"The wind came back with triple fury and put out the light for the last time. ... [T]he wind and water had given life to lots of things that folks think of as dead and given death to so much that had been living things. ...But above all the drive of the wind and the water. And the lake. Under its multiplied roar could be heard a mighty sound of grinding rock and timber and waters and timber and a wail. ... [T]he muttering wall advanced before the braced-up waters like a road crusher on a cosmic scale. The monstrous beast had left his bed. The two hundred miles an hour wind has loosed his chains. He seized hold of his dikes and ran forward until he met the quarters; uprooted them like grass and rushed on after his supposed-to-be conquerors, rolling the dikes, rolling the houses, rolling the people in the houses along with other timbers. The sea was walking the earth with a heavy heel."

But hurricanes are not engines of destruction only. In nature, they serve to clear away the old growth, making room for new life underneath, giving it the chance of exposure to sun and opportunity to build a new landscape. In much the same way, the Atlantic slave trade was a human-generated hurricane that blew away the old divisions among the captives crossing the ocean in the Middle Passage—family, tribe, kingdom, and language differences—and forced those enslaved millions to seek out things that were common among themselves. Out of that great storm was forged a people the world had never seen before, the people we now know as African American.

One of the elements of that blending was the creation of a natural healing regimen that combined the knowledge and experiences of the enslaved Africans with that of the indigenous peoples of their new land. This new system of prevention, therapy, and cure was deepened as many of the captives left the English-protestant Southeastern U.S., crossed the hills of Kentucky and Tennessee, and the fields and forests of Georgia and Alabama, and settled into the French-Catholic lands of the lower Mississippi Valley.

The first series of interviews in this collection follow that journey from the Southeast into the Lower South, with the descendants of those captive Africans describing the original African American healing practices that were handed down to them.

The Southeast

North Carolina, South Carolina, and Georgia were three of the major American slave ports-of-entry of the 17th and 18th centuries. The African captives brought with them vast traditions of healing knowledge and practices that had been building over the millenia since the dawn of humanity. These healing traditions rooted themselves in the southeastern coastline, quickly adapting to the new plant life and radically altering social life. This happened even as the captives themselves began shedding their old tribal identities and merging and forming themselves into a new people – the African Americans. From the plantation lands around Wilmington, Charleston, and Savannah, the traditions spread out north, south and westward, varying from east to west due in part to plant habitation and availability.

The following narratives are from interviews and relationships I had with healers from Georgia and the Carolinas, the overwhelming majority being from North Carolina.

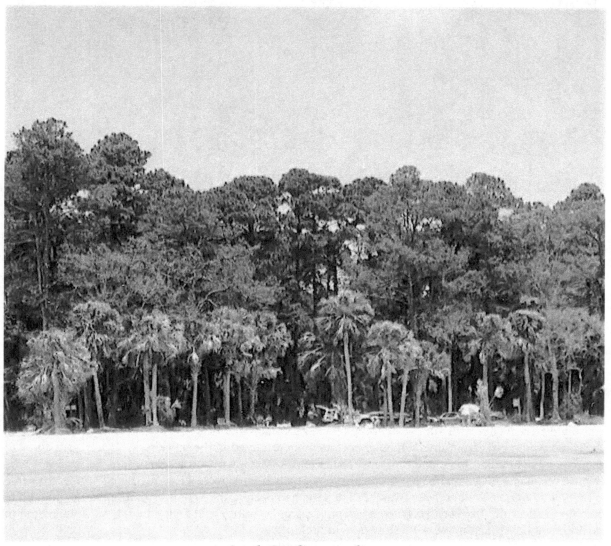

South Carolina coastline
Image I-2

Ms. Sally McCloud - *"I don't want this tradition to die out"*

Born July 17, 1910, North Carolina

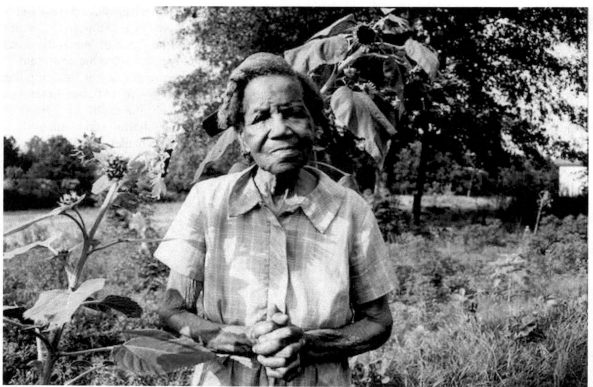

Ms. Sally McCloud
Image 1-1

When I first arranged to interview Ms. Sally McCloud in her home in Scotland County, North Carolina, folks had difficulty giving me directions that I could understand.

With an overall population of around 36,000 inhabitants[3], Scotland County sits on the South Carolina border far from the state's major urban centers of Charlotte, Greensboro, and the Raleigh-Durham area. While the county has five towns (Laurinburg, Gibson, Maxton, Wagram and Laurel Hill), Ms. McCloud lived in a community not claimed by any one of them, a nebulous area called the Sandhills. Local folks described the Sandhills as somewhere on the outskirts of the town of Laurel Hill, about 12 miles east of the "big city" of Laurinburg (the county seat), along NC Highway 74—the Andrew Jackson Highway.

I was unfamiliar with the area and all the long country roads looked the same to me. Besides that, except for the major highways and roads, no one remembers the name of any little street unless it's the one they live on. I was sure I'd miss an important landmark, make the wrong turn and end up in an entirely different county or state. I'm going to need a guide.

Three young girls from my own neighborhood where I lived in the outskirts of Laurel Hill agree to accompany me. Duke, Janie and Step are related to Ms. McCloud. At the time of this interview, Duke (whose real name is Daisy, like her mother) and her cousin Janie were 11, while Step (whose real name is Stephanie), Duke's older sister, was 12. The girls had been to the Sandhills before but not enough to be able to show me the way, so Duke and Step's parents, Bobby and Daisy Lee, have volunteered to escort us in their truck, while we follow behind in mine.

The ride to Ms. McCloud's house is long and beautiful. Every road is a picturesque landscape filled with pine and oak woods, farmland, or meadows accentuated with wild flowers and the majestic old oak or walnut tree. Homes are few and eventually, the further we drive, non-existent.

---

[3] Based on the 2010 federal census.

4

The final road to Ms. McCloud's house is a long five mile stretch that snakes through the countryside. We drive around the last curve through a patch of woods on the right. To the left is a field dotted with a variety of bottles on stakes. Plastic liter bottles hang loosely by string so that they swing in the wind; glass coke bottles and other miscellaneous containers, are strewn across five acres of unkempt farmland. Thin weeds and vines hug the bottom half of the stakes and the clumped bottles claim the top. Remnants of the previous year's farmed collards and corn grow wild and are randomly scattered across the field.

About 100 yards past the bottle field, a narrow dirt road barely eases out to the paved road we were traveling on. It's easy to miss if you don't know where you are going, but I'm with good guides. We turn left down the dirt road and drive about one half of a mile until we come to the authentic country home of Ms. Sally McCloud. It takes a full 35 minutes to get there from Laurel Hill.

Bobby and Daisy point to the house, turn their truck around, and leave. Duke, Step, Janie, and I are now on our own.

We walk through a modest sized garden with large sunflowers and other weeds and plants before we get to the house. It's a cute little wooden A-frame with a screened-in front porch. Four wooden steps that curve in upon themselves, sinking in the middle, lead to the porch's screen door. I open the door and step inside. Two more steps at the far end of the porch lead up to the front door of the house.

I knock on the door and there's no answer.

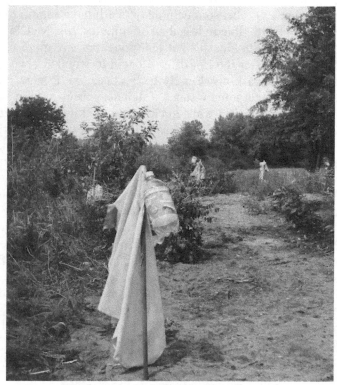

Bottle trees in Sally McCloud's yard
Image 1-2

We open the door, go inside the house itself, and I call out, "Ms. McCloud? You have visitors. Hello? Is anyone home?" It's dark inside and difficult to see since we just came in from the bright outside. A frail woman makes her way to us from the back of the house.

"Well I declare. And who are ya'll?"

"I'm Michele. Your brother, Mr. Red . . . "

"Hhhhhmmmm humph." She nods in acknowledgement.

" . . . sent me over here to ask you some questions about using the root medicines. . . "

"Did he now?"

"Yes ma'am. You know, the medicines from the woods."

"Yeeess, yeesss. I know them medicines."

Ms. McCloud looks toward the girls, whom I've not introduced yet.

"These are your grand nieces," I tell her.

"Iz they!"

The three girls stand there, smile demurely, and don't know what to make of Ms. McCloud.

"Hhhmmmm Humph! Ain't they pretty . . . they got long hair. And I'm their Ant!" Ms. McCloud declares this last with the satisfaction of knowing her bloodline continues.

I stay inside with Ms. McCloud while the girls return to the porch, where they decide to stay our entire visit. The three are normal precocious teenager wannabees. Step is dark brown and stands tall, slender and awkward, with an elegance waiting to blossom in another three or four years. Janie is a short, thick, sumptuous Mae West type with "high yellow" skin tone. Every child comes in with a gift from the other side. Hers is a natural sensuality that hopefully she will come to understand and use well.

Duke, brown like her sister Step, is the tomboy; a combination of both Step and Janie. She is tall, buxom, strong, tough and has a sassy mouth without the seductive flare of Janie's.

We chat for a while about preliminary things in that old Southern way before getting down to the reason I've come all the way out there: to talk about healing.

"Buttongrass is good for colds, you make a tea wit it," Ms. McCloud was saying. "My mother used to give us this during school. Wouldn't know it if I saw it, but my mother, you know, like when chil'ren be going to school, she use it for that. Of course all mothers along in there did it. Stay out the doctors office too. Pills cost so much today! Ya'll have sumtin to eat?"

For the fifth time in less than 30 minutes, Ms. McCloud offers Duke, Step, Janie and I something to eat or drink. She doesn't get many visitors any more or the chance to spoil them with her Southern hospitality. After the last offer, I begin to wonder if we are offending her by saying, "No Ma'am, but thank you for asking" Finally I say, "Yes, we'll have some water, please." Delighted, Ms. McCloud gets up to get us some water. I watch her shrunken, thin body shuffle from her cozy living room, which is about the size of a walk-in closet, to the kitchen. Old folks have a way of moving their feet without lifting them too far off the ground. Perhaps they instinctively know that they have more time behind them than ahead of them (here on Earth) and want to make sure their feet stay firmly planted on Earth energy. Lifting them too high off the ground may signal they are ready to fly.

"Do you need some help?" I ask as I get up and follow Ms. McCloud toward the kitchen. Allowing an elder to carry four glasses of water for young visitors is not in my upbringing. Also, I wanted to see the kitchen and whatever else was back there.

The kitchen was no more than four steps from my seat in the living room, and just as cozy. Ms. McCloud struggles to find four clean glasses amongst the dirty dishes piled in the sink, on the counter and on top of the old gas stove. A big propane tank sits off the back side of her house and feeds the old stove the gas it needs to fire up. To the right of the stove on the opposite wall is an old-fashioned cast iron pot belly stove. It's blackened from years of double duty heating and cooking before the gas stove arrived to relieve it. A rusty pot sits on top and a big pipe, just as blackened, extends from the top of the stove through the ceiling to the roof. I notice the once-white walls are dingy gray, and are particularly dark near the iron oven. "Does the pot belly stove work?" I ask.

"Oh Yeesss. That's what I use to keep warm in the winter. My son, Pete, chops me wood to burn."

"Does it warm up the whole house?" I ask wondering how the heat gets to the other rooms.

"Yeesss!" she answers It gets too hot sometimes. I close off part of the house and I only stay in this area." Ms. McCloud sweeps her hand in a circular motion to include the kitchen, the two small rooms off the back of the kitchen, and her little living room.

Her bedroom is behind the wall that supports the pot belly stove. I can only see a portion of it from where I am standing but I have a clear view of the small room catty-corner to the kitchen.

I feel Ms. McCloud can feel my sincerity and curiosity so I take a chance and ask her if she would let me into her personal space. "Can I see your bedroom?" She answers with her movement and shuffles over to her bedroom. I follow close behind. Though it can barely hold the furniture that fills it, the room looks much larger, open and brighter, from the inside. A full size bed with a beautiful wood headboard centers the room. An old-fashioned hand-made quilt covers the bed and an open Bible rests on the side, waiting to be picked up again. A small nightstand with an equally small night light sits to the left of the bed, with a matching six drawer dresser topped by an ornately carved mirror positioned on the opposite side. Miscellaneous odds and ends, stacks of paper, an old magazine and a hairbrush with a fine tooth comb straddled in its middle accessorize the top of the dresser. The only picture in the room is on the center of the wall right above her bed: a White Jesus with dirty blond straight hair and sad, piercing blue, puppy dog eyes. They watch my every move. I stare back and contemplate the layers of contradiction that cause so many Black homes to still accept the idea of a White Jesus as the son of God. The stare stand-off is broken as midday's summer sun/son shines through the only window in her room and catches my eyes. The rays bounce off the white walls and illuminate the entire space making it feel celestial and warm. The sun is the centerpoint of our existence here on Earth. Without it, we will cease to exist in our current state. Like Earth's sun, Jesus—the Son of God—is the center-point of Christianity; Christians believe that without Jesus, there is no life.

I breathe deeply and decide not to go through my full progression of inner thoughts with her, I declare only its conclusion. "Your bedroom is so beautiful."

She smiles at me, but whether it was in response to my compliment or whether she didn't hear it but was only being polite, I would never find out.

We return to the porch with the water, and Ms. McCloud immediately puts the girls to work shelling peas. As we sit down to begin our interview, she picks up a small can next to her chair and spits dark brown saliva into it. She's had snuff tucked away the entire time. Soon snuff dippin', spittin', pea shellin', a cacophony of bugs humming and young potent female hormones smothered by humid Southern air, become the sweet sounds and aroma of our visit. It's the end of July in rural North Carolina: hot, humid, sticky and insects singin' their relief song.

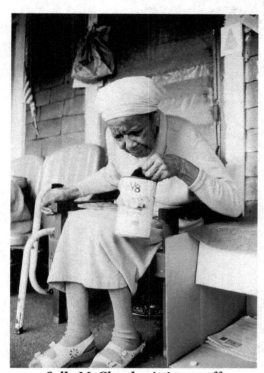

Sally McCloud spitting snuff

Image 1-3

I take out the tape recorder and put it on the table next to my chair.

"What is that?" Ms. McCloud asks.

"This is a tape recorder." I respond. "I want to learn about using the herbs and roots you use and your mama used when you were growing up. I'm writing a book."

"Is yah?"

"Yes ma'am. I don't want this tradition to die out because when you pass on . . . "

"… you carry that with ya." Ms. McCloud understood exactly where I was going and finished the sentence for me.

"I was raised down there near Baysville Church," she begins her story. "That's where my father and mother was stayin'. It's goin' towards Laurel Hill. My mama and my father raised us. My mama was Indian. Some of the knowletch about the medicines came along from the two of them.

"Yeah, they kep that kettle on in the winter time. . . kep the medicines made up, strained out and when one of us gets a cough, maybe once or twice, they go in that icebox and get that medicine . . . they say 'come on' . . . don't care how bitter it was or how sweet it was, you had to drink it . . . and they didn't carry us to no doctor neither . . . didn't have to . . . didn't have no money to pay no doctor. . . we had to try to keep groceries here, pay bills . . . no, we didn't have no money to throw away like that . . . thank God we made it.

"I got a brother down in there now," she says, referring back to Baysville Church. "Luther Stelly."

It's difficult to understand her thick Southern accent, and I lean forward to make sure I can pick up all the words. It's a sound of blended tones that undulates high and low pitches, drawls to a fade and then picks up again. I get lost in this song and hear no words, only the beautiful patois of Black diction, the drylongso from which we were all raised. It's the vibratory tone that matters, not the enunciation. This tone was the oral tradition that taught Black folk family matters: morals, respect, discipline, community, spirituality, strength, patience, faith, education, creativity, resourcefulness, endurance, resilience, determination, foundation, discretion, negotiation, medicine, good health, and taught us how to live successfully in two worlds.

I turn her mind back to the brother she mentioned, Luther Stelly, "You mean Mr. Red?" I ask. "He's the one who told me I should come talk to you about some of the old time medicine," I remind her. She suffers from Alzheimer's, and so her recall of her younger years is better than that of recent experiences.

"Yeah! Red that's what we called him." An excitement comes to Ms. McCloud's demeanor when I say "Mr. Red." I knew her brother and I knew what friends and family called him.

"Yeah Red," she reminisces again in a deep resounding voice. Those two words, "Yeah Red," unleash moments from her youthful days when she and Red were young and full of fresh, sustainable memories. I can tell on her face that she held those times close; they were real and then they were gone.

"Now who are these youngin?" She sees Duke, Step and Janie in the corner shelling peas and doesn't remember who they were.

"They're your grand nieces; your brother Red's grandchildren." I re-introduce them to her for the second time since we arrived.

"Iz they?" She responds with exuberance to know Luther Stelly and she have such fine looking descendants.

Then Ms. McCloud asks, "And where's their mother?"

She knows the important questions to ask, not where the parents are or the father, but quite pointedly the mother, bearer and carrier of life. I explain to her as simply as I can that their mother, Daisy Lee lives in Laurel Hill and is married to their father, Bobby, who is Red's first born child and Ms. McCloud's nephew.

"Sure nuf." She comments with satisfaction of knowing. "Well I'll say. These iz my grand nieces. Stelly's grand children. Yes they iz!"

My own family is related as well. Red (Ms. McCloud's brother) married Annie (Bobby's mother), who is the sister of my children's grandmother, Pearlie Mae, and that's how my children are related, through marriage. Leon, who is my children's father, and Bobby, who is Aunt Annie's, son are first cousins. And, Granny (Nora Dockery,) after whom we named my daughter, is Annie's mother, Red's mother inlaw and grandmother to all the children.

"I bet you don't know how old I iz," Ms. McCloud declares.

"No, I don't."

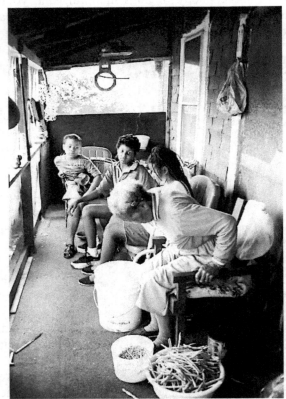

Shelling peas on Sally McCloud's porch
(l-r Janie, Step, Duke, Ms. McCloud)
Image 1-4

"Be 86, the 17th. July 17th is my birthday! Ain't come yet is it?"

"Nope."

"God Bless."

The sound of freshly shelled garden peas pours into a plastic bucket and draws Ms. McCloud's attention away from our conversation and toward the girls. Duke, Step and Janie stand up to stretch their bodies and put their hands on their hips to signify they are finished with this task, then bring the bucket of shelled peas next to Ms. McCloud. "Hhhhmmmm humph. Yeessss!" One could hear the satisfaction in Ms. McClouds voice. "Oh, they done shelled out! I reckon I have to give ya a few of 'em to let cha carry 'em home wit cha. You so nice to help me shell 'em. My son brought these up here to me." My young escorts are pleased that Ms. McCloud is pleased and don modest smiles of a job well done. Then one by one they saunter off the porch to the outside yard. I redirect the conversation back to the root medicine hoping Mr. Alzheimer will free her medicine knowledge for a moment.

"When you go out in the forest to find your medicines, do you go around here?"

"Sometimes I can find it around here. . . I got some friends over on the other Laurel Hill Road, they knows it. And, I just gotta get me some . . . yellow root. . . You know it?"

"No ma'am, I don't know it. Yellow root?"

"Hhhhmhumph. Yellow root . . . like yellow the color . . . gotta get me some. . . it's good for jus' 'bout anything . . . it cleans your blood, hmmmmhumph. . . you know your blood gets filthy and the yellow root sets the body good. . . if I had some here, I'd show it to ya . . . I'd let you see some . . . I ain't got none now . . . I done boiled up all I had . . . gotta get me some . . . you know where I can get it?"

Ms. McCloud pauses her words but continues to move her hands as if she were still talking about the virtues of yellow root. Her eyes eagerly wait for me to tell her where to get it. I desperately want to help but I don't know what yellow root is and don't know how to get it. We sit across from each other in an awkward silence except for her moving hands which I am increasingly drawn into. Her hands continue the story of her paused words and are full of the information that Mr. Alzheimer holds hostage. Osain[4] hands. Old growth forest hands. Aged tree limb hands that dance poetic lines and posture joyfully against Oya—the sky goddess. No, I cannot focus on words held hostage by Mr. Alzheimer. The land of impregnated ellipsis and dancing hands holds all the medicine knowledge. Somehow, I will have to learn this language to get to the priceless stored information.

"I can drive you over to one of the spots where yellow root grows and you can show me what the tops look like and how to pick it." I excitedly offer as a great idea.

"Yeessss." Ms. McCloud responds in a slow satisfying Southern drawl. "Not today . . . it's hot today . . . maybe on Tuesday . . . if it ain't stormin."

"How often do you drink yellow root?" I ask.

"Anytime you want to go and get it. . . see, it ain't got no alcohol in it. . . this is what kept me strong. . . it brought me a long ways. . . 'cause I went to the doctor about two months ago for the first time in 20 years . . . this is true 'cause I jus' slacked off my herbs . . . I was feelin' kina bad and I stay by myself . . . he gave me a prescription . . . I had it filled and I guess it helped me . . . he said I'm in pretty good shape. . . I told him I wasn't what I once was 'cause I'm old . . . nothin' lives forever . . . If I live to see the 17th . . . that'll be next Tuesday. Lawd! Lawd! I've seen an awful lot of changes."

"What else did you use for health and healing besides yellow root?"

"We used boneset for colds . . . it's a kind of real thin weed. . . calamus for colds too . . . I just mix it all together and its good for colds . . . Boneset, calamus and yellow root. . . if I get one first, then I save it until I can find some of the other ones . . .when I get all three of 'em . . . I put it all together then boil it and strain it out, sit it in the frigidaire and I just drink it when I need it. . . kept me goin' good 'til here of late.

"You can find all of these up in this place," she says, meaning up in the woods. "Boneset and calamus is a weed and yellow root is a root. It got a top. That's the only way I can find it by the top of it. It grows up and you can get the root. They say the root is better than the top. But the top is just as green as the root is yellow. And, you can break it and see the root, that's how I finds it. When I get a streak in the woods, I break it to see if it's yellow. That's it. I use all of it. I don't throw the tops away, the tops just as good as the root. I chop up all of it and boil it down. And, I don't make it all at one time. I make some of it and then I tie it up and save it and let it dry and if I need it again, or somebody else need some of it, I get it and give them some."

"This cleans you out and it's kept me healthy for 86 years . . .I haven't had any cancer or anything like that 'cept old age . . . old age honey, a little older, older and older and I'm still here.

"And that catnip, catnip tea. Yeah, they growed that 'round the house. Catnip was fer if you had a fever, boil that catnip and then drank it.

"We used the bark and the sap off of cherry trees for energy. Boil it and strain it off and set it where it won't sour. It's just like water, like medicine. See a lot of people would put whiskey in it. But I didn't. I just set it in the frigidaire and kep it cool like that. When I want it, I get a drink and that would be about every mornin.' I'd take me a good drink of that and I hadn't been to the doctor in over 20 years. You hardly see a cherry tree any more. It got a lot of medicine in it."

"Maybe they're choppin them down to make furniture?" I offer as an explanation.

"Do they?" Ms. McCloud says in a high pitch voiced sounding surprised to learn her medicine tree is being used to make furniture now. She shakes her head in disapproval.

"I don't eat much meat, mostly vegetables, but I eats mostly anything I want. Then keeps me a jar of the medicine in the frigidaire. . . get to feeling a little queer and I go there and get me a good drink

---

[4]　In Yoruba religion and mythology, Osain is the Orisha or saint of all the plants and trees in the forest and woods, the greatest herbalist who knows the power of all the plants. Oya is the sky goddess.

of it and it'll knock it out. This is stuff we used for a long time . . . it's God's medicine . . . God made the roots . . . He made them and we didn't . . . He made them so you don't have to run to the doctor for everything."

Duke, Step and Janie return from the porch outside and Ms. McCloud acknowledges once again their having completed the shelling task.

"I declare, ain't that so wonderful! I thank you girls. I don't got but one chile and they calls him Pete . . . he's in there now . . . I reckon he sleep now. I'm gonna wake him up right befo y'all leave ...let you know him."

Ms. McCloud gets up to awaken her son and introduce us.

"This is my son, Pete Smith."

Mr. Pete is the only one left to look after his mother, as she creeps toward her golden years. He has his own home and family but spends each night at his mother's because "she forgets to turn off the fire on the stove" or "she forgets to eat" or "she forgets to heat the house." Ms. McCloud no longer does mundane well or recognizes multi-generational relations other than her son, Mr. Pete or her brother, Mr. Red. No matter where he lays his head at night, Mr. Pete will rise and shine at 4 a.m. to begin his day as a farmer. What a gratifying life: fresh air; physical work; rewarding work; early to bed and early to rise.

Mr. Pete was born John Robert Smith to John Smith and Sally McCloud-Smith in the year 1929. He was named John after his father and Robert after his uncle. When John Robert Smith was a little boy his nose was always running and crusty. He'd often play in the open fields near his home and wander to his Aunt Beulah's house down the road. Aunt Beulah would see little John Robert playing without a care in the world, oblivious to his drippy, crusty nose. She'd call out to him, "Come here, let me clean that li'l ol' peaty nose," peat being that partly decayed, moisture-absorbing plant matter found in ancient bogs and swamps. John Robert would get his nose cleaned, eat some fresh baked sugar cookies, drink lemonade and then be on his way. After that, every time Aunt Beulah saw him, she'd call him Pete, feed him and clean his li'l ol' peaty nose and the name Pete just stuck with him.

Mr. Pete is one of the remaining few in a legacy of almost 200 years of Black farmers and sharecroppers in the South.[5] He farms in Scotland County, North Carolina and is famous in those parts for being able to grow a good crop every season regardless of too much or too little searing heat, drenching rain, asphyxiating drought or late frost that's infringed upon the summer/spring transition. Mr. Pete looks young for 68, which he attributes to an honest day's work. Each year he works 6 days a week for 9 months of planting, harvesting and selling. His tractor is old and sturdy, much like him. He is a man of few words saying only what he feels is necessary. It's obvious his best communication is with his crops in the field. Mr. Pete tends those crops like he's sweet sixteen and gone courting for the first time. He doesn't abuse his field and ask her to produce more than she should. He rotates his crops and lets fields rest after one season of laborious childbirth. And, he makes sure they are well fertilized before planting again.

Mr. Pete and I exchange cordialities. I tell him why I'm there and ask if I can interview him right now. He agrees, so I turn the tape recorder back on. This interview lasts for a good hour but continues on for another four years, blossoming into a friendship that still exists today.

Mr. Pete allows me into his world as a Black farmer and natural healer. "I grow produce down there at Sneeds Grove," he begins. "It's not my sto'. It's a White guy's sto', but some of the stuff I tend. We work it together on half and we sells a lot of stuff at da sto'. And I sells a lot of stuff right there in the

---

[5]   In 1910, nearly one million Black farmers in the U.S. owned a total of 15 million acres; by 1969 they held only six million acres. In 1920, Blacks owned 14% of the nation's farms; today, there are only 18,000 Black farmers, representing less than 1% of all farms. "The interesting thing about land is that in spite of the fact that we were enslaved, in spite of the fact that share cropping was a quasi form of slavery, between 1865 and 1910 . . . the African American community had acquired approximately 16 million acres of land. Now that's 45 years after slavery when we could not read, could not write, and for all intents and purposes did not know where a college or a university was at. Our ancestors owned more of this country on a per capita basis 150 years ago than we do today." Thomas Burrell, president of the Black Farmers and Agriculturalist Association Inc.

field too. Folks can pick their own bushel and I knocks the price down. So by him havin' the sto', we jus' got a place there where we can sell it when I'm not out here, ya know. And dat helps both of us out. I got probably about 25 acres. Peas, butterbeans, okrey, growing watermelons, cantaloupe, cucumber, corn, but da drought 'bout worked on the corn this year, everybody corn really. I got some of all dat stuff and a good bit of it. I reckon we take a hundred bushels[6] of peas this year. I had to give a guy ten bushels of peas this morning. He must be down dere makin' church. There was a woman yesterday went to two different places lookin' for peas.Couldn't find any 'til she came to me. She gonna take dem back to New York. You cain't get dem up dere."

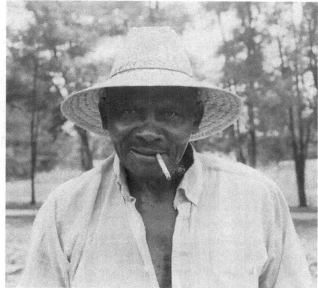

Pete Smith
Image 1-5

The conversation turns to healing and health, and how people in his community handle it.

"When you get sick, folks just got to go to a doctor," Mr. Pete says. They don't know they makin' the doctor rich. Once you go, he gonna wear you out. Keep you comin' back every two weeks; comin' back for those pills and they change up pills on ya. What da doctor doin' when he tryin' all dat kind of stuff, he tryin' to get you hooked. They tryin' to figure it out if they really don't know, but they still getting' money outta ya all da time. I know people went to da doctor and got medicine from da doctor and it didn't do 'em a bit of good. Well, he told 'em to come back and when dey went back, 'Well, I wanna see you again in two weeks.' You see how dat work? Alright, you go back dere in two weeks, well he may change dem pills or medicine on ya and he say again, 'I wanna see you back in two weeks.' Dat doctor got a book dere with everybody name in it. He know jus' how many patients dat he got. He know jus' 'bout how much money he gonna make because he havin' you to come back every two weeks. And he jus' got money rollin' round da clock, round da clock his money is rollin'. I been learnt dat for a long time. I've been learnt dat for a long time because when I was bringin' my chil'ren up sometime you have to carry a chile to da doctor. Some time. But you don't have to carry 'em as much as I see dese younger people doin' now. Now doctors is good for a lot of thangs. You don't wanna die. Well da Lord put 'em here and give dem knowledge in how to go about to do dese thangs, but like I say, a lot of time, dey tryin', dey practicing. I don't like to go to doctors. But jus' like dey try different medicines, sometimes you have to try different weeds and roots to see what's gonna work, but it better for you."

"So what medicines do you use from the woods to stay healthy?" I ask him, and he provides me with a quick list.

"Buzzard weed is a good medicine. Take rabbits tobacco and pine tar with dat buzzard weed, put it all together in a pot, poor water on it and boil it and drink it and that's good for colds, pneumonia, influenza and all dat stuff. It'll jus' cure ya. You can find it right around here. You don't have to go out in da woods. I get some stuff from the woods still but I don't do it as much as when my chil'ren was comin up. I go out and gets stuff for my chil'ren when dey get sick, you know, but since dey grown up, I don't do much getting much stuff like dat now. Sometime if I have a cold, I get pine top and a li'l buzzard weed and rabbits tobacco and boil it and drink it.

"Sassafract," he adds, meaning sassafras. "That's a bush grows out 'round da nape of da woods where da fields and thangs iz. That's good for measles, a child havin' measles. Got to get the red kine of sassafract. The white will run ya blind. They two kines of it. But you peel the bark on it and you can tell whether it red or white. And if it white, don't bother it. Get one dat got a red color to it, like dat

---

6   Bushel: a unit of dry measure for grain, fruit, vegetables, etc. equal to four pecks or 32 quarts.

water down dere under the rine, and dat good for measles.[7]

"Sardines good for mumps. You have to rub them up. Rub the juice and then catch 'em under da chin and den tear it up. That's good for mumps. When we was comin up, this is how we cured it. Now, we didn't go to no doctor. 'Bout the only thang you go to a doctor for is you break a limb.

"Lion's tongue is a good medicine. It's another weed that grow out in da woods like the ones up yonder. A li'l ol' bush dat get 'bout so [6 inches] high and dey jus' be a patch of it. We used to take dat stuff and give it to our mules and cows and thangs. And if they was feelin'sick, it would cure 'em too. You have to boil all dat stuff to get da results out of da stem and root part of it. See, dat's where you got your medicine. You take da root and da stem and da leaves. I learned all of dis from my mother. When she was givin' me dat stuff, I was learnin' then, what it was for and then what they say I had. Den I was learnin what dey givin' me and dat's the way I knew what it is. And it pays to know."

After listening silently all this time while I was interviewing her son Mr. Pete, Ms. McCloud chuckles and adds her words of approval. Mr. Pete continues.

"My chil'ren, dey know when I was givin' dem dat same thang my mama and granma give me. I gives it to my chil'ren and I told dem what I was givin' 'em and what it was for and what dey had. My Uncle Red should have passed it on to Bobby [Red's oldest son] cuz he know. And den Bobby should have passed it on down to his chil'ren. It's got to be handed right on down through the generations in da family. So Red would have passed what he know on down to Bobby, and Annie [Bobby's mother] should know somthin' 'bout dat stuff by her mama and pass it on down to Bobby too. 'Bout all parents were dealin' wit some kind of herbs and stuff."

Mr. Pete goes on with his list of medicines.

"Boneset. I done drunk a many bunch of boneset. It good for colds and draw da fever out. It's good to drink if you got a broken bone; it helps to set it back. Back den, most all da old people, dey have a bush of it and grow it 'round dey house and da yard and stuff like dat. Most all da people had a bush of it and if dey out, dey go to da neighbors and get a lil piece from it and bring it back home and grow dem a big bunch of it. I had it at my house when I was bringin my kids up. I don't have one at my house now, it died. I don't know what really happened to it. I think da dawg destroyed it. That's what I think destroyed it.

"Yellow root is like yellow da color. You go out in da woods and it grows in certain places. I knows where most of it growin 'round here. I don't know yellow
root dat good in the woods. I been talkin' to my mama and got to learn it."

"All you got to do is get in the woods where it supposed to be at and break it, and if its yellow, you can dig dat root up." Ms. McCloud instructs her son.

"I been tendin' to do dat in da winter months when da snakes an thangs ain't so bad," Mr. Pete replies. "I plan to go out with Willie Monroe in Laurel Hill. He knows yellow root, exactly what it looks like. I was gonna learn by him, the color of the bush and everythang and then I will know. He said there's a place on the backroads goin' to Hamlet where it used to grow over there, but somebody knowed it and dey went in dere and dug up all the yellow root. Dug it all up! He couldn't find a lick of it. It grows in beds and certain spots. I hear tell of another place up here on Marston Road back where Curly Morris and dem used to go get dat yellow root. Then Mama was telling me about another place on the other side of Hamlet, there's a spot over there on the left side of the pond, behind the house just built back there, there's a patch of yellow root. But you gotta ask them people in dat house could you look for it. So that stuff grows in certain spots. Maybe we can dig up a good bit of it some durin' the winter month and then make you a bed out of it and take care of it and all and just let it grow and multiply. This winter when it gets cold enough and the snakes goes in, me and him gonna get together and go where it is."

As is common in rural Southern conversation, Mr. Pete's talk begins to wander off into a side path, this one about one of the Deep South's favorite creatures to avoid.

---

[7] An important warning note about sassafras and safrole: Sassafras contains safrole, which is known to have harmful effects if ingested over a period of time in large and concentrated quantities. See warning and instructions in the Sassafras section on pages 319-320 before using.

"Snakes is a real problem in da summer time. Sho is," he says. "They hang around places where they can get water."

Ms. McCloud agrees nodding her head and says, "They got to have water."

"Yep, they got to have water," Mr. Pete says. "All life got to have water."

We talk a little about farming, and I tell him I have been longing to get my hands down in some dirt. He promises me that when I come again sometime, he will certainly put me to work in his vegetable garden. I intend to hold him to his promise.

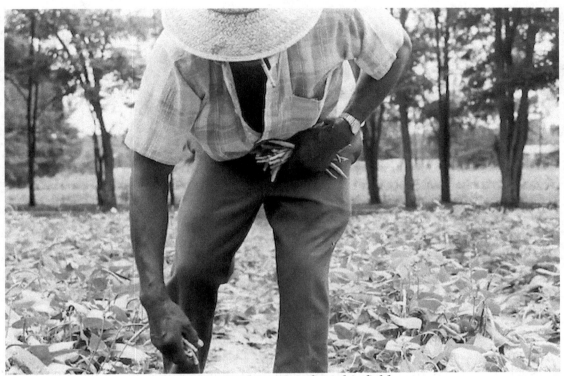

Mr. Pete picking peas from his field
Image 1-6

Romancing the Farm: A Day in the Life of a City Girl Picker

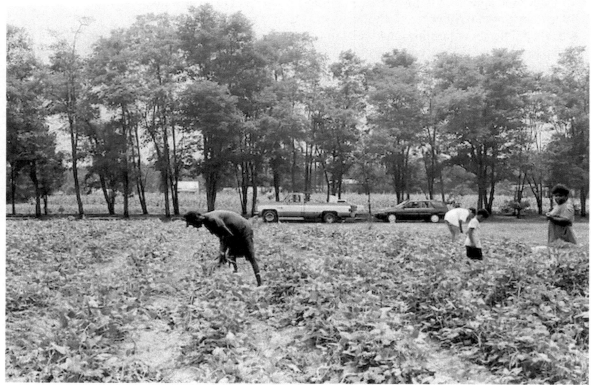

Pickers in Mr. Pete's field
Image 1-7

A couple of days after my first meeting with Mr. Pete, I visited him at his Sneeds Grove farm. Three young people were in the field when I arrived, bent over filling their baskets with a ripe harvest of vegetables. They were part of the group of young local folks ranging in age from 6 to 14 who Mr. Pete hired every year to help pick crops during harvest and selling time. These were from mostly poor Black and Indian families who sent their children out to labor in the fields and earn extra money. Mr. Pete paid them $3.00 for each bushel they picked, then turned around and sold the bushel for $7.00 in the field or $9.00 in the store.

In a way I envied, albeit naively, these young pickers. They worked in fresh air. When it got too hot, their bare feet on the cold, moist, soft soil kept them cool. Their bodies moved all day long and worked out the kinks of stress and stiffness that can accompany city jobs. A physical honest day's work translates into a great sleep particularly in country quiet.

These young souls had endurance and tolerance. They knew how to regulate and preserve their movement within the heat of the day. But how hard could it be, I thought? So, I arranged with Mr. Pete to pick in his field one day. I needed some extra money anyway and didn't want to work in a local factory as a temp as folks my age had advised me to do.

At first Mr. Pete laughed at me and shook his head, but when I continued to insist, he agreed. "Be out heah on Tuesday," he said. "I'll pay you $3 a bushel for peas and okra, bring a long sleeved shirt and wear long pants."

"But it's gonna be hot." I protested about the clothes covering.

"You don't wanna pick okra without any sleeves." That was all he said.

Excited, I rushed back to Granny's house in Laurel Hill, Scotland County's smallest township, where I was staying during my visit. I zoomed down several long country roads and finally turned into the dirt driveway that leads to Granny's cozy, two bedroom home which sits in the middle of her lot of just under an acre.

"Guess what, Granny? I'm gonna pick some peas in Mr. Pete's field and I need to borrow a long sleeve shirt." I proclaimed to her with great exuberance and flair.

"Huuuh, huuuuuh, huuuh, huuuh," Granny bellowed her laugh. "You can have it. I had all the pickin' days I'z gonna have."

Granny had plenty of overdue stories about pickin' cotton by the pound for next to nothing. "Overdue" meaning she hadn't talked about this in a long while and was eager to share and glad someone was eager to listen and learn. She earned no workman's comp, no unemployment, no social security, no minimum wage, no health insurance, no vacation time, no sick leave, no personal leave, no maternity leave, and no retirement. Working from sun-up to sun-down, body bent over all day, in the humid heat of a southern summer and earning $1.00 per one hundred pounds of cotton was nothing to romanticize and get excited about.

One could live well while living poor in Scotland County. Land was inherited or affordable to purchase if you didn't already have it, and the soil was fertile. Underground water springs abounded and a labyrinth of creeks, branches and swamps hydrated this region known as the Sandhills. It is a land of fertile sand, where torrential and frequent downpours rarely resulted in a flood. Instead, rain drops would hit the topsoil and go straight through to the underground water springs. Vegetable gardens were plentiful, salt pork was cheap and turtles, frogs, squirrels, coons, possum and deer were free for the hunting or catching and eating. Poke sallat grew wild as did grapes and walnuts. Nature provided and few went hungry. Winter cold weather was durable without central heat, but most folks had wood stoves or a fire place if they lacked the modern comforts of warmth. Fall and spring seasons were wonderful and perfect. Only summer in the Sandhills was a problem.

Summers were unbearably hot for those who forgot and even for those who remembered that air conditioning is a new "thang." Before air conditioners, most people did not have the luxury to stop working during the heat of the day and seek refuge under a tree that cast a wide berth of shade, fanning oneself. The heat was brutal and stifling. Enslaved Africans and sharecroppers worked on the average 15 hours or more, from sunrise to dark and with only one short break to eat at noon. Eating watermelons cooled and hydrated their bodies, quenched thirst and provided a good source of vitamins, minerals, and electrolytes. Keeping water in clay pots kept the water cool. Cabins, shacks and quarters gave no relief from the heat, as they were either too hot in the summer or too cold in the winter.

For that new generation who never experienced a summer without central air, summers are an indoor affair. The thought of doing anything outdoors during the heat of summer's day is completely out of the question. Work begins at sunrise or shortly thereafter and ends at midday, possibly picking up again in late afternoon as the heat wanes.

Granny, aka Nora-Lee Gay-Dockery is my grandmother-in-law and my daughter's namesake. She has experienced life before central air and now thoroughly enjoys it in the comfort of her own cozy home. Granny has lived in Laurel Hill all her life, just like her parents and grandparents. She says she is half Indian (Lumbee/Tuscarora) ancestry and half African American. The one room shack she lived in with her mother and sister is still sitting, a sturdy lean-to on Sneeds Grove road. It's been hugged by vine and ivy since the family long-since moved away, and more than likely squatted by a den of healthy rattlers. I don't know anyone who would go in there now without an earthmover.

Granny was blessed to bring eight healthy children into this world. One year after Granny's youngest child was born, her eldest, Pearlie Mae, delivered birth to Leon, my children's father. That was in 1958, eighty three years after the end of slavery and the beginning of slavery's own child, Jim Crow. Pearlie Mae was seventeen and hoped to marry the man she allowed to swim in her juices. But this didn't happen. He reneged on his promise and had other plans which didn't include a new wife and a baby boy.

"Mama, there ain't no future here for me. I ain't gonna pick in these fields or work in these factories for slave wages," Pearlie Mae pleaded her intentions. And six weeks after Leon was born Pearlie Mae went to find her grown-up life up North in Piscataway, New Jersey. She left little Leon with her mother, his three uncles, four aunts and crazy Mr. Jake (the man Granny loved to hate) on the promise that Pearlie Mae would come to get him when she got on her feet.

Granny and her kin all lived in a two-room shack on the corner of Archie Bunch's property in the land where the Tuscarora and Lumbee Nations once thrived. They slept three to a bed and used rags to plug up the open spaces in the wall to keep the cold out. There was a sink, a wood burning stove for cooking, and a wash-tub for bathing. They used the outhouse or went in the woods to do their personal business, and used leaves to wipe their asses.

"We weren't poor; we just didn't have a lot of money." This was how my Leon described the richness of his upbringing. They lived off a diet of spring water, fresh garden vegetables, beans, squirrels, fish, turtle, sparrows, coon, venison and homemade biscuits sopped in fatback gravy or molasses. The treat was going to Ms. Ola B's store for sugar cookies and fresh lemonade. Ms. Ola B's was a store by day, but turned into a foot stompin', booty shakin' juke joint by night. Fish fry's were commonplace when Leon was coming up in the '60's and '70's, and everybody had a little bit of their own creek liquor or homemade wine made possible by the hearty supply of wild grapes. Hot dogs were a rarity and a luxury reserved for occasional visits into Laurinburg, the big town where the county held its seat.

Leon often shared his wealthy memories of youth with me: fearlessly treading through the forest any season, barefoot and almost naked, catching bite-size fish in ponds with bamboo poles, building smoke houses and lying under the Carolina night sky where dark baptizes your soul and the Creator sends endless blessings of shooting stars.

One day, Granny showed me Archie Bunch's field. This is where she lived when she left her mother's home, and where she, her children and grandchild, Little Leon sharecropped. This is where their two room shack eventually burned down. Granny never went to school and her children rarely attended school for a full year. Education was a seasonal thing, a privilege not extended to sharecroppers. All hands were needed during the planting and harvesting season. At four years old, Little Leon was too young to help make a difference and too old not to, so he played his own games between the endless rows of cotton bolls while everyone else worked. His uncle Eugene, who was 6, was considered old enough to make a difference. He did not have the luxury of days of play, and had to put in his time in the field with his older siblings.

Eleven years after Leon was born, his mother Pearlie Mae kept her word. Little Leon left Laurel Hill and all he knew to live in Piscataway, New Jersey with his mother, step-father, two brothers and sister. His new life was filled with fear and excitement but even at eleven, Little Leon knew the South had no opportunities for folks who looked like him.

Granny brought me out of my memories of Leon's past and back to the task at hand: preparing for my day of work in Mr. Pete's vegetable field.

"When do ya need the shirt? she asked. "You ain't fix'n ta pick right now, iz ya . . . it's 'bout ready to rain. Dey say a storm comin disaway."

"No Granny. I'm going out on Tuesday morning."

"Good. I ain't tryin to tell you what to do, but I think you should just stay here 'til the storm passes."

Thunder and lightning storms always command ominous respect from Southern folk. In the old days when such weather would come up, Granny would give out a call to the crowd of young folks working or playing outside. "Ya'll chil'ren come on in heahs," she would say. "It's fixin' to storm."

Sky's belly ached and pulsated from the fullness of rain. It beamed a dark grey-blue, deep with passion and sincerity. Soil and all its inhabitants on top and below were thirsty. Burst was imminent. The downpour would be immediate and absent of warning drops. If you were caught in it, you'd be drenched. When all her children were safely in, Granny would command:

"Ya'll sit down. Quiet. Fold your hands. Don't move. Let the storm do its business and stay out da way. Lighning is lookin' for someone to strike and take back and she ain't gonna get none of mine."

Everyone would sit in her little living room on the floor, dark, still and quiet. In the days of kerosene lamps and cookstoves, that was enough to satisfy her. But when the electrical lines came out to her house on Bunch Road, Granny would also shut off the electricity and unplug all the outlets because, as every good Southerner knows, lightning and electricity are close cousins, and seek each other out.

Granny's habits have not changed with the years. She does the same with the outlets today. We sat in the living room in the dark with the television now blank and quiet—Granny and granddaughter-in-law waiting for the storm to roll in. Thunder's sonorous roar exploded a yell from Sky's center; the same place that leads us to the other side—wherever and whatever that is—when we pass away.

It sounded like one million mothers groaning from labor pains.

It sounded like 10,000 bass tones maximized on an equalizer. It sounded like two million lion roars. It felt like 360 million Africans wailing slavery's song. This was the way southern thunder spoke as lightning lashed through the sky daring someone to love her.

The storm came and went without causing any damage.

"Mashell, Mashell. Go get me some goofadus[8] from the sto' down yonder in Laurel Hill."

"Some what Granny?" I ask, very confused.

"Huuh huuuh huuuh huuuh." Granny bellowed her hearty laugh again. "Some goofadus. You aint's heard dat befo? Girl you been livin' in dat city too long." Then she brought out a small blue and gray cylinder can and instructed me to "Jus' axs dem for dis kine, not the green or red kine, dis kine. And if dey ain'ts gots it dere, check over yonder at Sneeds Grove."

Granny waved her hand forward when she talked to emphasize her point or show me a direction.

I took the can and examined the words on it. It read:

"Tobacco Snuff: for your dipping pleasure." I repeated these words in delight to know what I was purchasing. "Can I take the can with me."

"Yeah, and when you gets back, I'll have da shirt fer ya."

"I appreciate it, thank you Granny."

"You're welcome. Anytime."

I head out the front porch, through the screen door and into my car to "fetch" some "goofadus" for Granny. I'm not sure whether it was the storm or something else which prompted her request at that particular time, and I don't ask . . .

Tuesday came quickly and I started off to my job with Mr. Pete. Granny advised me to keep my shirt on in the okra patch because the okra leaves are sticky and will irritate my arms, to keep my hat on to protect me from the hot sun, and to use the handkerchief to wipe my face from the sweat. I drove away, keeping Granny's advice tucked close in my shirt pocket, next to my heart.

Working a rhythm between the rows

I met Mr. Pete out in his field around 9 a.m. I took his advice and wore long pants, the long sleeve shirt I had borrowed from Granny, as well as a scarf she had also insisted I take. The temperature was already 77 degrees so I knew it was going to be another blistering hot day. Three young folks were already in the field picking: a young Black boy who looked about 7 years old, and two teenage girls, one Black and one Indian. I saw that none of them had on long-sleeve shirts; so thankful that I wouldn't have to be bundled up in the heat, I left mine and the scarf in the car and came out wearing just a tank top and my work trousers.

Mr. Pete gave me an empty bushel and showed me how to pick the garden peas. I followed close behind him in the field and watched. "You work up a rhythm between the rows," he explained. "You pick all the peas on this bush that's ready with the right hand and this other row over heah with the left hand." With just one step forward, he had already picked quite a few peas going down the center of two rows. His large hands held a nice bundle before he dropped them in the bushel bucket. He showed me how to tell if a pea is ready to be picked and where to snap it so more could grow back. He made it look easy. No problem, I thought.

"Now you do it."

He observed me for a moment, chuckled and went back to the edge of the field where he had parked his truck, which served as his office during harvest time.

Two hours passed and my rhythm never came. I struggled to break the peas from the vine crisply. I couldn't coordinate working two rows at the same time, one with the right hand and the other with the left. My hands couldn't hold that many peas at once. I wasted a lot of time dropping just a few peas in the bucket. I scrapped the effort to pick two rows simultaneously and focused on doing one at a time. This was better, but I still struggled. At one point I actually sat down cross-legged between the rows and comfortably picked the peas within my reach and then moved down to the next section and picked

---

8   Goofadus or gooferdust generally refers to any powder used to cast a harmful spell or connotes natural ingredients that can be used to harm. Often used in hoodoo practices of African Americans in the South, the word "goofer" comes from the Kikongo word "kufwa," which means "to die." In North Carolina, the term "goofering" was a regional synonym for voodoo, such as, "She goofered him."

those cross-legged.

Three hours passed and, while my young comrade laborers were on their second and third bushels, I hadn't even picked one. At $3 a bushel I'm not even making $1 an hour. At this rate, it would take me all day to pick one bushel.

I grabbed my paltry effort and humbly walked over to Mr. Pete's truck on the side of the field. He was conducting business with two customers. One was on his way back to New York City early the next morning and wanted to purchase two bushels to take with him. Mr. Pete glanced over at my half full bushel and told the customer that he'd have to wait to get the order filled. "I had to give a guy 10 bushels of peas dis morning," he explained. "Gave it to him at church. He goin to take dem back to New York too cuz he cain't get dem up dere." He told the customer to check back at the end of the day, right near sundown. Both customers left and Mr. Pete and I stood there alone with the half empty bushel between us.

The silence was awkward, and then I blurted out a litany of excuses:

"This is harder than I thought . . . I can't seem to get a rhythm. . . I worked on one row instead of two. . . some of the peas weren't ready to be picked . . . I couldn't find many peas . . . I was in the wrong row, someone must have picked here already. . .I couldn't grab enough in one hand . . . I got tired of bending over . . . This is hard!" I gasped, eyes conceding that if I had to feed my family off of this work, we'd starve. Mr. Pete was nice as he chuckled.

"Weelll, you just need more practice."

I realized pea picking is a rhythm, a mantra, a long, arduous back-bending southern ballet that requires speed, accuracy, fluidity and keen sight. I made it look too hard.

"I'll try picking some okra," I said, thinking maybe I might do better over there. "Will you show me how to do it?"

"You bring anything to cover your arms? Mr. Pete asked.

"It's in the car . . . I borrowed a shirt from Granny Nora." I trotted off to my car to get the shirt, still not clear why I'd need it in the okra patch but not in the pea field.

We walked to the okra patch behind the truck right over yonder. I would be there by myself. The okra vines were taller than me. Good, no bending over I thought. I followed behind Mr. Pete again. The rows were not as discernible as in the pea field. The okra vines grew out and every which way like briars. I'd have to use my body and arms to push the vines back and move through the rows. Being in the middle of an okra patch feels sticky and stingy—as in "full of stings"— and I was immediately grateful for the long sleeved shirt and long pants. Mr. Pete glanced over his shoulders and said, "If you have a scarf you should wrap your head." I pulled out the scarf from my back pocket that Granny had fortunately insisted I bring. I took a moment to tie my head, then I was ready!

Mr. Pete showed me where to snap the okra and which ones were ready to pick.

"If they too long, like this one heah, it gonna be tough and stringy. Don't pick that. Pick em if they small or medium size. They easier to cook."

Seemed easy enough, I thought. Better than the peas. Mr. Pete left me to the job. One bushel, $3.00. For certain, I'll do better in the okra patch. The okra is bigger and will take up more space and it's easier to snap from the vine. But an hour passes and I barely cover the bottom of the wooden bushel bucket. The okra doesn't snap easy for me. The overgrown okra is easy to spot but the ready-to-pick ones are not in sight. The same thing happened in the pea field. Either Mr. Pete and my young co-pickers could spot more peas and okra on the vines because they had more experience, or the peas and okra hid from me and revealed themselves to these people who are indigenous to this land. Perhaps I hadn't earned the right yet. Nevertheless, it was almost 1:00 p.m., I'd been out there for four hours and barely picked a half-bushel, total. I'd say I earned almost $1.50. My pickin day was officially over!

Mr. Pete graciously offered me a "lil change for my trouble" and told me I can keep the peas and okra I picked. I thanked him for his time and the peas and okra but declined the money. When I got back to Granny, we sat on her porch and shelled peas while I told her all about my day working in the field.

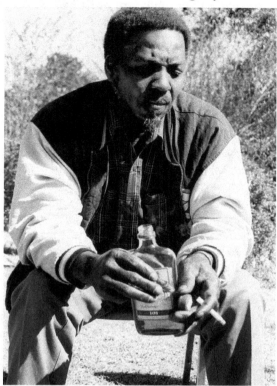

JoeHayes
Image 1-8

The air was thick, hot and humid, in that order, around our home in Laurel Hill, North Carolina in the summer of 1998.

His coal black skin offered relief from the blinding glares the sun reflected on the white sand, a fertile sand whose color epitomized the name "sandy white." His shirt was off. Sweat mixed with his natural body oils to moisturize his dark complexion. It was the kind of dark that saturated every layer of skin and reached way down to his soul and mine. JoeHayes was a provocative sight as he worked in midday's sun to strike water and dig our well. He stood erect, assured and oblivious to being watched. Broad shoulders and sledgehammer arms effortlessly swung the heavy pickaxe high above his head and then brought it down mightily to pierce the soil again, again and again. He dropped the pickaxe, picked up the shovel and rammed it forcefully into the beginnings of his well hole. He stepped on the shovel blade hard and pushed it in further with brute strength, then scooped up about two feet worth of sandy soil and deposited it to the side.

JoeHayes was stronger than the average man. I enjoyed watching his agility and precision of movements that made his muscles bulge. He dug a hole about four feet deep and four feet wide before he paused.

I was standing about fifty yards away and waited for that pause in his work before I approached him. JoeHayes sensed I was coming and turned around. He watched me as I neared and when I got close enough for him to hear, I smiled and said, "Hi. You're JoeHayes. I've heard so much about you."

His guarded but hospitable look turned to relaxed familiarity after I mentioned my relation to Nora, Pearlie Mae and "little" Leon. JoeHayes' deceased Uncle Jake was Nora Dockery's main man and father to three of her nine children, so he and I were practically family: twice-removed cousin in-laws to be exact.

JoeHayes nodded his head to affirm our distant familial connection. Then, he gave me a big warm smile that showed off a set of strong teeth. A gold tooth on the left side of his mouth twinkled in the bright sunlight. Ordinarily, I'm not attracted to a man who decorates his mouth with a gold tooth, but it made JoeHayes gorgeous. I savored the sight of this ebony Adonis and melted right into his subtle intense gaze. His reputation of being a ladies man preceded him. In his first words to me, JoeHayes declared, "So you Leon's wife." I remembered I was Leon's wife at the time.

This was the Sandhills region of southeastern North Carolina, an area folks called "the country," about six miles outside of the rural agricultural town of Laurel Hill in Scotland County. What had been an ancient sea that existed millions of years ago is now characterized by a land of fertile soil, with long-needle forests of majestic pines—whose needles reach as much as 18 inches long—set amidst a plethora of creeks, rivers, ponds and underground fresh water springs.

JoeHayes, Nora Dockery, Pearlie Mae, and Leon were all raised in this part of the country. Their ancestors had been there for generations, descendants of enslaved Africans, local native tribes and the Scottish colonizers for whom the county is named. Double-wide and single-wide settlements are modestly carved out within the landscape along with an occasional brick home for those who are better off. Endless rows of cotton, tobacco, soybean and corn fields dominate the agricultural landscape and the economy, many of these pesticide-ridden fields right next to public schools.[9]

Laurel Hill and the surrounding county look beautiful particularly in the springtime when dogwood blooms tickle the eye. But Laurel Hill is most famous for being the town next to Hamlet, which is famous for being the birthplace of John Coltrane.

Locally, it was also famous for being the home of JoeHayes. I had heard many stories that painted JoeHayes' five foot seven inch frame larger than life. Legend tells that he would regularly snatch water moccasins from a pond, swing them wildly above his head and then flicker them back to the pond from whence they came. He was a waterwitch, a snake dancer, a healer, a husband and father, a consummate hunter, a great cook, a ladies man and, most important, the one who preserved the traditions of the community in the midst of modern society.

I never formally interviewed JoeHayes. I spent time with him over the course of 4 1/2 years. We developed a strong kinship and respect for each other. During these years I learned snippets of JoeHayes' life that he chose to share with me. One of those stories was about how the ancestors gave him a gift that changed his destiny forever.

JoeHayes lived in the Paradise settlement off of McFarland Road in the outskirts of Laurel Hill. Paradise got its name from the Black sharecroppers who left their one and two room shacks and outhouses over yonder for Jim Walter Homes[10], single and double wide trailer homes, or the do-it-yourself cinder-block houses. These homes provided their first taste of indoor plumbing, electricity and walls that didn't creak, leak or require stuffing during the winter. It was Paradise.

In 1968, JoeHayes built his one room gray cinder-block house himself. It was snugly ensconced behind a clan

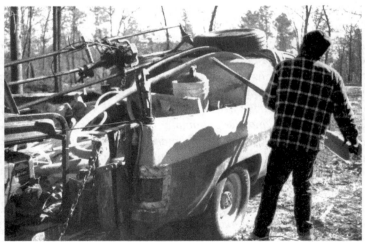

JoeHayes and his work truck
Image 1-9

of long-needle pines at the curve of his U-shaped dirt driveway. One side of the driveway led to the front of the house and the other to the back. His work truck, which was the only vehicle he owned, was always parked on the front side. Not many folks had seen the inside of his house. The few times I went

---

[9]   Today, solar panel farms have replaced many of the vacant agricultural farm acreage.

[10]   Jim Walter Homes are affordable "shell" homes that were water tight on the outside. The customer would finish the inside with their own labor. The only requirement for buying one of these homes was the customer would have to own the land on which the house was placed.

by and knocked, JoeHayes opened the door just wide enough for him to slip out and for me to catch a glimpse of the inside. There wasn't much to be seen, because a dim-watted light bulb rigged from the ceiling illuminated nothing except itself, much like a firefly. Everything else around it was dark. The bulb's juice came from a cord that stretched all the way to his daughter's trailer several yards behind his. Folks privileged to have seen the inside of his house say he had a wood burning stove which he only used for heat, an old fashioned hand pump for water, a dual purpose mattress-couch which had seen better days, and an icebox and cooler that stored perishables and beer. No one had ever seen the bathroom.

Joe would visit with me in his yard on the days I came by, and we'd sit on tree stumps arranged in an intimate circle for socializing. Deer heads from his hunting kills were posted trophy-like in the trees next to the sitting area; it was a surreal décor that Marcel Duchamp would have appreciated. Come Christmas time, JoeHayes strung colorful lights around the tree and deer heads. It was a sight to behold.

Anyone looking for JoeHayes only needed to find his work truck and he was close by. If it wasn't parked on the front side of his house, he was out in it some-

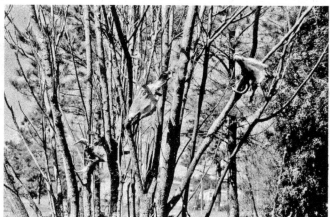

Deer heads on JoeHayes' trees
Image 1-10

where making money with it. The 1970's beige two-toned wide-bed Chevy had served him well. While the truck was old and overused and looked like it could break down at any moment, it was strong, dependable and durable, much like JoeHayes. It was infamous for carrying all his well-digging equipment in a disorganized pile that sat higher than the truck itself. That heap made the back sink to only a few inches above the ground while the front end reached toward the heavens. All his equipment was randomly thrown in, making its own order on top of the generator and 500 gallon plasticene water tank which were always placed in the back of the truck with deliberate care. Hoses were intertwined with shovels, pick axes, saws, buckets, pipes, sledge hammers and the usual assortment of basic tools. Some tools looked fossilized from the years of work encrusted on them. An eight-foot heavy-duty metal earth drill that required manual operation straddled the top of the pile. Sheer gravity held the equipment in place but JoeHayes tied the mound down with a rope anyway.

Everyone in Scotland County knew JoeHayes' truck. It was easy to spot. People could be driving, walking, working in the field or just sitting on their porch and when they saw his truck go by they'd point and say, "There goes JoeHayes." Or they'd shout at him, "Hey Joe," or simply call out his name, "JoeHayes," and wave their hand, and he'd give a honk back with his horn.

If you were looking for JoeHayes and couldn't find him, all you had to do was drive to any one of the small towns in Scotland County, ask anyone, and then follow the leads.

"You seen JoeHayes?"

"He been heah 'bout an hour ago . . . he's out there near Hamlet."

"Seen him drive towards Gibson while ago."

Or, "He was heah early to get a sausage sandwich then took off . . . said he had to drill a hole in Wagram. . . should be back heah later on. You can go on up dere and ask fer yo'self."

JoeHayes had the reputation of being a good cook before his wife and childhood sweetheart died from complications delivering the last of their three children, whom he raised afterwards with help from members of his family. He hunted and grew vegetables to feed his family and worked at a local factory job. He was a good and disciplined provider, even though he did always refer to his work at the factory as "doin' time," as if he were in jail. He took regular swigs of cod liver oil (which he always kept in his jacket's pocket) and sips of root medicine for his health maintenance.

But the tragedy of his wife's death almost sent JoeHayes over the edge.

He stopped cooking and instead, ate daily at the greasy spoon just two miles down the road. He started drinking more Wild Turkey whiskey than water. When he wasn't working, he spent most of his time in the woods, and told folks he was just "goin' huntin'." He'd leave before sundown to stake out a spot in the only environment where he felt comfortable along with his shotgun, Wild Turkey, a pocketful of jerky, and his two nameless hunting dogs he called sooners because they would rather sleep on the porch than hunt. He'd return by sun-up and night's end with no kill, empty handed except for the things he left with. Folks say he really went to the woods to scream, bellow, cry and damn the world for his loss hoping to get some reprieve from his impenetrable heartache.

But only JoeHayes knew why he was there. "I was huntin' for direction, forgiveness, peace of heart. I also didn't care if I became the hunted."

After his wife's death, JoeHayes felt he was being punished for all the daddy deer, brother squirrel, mother coon, cousin rabbit, sister possum, auntie turtle, uncle bird, grandma snake and even the road kill life he had taken since he was a boy. "Life killed my wife, and I will never kill life again. It was bound to happen because energy finds energy."

What he meant was that because he had hunted and taken the life of many animals, who came from families themselves—the life of one of the dearest of his own family members had been taken from him. It had been an exchange of energy.[11]

"Energy finds energy." These were JoeHayes' prophetic words that changed his life.

His downward spiral escalated when JoeHayes and the Scotland County Volunteer Fire Department (VFD) wrestled a fire half the night trying to save the house in Paradise where Miss Ola B lived and operated her two businesses. By day her house was the store where barefoot children bought three sugar cookies for a penny and by night it became the local juke joint. The fire at Miss Ola B's house was particularly close to JoeHayes' heart since after his wife's death, he began spending many of his evenings there.

The morning following the fire that ate Ms. Lula B's house-store-jukejoint was the morning that JoeHayes took the first step toward his new life.

"One frigid mornin' at the start of the huntin' season I didn't go to work," he told me. "I had been up half the night wrestlin' a fire at Ola B's house and certainly didn't want to do my time at the factory. I was sick and tired of doin' work fit for a monkey that called for no brains and was repetitive. I needed the outdoors. I said I was gonna call in sick. It was six a.m. I took a swig of liquor to give me the courage to make the call. I took another swig after the call to congratulate myself for callin' in sick. The third swig I took to cut the bone cuttin' chill in my body. The fourth, fifth, and sixth swigs I took to shake my head awake and be ready to go, anywhere. I took my last swig of liquor for courage to move forward and out of the factory cuz I wanted to set an example for my children. I grabbed my shotgun, put on my jacket and headed for the woods. I didn't take my truck and I didn't take my dogs but I did take my jerky, my flask and my cigarettes."

Joe walked for hours in the woods that day, woods he knew well because he'd trekked them since childhood. At midday, he stopped below a hunting post in an old oak tree. He climbed up the primitive ladder made out of wood branches to reach the 4' x 4' plywood post on top. He sat down, leaned back against the wall and unstrapped the shotgun that had done the killing for him for the last 15 years. He carefully laid it to his side and began stroking the barrel. Hunting had been a part of JoeHayes' life and culture for as long as he could remember. He was raised to think of hunting as a necessity, not a sport. Now he questioned the validity of that reasoning. Was it really a necessity? Did his wife really need to die? In the midst of his reflections, JoeHayes ate jerky, sipped Wild Turkey for courage and watched as huntable creatures began to reveal themselves around him, more often than they usually did on his hunting trips. Somehow, they knew he was not there to take life but to regain his own.

Time passed. The sun was setting and dampness from the surrounding wetlands rose along with the sound of night's creatures. JoeHayes dozed off several times, allowing himself to recover from his Wild

---

[11] JoeHayes had a life's philosophy that was atypical for someone who had been raised in the rural South with little formal education. He did not see and define life through the lense of a typical Southern Christian. He understood that the laws of science intersected those of spirituality, and many things he told me in our interview could have come not from the pages of the Bible, but from "*The Tao of Physics*," a 1975 book by Austrian-born American physicist Fritjof Capra exploring the parallels between modern physics and Eastern mysticism.

Turkey and escape his woes. Finally, after napping for the last time, he climbed down from the hunting post and began gathering food while there was still some light. Grapes, nuts and edible roots were plentiful for those who knew what to look for. A protruding root at the base of the hunting post oak offered a seat; he rested his back on a patch of moss that cushioned part of the trunk, then feasted on his gatherings and the last of the jerky.

Darkness hovered in the woods and would soon conceal the things daylight had revealed. JoeHayes sat on the tree root and listened as night's sound became louder and bolder with day's retreat. He stayed there for another hour after nightfall, finished the last of his Wild Turkey and then headed back to his one room home in Paradise. As he made his way out, he didn't think of his life's past, present or future. He strode in the balance of the moment.

For most people, it would have been difficult to see in the dark of the woods, but for JoeHayes it was easy. He had explored every inch of this area since he was a boy. His people had a long and intimate relationship with those woods and had been buried in its soil for the past 400 years. One could easily call JoeHayes' familiarity second nature and intuitive. He ate what grew there, what lived there and found protection and solace there. In a way, JoeHayes and those woods shared the same genetic coding and memory. The woods were himself and he could not be afraid of himself. He could see in the dark in the woods the same way he could vision himself with the lights off.

But this night was different.

One hour passed, two, then three. JoeHayes was still searching for his way out. He thought the Wild Turkey might have disoriented him, so he took out the cod liver oil from his pocket and swallowed a couple of hefty gulps. It went down slimy, thick and sticky. It stuck in the middle of his throat. He coughed, choked and gagged on it, trying to keep from vomiting. He wished for cold water, an orange or a lemon to chase the oil down. He searched frantically for a nearby creek or pond but found none. His stomach jerked and hiccupped. His throat swelled. It was coming. He wanted it to come. His torso lunged forward, Aaarraaaghh. Out sprayed the slime. His stomach tightened and heaved in readying for the next expulsion and aaarraaaggh. Breath. Aaaarraaaghh. Breath. Aaarrraaaghh, aaarrraaaghh, aaaacck, aaacck. Breath. Breath.

On the ground lay chewed jerky, grapes, nuts, and roots in an acrid Wild turkey and cod liver oil stew. JoeHayes looked for fresh water to renew his face and to wash out his insides. He was walking in muddy wetlands. Moisture was everywhere, but no open pond or running stream of drinkable water was in reach. He bent down, scooped up the wet mud and spread it on his face and neck. The coldness felt good and refreshing. The rich smells of the soil held his childhood and every cell and vessel in his body was opened. He nibbled the soil. It tasted good and brought him to his senses. JoeHayes found a dry spot to rest and muse over his predicament.

It was well into night and the darkness was heightened to its fullest. JoeHayes surveyed his surroundings, certain he had tread this ground before and missed his cue, his way out. Then, in the far distance, he heard the faint sound of steady and deliberate steps coming his way. The average person wouldn't have heard this but JoeHayes had canine hearing, especially at night. "Ain't no mo' bears in dese parts," he affirmed outloud for himself and for who or whatever was fast approaching. He grabbed his shotgun and pointed it in the direction of the oncoming steps. A dense mass about half an acre away emerged out of the dark and headed directly toward him. He squinted his eyes to see it better. He had owl vision, but the figure looked blurry to him, and he could not make it out. The mass neared quickly and he knew contact was imminent. JoeHayes steadied his shotgun and continued to aim, ready to shoot if necessary. But he was not afraid, not like he'd been when he had to watch his wife die without being able to do anything about it. That was the only time in his life he'd ever felt fear.

Amidst the chorus of nocturnal sounds he heard his name sung across the air:

"JoooeHaaayes."

He didn't answer. The mass moved closer, but was still obscure to his eyes. Again, he heard:

"JoooeHaaayes." It was now twenty yards from him. Again:

"JoooeHaaaayes." Ten yards. Still coming.

"JoooeHaaaayes." Five. . .

The figure now stood directly across from JoeHayes and his shotgun barrel. It looked smaller than it had in the distance and wore a dark cloak that melted into night's background. Up close, it still looked unformed and dark, especially the face. Only the eyes were clear. They conveyed a visceral connection. JoeHayes felt kin to this amorphous creature whose gaze pierced his soul. He put his shotgun down and stood before the being with nothing in-between.

Night's song carried words to JoeHayes again:

"Jooooe Haaaayes. I'm going to give you a gift that will change your life forever."

This time, JoeHayes answered back. "And what's that?" He questioned with guarded curiosity. He had become cynical about hoping for good things coming out of life after his wife's death.

"Oh, I think you will want it," replied the figure. "But you will have to come with me. It's something I need to show you, not tell you. We won't leave the woods, but we do have to take a little journey."

The figure gestured for Joe to follow and spoke one last time. "To get your gift JooooeHaaaayes, follow me. I am Ayamey." And suddenly, the figure that was Ayamey turned and headed back into the trees from where it had come.

JoeHayes hopped to his feet and struggled to keep pace. He followed the figure called Ayamey across creeks and through swamps JoeHayes had known all his life, but somehow they seemed different now. The majestic oaks, pines and walnuts were rooted firmer into the ground and reached higher and broader than he remembered. The vegetation was thicker and carried more life. Cricket clans resonated high-pitched mantras as bullfrog songs pulsated loud and plentiful. Rabbits scurried across the path to the nearest underbrush. Owls hoo-hooed and the Bob Whites shared their love songs. A vision came to JoeHayes of the storms of his youth where thunder rain deities invited frogs to hop in yards and dance wildly, and the snakes had a field day and ate well. He felt himself flowing through the life veins of the woods from the times of his boyhood that had disappeared as he had become a man.

JoeHayes' excitement grew as his night vision became keener. He could even see the top of root medicines as he passed them, root medicines his mother and grandmother used to doctor their family. He had not found them in a while, and he had thought they were all gone, overharvested and missing even from these places tucked deep in the woods.

After a long while, Ayamey stopped far ahead of JoeHayes. Joe hurried to catch up and stood next to his mysterious guide who gazed straight ahead into the dark of an open clearing in the midst of the woods. Joe did not know this spot. He stared along with Ayamey and looked for a form he could identify, anything. All he saw were the dark silhouettes of tall pines that protected the forest surrounding the open clearing. JoeHayes and Ayamey stood side by side and stared for a long while. Just when Joe felt he could stare no more, two forms melted out of the woods and moved toward them. The figures were shrouded in a darkness that blended into the night, as when JoeHayes first saw Ayamey. He heard no footsteps. They seemed to float through the air and moved swiftly.

"JoooeHaaaayes. We have a gift for you." Joe looked around as these words whispered in his ear, coming from the approaching figures. "Use this gift well and you will become indispensable to your people. You will never have to work for anyone else and never want for anything." The two figures were now in front of him. Joe turned to Ayamey to look for answers but Ayamey was gone. The whisperings continued:

"There are water ponds that lie deep underground. We will show you how to find them and bring the water up for your people. Knowing how to bring the water up is a mechanical skill much like working the machines at your factory and will not make you successful. You can learn this anywhere. The gift we give you will open you up to receive all life, especially water, wherever it is. When your wife died, you said energy finds energy. This is true. And the energy you find is also you and you will know it like you know yourself, your children, your parents, your brothers and sisters, just like you knew your wife, and you will treat it with respect. Water will know this about you and will look for you and claim you."

JoeHayes showed little emotion on the surface but was intrigued by what he heard and deep down excited at the possibility of being able to quit the factory and create his own livelihood. He had nothing to lose and was ready. He simply said in a matter-of-fact way, "I'm ready, What do I need to do?"

And at that moment, a hand from one of the figures swept across his face and gently closed the lids of his eyes. "Just watch," the whisperings instructed.

He saw a vision of himself on someone's land, land that was cleared to put a house on. A voice said, "Find a fruit-bearing tree or vine and break a branch off 'bout yeah big." Joe saw himself walk over to a grape vine and break a branch off.

"Leave the grapes on and bend the branch so it has an arc. Extend this out in front of you; make known your intentions to find the best underground pond, and the branch will lead you to the perfect spot. You are doing nothing, except being led. Remember, you are only the vessel."

In his vision, Joe saw the branch bend to the left and his body pulled in that direction; then a hard right; a hard left again; a few more feet to the right and then the branch stopped its pull, bent itself down stiff toward the ground, and stayed pointed there. Joe's entire body bent with it. The voice returned. "Now raise the branch up and tap it hard on the ground and count how many times it pops up and down."

Joe counted as the branch popped up and down forty times.

"Dig your well here," the voice said, "forty feet down to get to the water pond. The water you bring up will be water from the days of your grandmothers and grandfathers."

The voice faded and the vision slowly disappeared. JoeHayes continued to keep his eyes closed to digest the vision. When he finally raised his lids, the figures were gone. He ran across the clearing, into the woods to catch up with his night prophets but they had left no trail, nothing, not even a footprint or a scent. At last, realizing his search was futile, JoeHayes gave up and stopped. "It's time to find my way home," he assured himself.

JoeHayes walked out of the woods to the clearing where he had the vision and looked across the way. Night was ending her reign and sun-up was near. The open space had changed. It was no longer surrounded by dense woods and for the first time, he saw McFarland Road, the road that would lead him home, to Paradise. He realized he was on the other side of the forest from where he entered almost twenty four hours ago. JoeHayes didn't think about how he got there, or that just a few minutes ago the clearing was surrounded by woods, he was just glad he knew the way home.

Out of habit, he patted his side to feel his shotgun. It wasn't there. He realized it hadn't been there since he ventured off with Ayamey. "Must be restin in the huntin post at the old oak tree," he muttered to himself. He turned to retrieve it and after a few feet, he stopped. He thought about his wife. He thought about the gift he was just given and water claiming him. "Don't need it. Done enough killin' to last a lifetime," he declared. JoeHayes turned around and walked toward the road to Paradise with the best hunt trophy he'd ever had—the start of a new life.

After his vision quest in the woods, JoeHayes quit his job and began making a living as a water witch and well digger. His first clients were from the comfort of the Black community. Word quickly spread that JoeHayes could find the best springs and he wasn't going to charge you an arm and a leg to dig your well. Even White folks started calling on JoeHayes. This usually happened after they had spent a lot of money to have a big company bring their state of the art equipment to find good water, dig a sound well and then—for some unknown reason—failed. Good water was water that came up clear with no sand residue and a good well was one that did not have to be abandoned after a few years. JoeHayes would show up with his rudimentary materials: a pick axe, shovel, manual drill and a branch from a fruit bearing tree, which would lead him to the spot. That was all he needed. For the next thirty-two years, JoeHayes was self-employed and earned a sound reputation as the wadastick man.

In 2001, the government required all water witches and well-diggers to prove they were qualified. This meant passing a test filled with mathematical equations and questions on geology and hydrology. Thirty-two years of experience invalidated by the stroke of a pen. One can still practice without a license but those caught are fined heavily. Governments pass laws to contain people they fear and maintain control and power. But the traditions of a people and the gifts from their ancestors can never be contained or destroyed. Traditions are the life breath of the people. It is how we have survived; it is why we have survived.

The stages of finding and digging a well

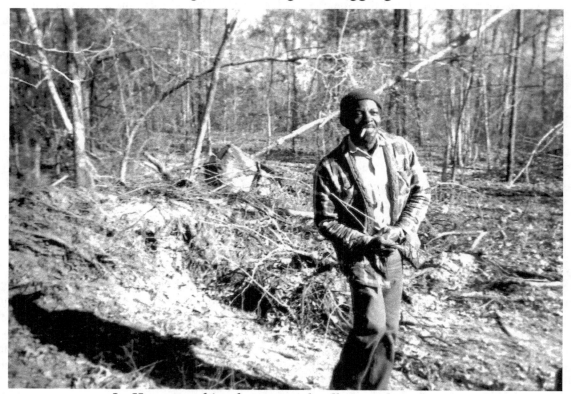

JoeHayes searching for potential well site with wadastick

Image 1-11

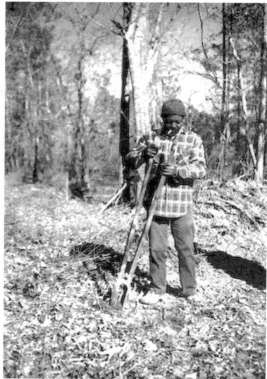

First diggings with post-hole digger

Image 1-12

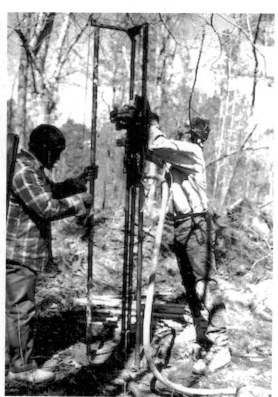

Finishing digging with well-drilling machine

Image 1-13

That Which Exists In-Between State Lines: Searching For Yellow Root

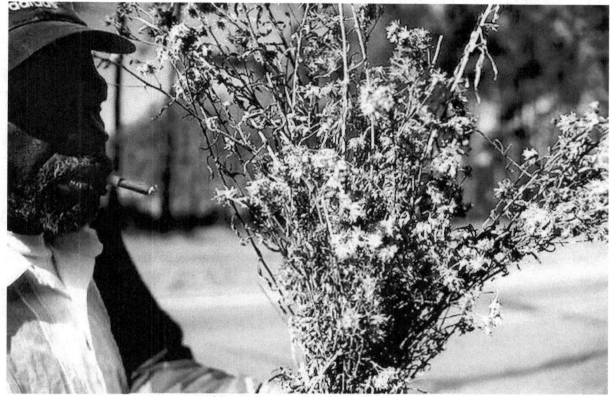

Eddie Nelson with rabbit tobacco
Image 1-14

A conversation and journey with Eddie Nelson and Mr. Bears

In 1663, the province of Carolina was created spanning the region between the current states of Virginia and Florida. This lush, fertile homeland to the Tuscarora, Waccamaw, Cheraw, Yamasee, Catawba, Saponi, Meherrin, Occaneechi, and Mattamuskeet Indians[12] would now have to be shared with the European colonists, forcibly and violently on the part of the colonists. Sixty-six years later in 1729, the southern region of Carolina separated and became its own colony, hence, South Carolina. This action set the stage for what eventually became state number 8, South Carolina, in 1788 and state number 12, North Carolina, in 1789.

Boundaries have always been used to separate and segregate. That illusive line which humans draw to set one apart from another contains in itself an existence. To which side of the line does one belong?

It is here, along the line in-between, in an area that is claimed by both sides yet in actuality is outright owned by neither, where I would finally find the potent strong medicine, yellow root. It was apropos because no one really owns the medicine or the root or the land, just like the state line. It belongs to the people, the animals, the plants, the water, the sun and the moon. Humans set up these archaic ideas of boundaries out of fear, the need to control, greed and a general feeling of not being connected to other humans, Mother Earth and the universe. Yellow root belongs to us all.

During my first three years of researching and documenting African American healing traditions everyone I interviewed had unequivocally extolled the virtues of yellow root medicine. I had gone out with others to find it, but the golden plants are no longer rooted in the easy-to-access places near creek beds and under bridges. A couple of folks shared with me what little yellow root they had in their freezers, but it wasn't the same as harvesting it fresh and seeing where it originated and lived. Finally

---

[12] This is only a partial list of Native American nations in that region.

in 1999, I was introduced to Eddie Nelson, with whom I shared my desire to find yellow root in its natural state. To my delight he answered, "We gots plenty on our property."

Two hundred years after the separation of the two Carolinas, the property owned by Eddie and his 90-year old father, Nathaniel Bears, was situated on 52 acres that literally sat on the boundary line. The Nelson-Bears homestead is located in-between Gibson, North Carolina and McColl, South Carolina, but is part of neither. The household has a South Carolina telephone area code but a North Carolina address and zipcode.

The drive to their property took me down long, isolated country roads lined with stately pine and oak bush forests draped in Spanish moss and the occasional corn or tobacco field. Flocks of wild turkey ran free across fields without fear of winding up on someone's dinner table. I had to swerve more than once to avoid smashing hefty pond tortoises who took their time crossing the road. Obviously, these turtles rarely expected any metal four wheeled contraptions rolling through "their" parts. The road to the Nelson-Bears compound started off paved, and then became gravel and finally dirt. Eventually the street signs disappeared and I had to rely on landmarks such as "turn right at the second crossroads with the tree stump next to the big walnut tree."

I was ready for my trek into the backcountry with Eddie Nelson. I had heeded his words of advice, his only advice, to "wear some strong boots and cover up." But while I waited for Eddie to get himself ready to take me down into the yellow root woods, I got the chance to talk to his father, Mr. Bears.

Mr. Nathaniel Bears' skin tone was a rich, dark chocolate brown that glistened from the sweat that graced his face because of the hot, humid air. He stood about 5'5 inches tall and slightly hunched over because of his age. When I first saw him, he was sitting in a chair in his yard under a big shade tree which offered only cosmetic relief from the heat of this late summer day. He offered me the chair at his side and we sat on the porch as he talked about his long life in rural North-South Carolina and the philosophy that governed it.

The Father: Nathaniel Bears

Nathaniel Bears is my full name, B-E-A-R-S (pronounced Beers). I was born and raised in South Carolina, Bennetsville. I stayed arounds there, with my two half brothers first of all, and after them, my daddy. Been here a long time.

My birth date is November 29th. I can't tell you what year I was born in but I'd have to go and count back. I'll be 90 on my next birthday. I was born in 1905 or 1906.

I done so many different kinda work. I farmed some. I worked the fields. I was workin' for 50 cents a day pickin' cotton, all day long. But then, they (the White land owners) weren't satisfied. You had to take your money and pay it back to them for rent. You had to go and buy your foods and thangs from them too.

I had good luck and bad luck in my time. I went to the city and worked at the steel mill. All the mills struck and went down so I had to come back down here again because I couldn't get a job nowhere. Everybody had been cut off for jobs. The town was full of peoples. Whoever work in the mills, they go down every week and get a truck load of groceries, this would be given to each one because nobody had any money. So I come on back down here.

I worked servin' for Uncle Sam in Second World War. I didn't go over to Europe. I stayed on this side. I was in Fort Bennet down here, then after that come Fort Bragg, then after that was Louisiana and after Louisiana I go to Boston, Mississippi, I mean Boston, Massachusetts, and then I was discharged. I was glad I was. I was loadin' boats.

I have 52 acres here.[13] I used to farm it. It's more than I can step on. This whole area used to be Black, but some left this place to go up North. Some sold their land. Some died out. So I say, I have to stay here and let us be and they can do what they can do with it. But now, people tryin' to live like other people, so we have had our time.

I had one girl and four boys. I got one son in Gibson. I lost my wife and went and got me another one. I lost her and said I wasn't gonna marry no more. I was old and nobody want old. When you get old, it's hard to find nobody my age.

---

[13]   Inherited from his father, I believe.

When I was comin up, my parents got most of the medicine from the woods and didn't fool with no doctor. It's a shame and scandalous that a person don't try to take after the older folk and don't try and learn nothin'.

Now when my wife died, I didn't e'en know how to wash clothes. Didn't' know how to do nothin', cook and all that. She had stomach trouble and I had her under a doctor for I don't know how long, and the doctor wasn't doin' nothin'. My wife couldn't even stand around and walk across the floor. She was real sick so the root doctor lady came in the house and tells her what herbs to get. That root lady got her up in 'bout three days and had her walkin' and showed her what kinda medicine to get from the woods that do that work. I didn't look to see what it was. And so, after my wife died, I didn't know nothin' and I still don't. The woman who took care of her died the next year after she showed my wife what to do.

We would use rabbits tobacco and get it and smoke it, but most of the time my mother would make the teas. Yellow root, buzzard weed and pudgegrass is good for stomach problems just like castor oil. Pudgegrass is tough, it's a li'l grass. You make a tea outta it and boil it. It cleanse you out. You gotta know the top of yellow root in order to pick it. Mullet grows good around heah. You boil it and wash your leg down in it. It's a big wide leaf. Poke sallat grows around heah too. It cleanse yo blood. Don't eat the berries, the berries will kill ya. You eat the leaves and you parboil them and you pour it off and the water be real green, and you pour 'em off, then you boil 'em again, then you cut 'em up. Some folks say the poke sallat root is might strong medicine. I ain't seen no pudgegrass in a long time. Cain't find no buzzard weed anymore either. We used to feed lion's tongue the hogs to help keep them healthy. We chop up the leaves and put it in the feed. You can take lion's tongue and boil it and drink it yo'self. But that yellow root, you got to go way down in the swamp and when you come out, you be all bugged up. Eddie gwonna take you down in dere.

The Journey Begins

"Dem da boots you bought? Eddie asks me before we head out.

"Yeah, are these good enough?" I stick out my foot to show off my California style hiking boots.

Eddie and Mr. Bears laugh at me and, Eddie simply says, "Nope. It won't work to get da yellow root."

"Why not?" I ask persistently.

Eddie looks down, shakes his head and chuckles. "Cuz you need sumtin like dese heah," he says. He points to the boots he has on which reach up to his knee. "We got to get in this stuff way, way back through the swamp to the pond where the yellow root grows."

I offer as a solution. "Can I put some plastic bags over my feet and hold the top in place with a rubberband?" I was determined to go and thought my quick-thinking ingenuity would impress them.

Eddie shakes his head again no and instructs me to "Wait here." He turns and goes into the front porch of his house which resembled an old wooden screened-in shed. After a couple of minutes he returns with a pair of rubber swamp boots and says, "Heah, try dese."

I put my right foot in and the boot fit perfectly. I put on the left boot, strut around for a moment, give a great big smile and declare to both men, "We're good to go. I'm in."

They continued to get their last bits of tease on me before we head out. "You not goin' down in dere. You not goin' to get any yellow root. You get stuck in dere and we have to come get the tractor to pull you out. Now don get caught up in dere."

"Let's go, Let's go. I'm ready." I jab back at them.

Along with the boots, Eddie has brought his shot gun and little beagle hunting dog, which trots close behind him.

"I wanna see if I could shoot sumtin. My dog heah, she jus' a puppy, she need trainin'. This'll be good fer her. Wanna see what she can do."

"Sho her dat rabbits tobacco, too" Mr. Bears calls out to remind Eddie as we walk away across the field.

First we survey the property to look at the medicines around their house. The land is expansive. "We got all kines o' trees out here: pear, pecan, apple and walnut trees, the kine people buy at the sto, and they shell and make dem walnut cakes out of."

I imagine what it looked like when they made their living full-time farming on their 52 acres. Perhaps endless rows of cotton, tobacco, corn and peas; fenced-in acreage with cows grazing on one side and horses on the other; hog pens, chicken coops, a couple of "sooner" dogs,[14] a couple of full-breed hunting dogs, and of course the fruit and nut trees which still stand and bear gifts.

Today, rabbits tobacco (aka rabbit tobacco) covers the field and way back yonder, behind it, is the dense brush that surrounds the pond where yellow root flourishes. Eddie shows me rabbits tobacco when it's green, with the flowers on top. "It ain't ready yet. We wouldn't smoke it now, it gotta be dry. It don't get us high or nuthin'. It jus' like you smokin' a cigarette. You can smoke it good in a pipe. But what we did wit it when we wuz kids was roll it up in a paper bag and smoke it. Sho did. See now you had it good. You was smokin' cigarettes, we wuz smokin' dat rabbits tobacco. It's not a bad taste."

I offer a positive twist to what he thought he was lacking. "I'm sure rabbits tobacco is a lot healthier for you than cigarettes."

We continue on across the property. The further away from the house we get, the denser the trees become.

"We got yellow root, mullet, rabbits tobacco, buzzard weed out heah. There's even cactus out there." Eddie points to a bed of flat leaf cactus that hugs the ground.

It's a late summer afternoon in the Carolinas. Not the best time to go through dense brush or a swamp. The air is hot and the humidity hangs like molasses on our skin. Everything is covered except our hands and face—fresh meat for the mosquitoes. They feast on me where they can. I move the scarf on my head to cover my face, hoping the mosquitoes won't recognize me. It doesn't help.

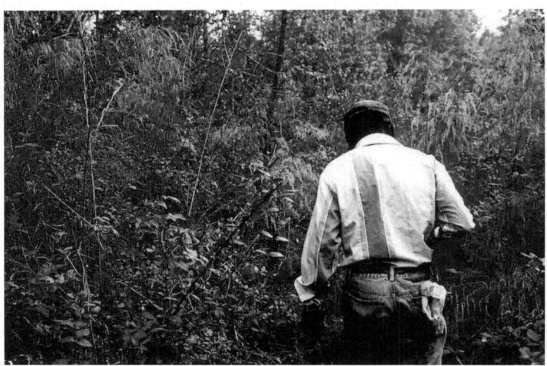

Following Eddie Nelson into the brush

Image 1-15

The way to the pond is protected by thick, thorn-infested briar brush rooted in swamp. Eddie leads the way with an axe that is mildly effective. I follow behind, a far second, making sure I place my foot steps in his, exactly. If Eddie had stepped there and nothing happened to him, then there's no chance of being bitten by a copperhead or a water moccasin or a rattler.

(Later, when I replayed the sounds of us struggling through the brush on the tape recorder, those sounds come out with great clarity; swishcrush, snap; swishcrush snap, swishcrush, snap. Our

---

[14] For a long time I thought a "sooner" was just a name for a mutt, but it's more of an attitude of a dog, a lazy dog, who would sooner nap than hunt, or pee on the carpet as opposed to a tree.

conversation can be heard faintly in the background, second to the language of swamp briar brush. The brush's inhabitants must have been alerted by our alien-ness and awkwardness and pumped up their volume as well. No human had been back there in quite a while.)

"I didn't know it growed up like dis." Eddie commented. "We got the kettle mixed up real deep. I guess we ain't stirred it in, I don't know how long."

The "kettle" Eddie is referring to, I understand, is their swamp, the dense brush that they haven't tended to in years, so that it's become thick and congealed and difficult to stir your way through. But instead of perceiving these matted acres from the point of view of someone who has to traverse and manage and work them, I look at them romantically, with city eyes. "See how, free, fertile and strong things can be if untouched by human intentions." My urban perspective draws only silence from Eddie. "Yellow root must be some strong medicine if it's way back up in here," I add. I certainly had not expected to be trekking through a thorny swamp for over an hour to get to it.

Laughing and waiting for me to say when, Eddie asked, "You wanna go back?"

I answered, "No, it's just if folks have to go through this jungle every time they want some yellow root, it must be a cure all."

The dog Betty, a puppy, trails behind us, struggling to find her path down below the level of the brushline, whimpering every now and again.

"That dog ain't worth a shit," Eddie Nelson declares. He continues on about the yellow root. "Used to be you could fetch it near the creek beds or back over yonder near the mill," he said, "but as of late, I ain't seen none. See, folks gets greedy and they sells it up there at that flea market in Rockingham. They finds a spot where yellow root be at and then they pick all of it and don't no more grow back."

"How much does it cost at the flea market?"

"Bout $5 for yeah much." He uses two fingers to make the shape of "yeah much": a small bundle about 2 inches in diameter.

"Wow. It must be good if folks are gonna pay $5 when they used to get it for free."

Yellow root: the new darling of free market democracy which eventually devours its victims. During my many interviews, I'd often hear Southern folks say, "Gotta get me some yellow root. Got any? When you go get some, bring me by a bit." There was a community consensus that you couldn't find yellow root anymore near a creek bedside, under a bridge or nestled in a nearby swamp. But one could easily find it at the Rockingham, North Carolina, flea market for that $5 a bundle. Yellow root has fallen prey to the vestiges of the free market and is now an endangered species. It's retreated to the place where few two-leggeds tread, or perhaps yellow root only reveals itself to the un-infected. Once a staple in Southern folk medicine, it is now a rare and valued commodity. Most poor southern folks can't spare the $5 to get a small bundle from a flea market vendor. It had never been exchanged that way and I think to do so would make its medicine less potent and the exchange impure. Yellow root, aka goldenseal, now fetches a whopping market driven price of $27 for a bottle of 100 capsules at your local health food store.

He changes the subject to talk a little about his family as we push on through the brush.

"My granddaddy was a root doctor. Hmmmhumph. Say he was good, too. My daddy say he was real good. He cured a bunch of people. Back den I didn't ask no questions. My grandfather, I say he was a pimp. He was hustlin' a lot. He bought a lot of land, used to own a hunk of land. Used to own dem woods all down in Bennetsville, Cheraw."

All the while he's talking, Eddie easily hacks a path through the web-like brush with his axe, but the thorns still pull at our clothes and nick the surface of our skin. I notice little cuts on my hand and all the flying insects they attract.

"See what I'm talkin' 'bout. Dem briars will tear you up. You ain't run into nuthin' yet. This is jus' light action right here," Eddie portends. "Befo we get to that yellow root you might wanna turn an go back."

"Nope." I say with determination. "I been on this search for pickin' some yellow root for almost three years now. I'm not turning back."

I grow silent and dedicate all my energy to push through the briar thicket that is intent on making my journey tenuous and painful. I watch and mimic Eddie's every move through these parts. It's an improvised choreography with two props: a hatchet and a shotgun strapped across his body. He's mastered negotiating his body to slip over, sideways or under each briar confrontation. Low brush and thick branches moan as they are pushed back. The hatchet is used to facilitate. He chops with it only when absolutely necessary, returning the tool to its place in a holster belt at his waist when not in use.

He is about five feet ahead of me. At times our distance is even greater and he waits for me to catch up. The ground is all swamp now and my feet sink with each footstep.

"Oooh my goodness, we're gettin close to water," he excitedly declares. "Dats why I told you to put those boots on."

I now understand. Visions of vicious water moccasins attacking my feet consume my thoughts.

We struggle forward in silence for about 20 more minutes, Eddie, myself, and the little dog. I can feel we are in deep. The ground becomes gradually wetter and the sounds become distinctly louder. Crickets, skeeters, hoppers, junes, flies, and bees chant their mantras in unison, simply saying, "Thank You Creator for this sweltering, dripping, heat-full day." Their choral is the heartbeat of this habitat.

My face has become a mosquito's feast: fresh Yankee meat. I do an occasional wipe of my entire face with the palm of my hand just to let the ravenous mosquitoes know their entree is not without a price. Each wipe takes out a few of their brethren. Eddie laughs at my determination to press on.

"Did you ever bring your wife up in here?" I ask.

"No, no. My wife hadn't stayed down here none. My wife was a city girl. She didn't even want to stay here. She from Winston-Salem. Dat's her home and she right dere now. We not together. We wasn't together when we was together. She rather stay with her daddy than to stay with me."

He stops in his tracks as we move through a clearing. "OK wait a minute now," he says. Protruding out of the ground up ahead is a mound about two feet high and two feet wide.

"OK, watch dem fire ants, see dem fire ants. Dem bad boys will bite you hard too. Come on." Eddie gestures for me to follow him.

We walk for a while in an area with little brush. Without breaking stride, Eddie gestures his hatchet towards the left and says, "dat right there is the barrel my daddy used to make creek liquor back in da day." The barrel, which must have seen much use in its time, is almost entirely surrounded by vines. Its once-smooth and shiny exterior is now charred by rest and marked by several bullet holes. Eddie told me that after his father retired the barrel from distilling liquor, Eddie and his young freinds used to use it for target practice.

We continue on past this dying relic of old times. Before long, we come to

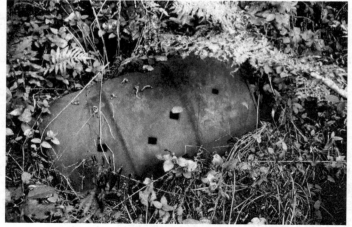

The abandoned liquor-making barrel
Image 1-16

the next dense thorny entanglement we must move through to reach our destination. I'm getting tired and cut up. Every step is a struggle —stomping, hacking and then pushing briars out of the way. It takes much effort and the worst is yet to come.

"Did you used to come up in here when you were a boy?" I ask, making conversation to make the trek seem less arduous and long.

"Yeah, we used to plow all back heah. We had corn and watermelons. This was part of our farm, but it growed up now. It used to be worser than this, before daddy had the timber cut outta heah."

"You tellin me." I agree.

Eddie suddenly stops again and stretches out his arm to stop me too. This time we're not faced with vicious thorny brush but a colony of several alive and active red ant mounds just like the one mound we saw earlier. This now determined our path. Each mound was separated by a space a little larger than my foot. It is difficult to pass.

"I've never seen anything like that." I say in amazement.

"They big ones, ain't they?" is the only thing Eddie replies to me about this oddity of nature.

I stand still and in awe, then proceed with a conscientious step, the little dog trailing even further behind me than when we began.

"That li'l dog is right wit me," Eddie says. "This is a test for her and you. Yeah, here she comin'. This dog ain't never been back up in heah befo. She doin' alright for a puppy. You be alright, too."

The sounds of moaning brush, thorny briars and snapping twigs are amplified ten fold as we enter into thick briar territory again. This brush is thicker, woven tighter and cuts sharper than before. We're getting scratched and tugged from every direction. It becomes more difficult to move with each step. Eddie begins to look around for a way out. Is he lost? The swamp floor grows wetter and our feet sink far into the muddy water halfway up our calves. I look down and watch every step to make sure I don't step on a snake. My thoughts travel to slavery times when some of our folks escaped, barefoot through these woods and thorny swamps. I'm sure it was "growed up" more then, but some of the escapees endured and survived. We are a strong and determined people.

I start thinking about the creatures who live here. "Do they have fox in here?" I ask.

"Oh yeah. Bobcats too."

I look up to see that both the dog and I are far behind him. The sounds of us moving through these woods muffle Eddie's conversation. I'm stuck and start to panic because I can't see Eddie anymore. My only prayer is to make it to him without stepping on a snake. I hear him push forward with one goal: to find the way out and the clearing to the creek that leads us to the pond where the sacred yellow root lives.

Eddie waits for me. But as I catch up again, he stops in his tracks, cocks his head and says, "Be still. Be still." I do as he urgently commands and watch for any indication of snake, bobcat or fox. "Heah da wada? Heah da wada?" He finally says.

I relax and listen through the cacophony of bush sounds. "Yeah, yeah." I finally whisper with delight as I discover the sound of water for the first time. I know we're almost there.

"Gettin' close. We getting' close. Dese are my woods, but I don't travel 'em unless I'm wit somebody."

"Why is that?" I wonder.

"Cuz sumtin can happen and den you be stuck out here."

We continue forward and with lighter energy, happy we're almost to the pond.

Just when I think we're at the end of our morass, it gets even thicker. This time, I feel like a fly caught in a spider's web struggling to get free. These woods, or rather this jungle, has a tight grip on my movement. Vines, briars and trees whose branches extend far, engulf me. I don't feel trapped, just caught, unintentionally or perhaps I'm being held until my credentials check out.

He turns back to check on me. "I'm alright," I assure him but he sees that I'm stuck yet again. He uses the hatchet to cut the briars, vines and branches in front of me.

Once my path is clear, Eddie points ahead to a gigantic briar with monstrous thorns. "That's what you call a bamboo dere. That'll cut you like a razor. Yeah, that one will get ya. I'm lookin' at those big briars and I didn't bring no machete like I should've." He changes our direction again as we face an impenetrable wall of vines and colossal bamboo briars with razor sharp thorns. We head up an incline toward more razor sharp bamboo briars. If this is a good direction then I'd hate to see the bad.

I turn off the recorder, put it in my pocket and cap my camera lens so nothing can impede my already strenuous move forward.

We move through another dense area and just as I'm feeling that the path we've taken is endless and we'll never actually get there, we break through the last bit of thick brush and come out into a clearing. Beyond it, just in front of us, is the pond.

I am in the heartbeat of the woods.

"The yellow root is over yonder just under those trees." Eddie points toward a group of towering long-needle pines that sit at the far end of the pond. He moves quickly, toward the trees, but I don't move. Instead, I watch him through a small opening of the brush at pond's edge. He gestures for me to follow him and I start forward, making my way through the brush along the perimeter of the pond. I finally reach him where he is standing in a clear spot, just out of the brush.

"Here it is. You knows it by its top." He holds the leaf gently in his hand like it's a precious stone. It's smaller than I had imagined and vibrant green.

"You gotta pull it up and check the root, break it open and make sure the color is yellow." Eddie grabs the yellow root by the stem and gives it a gentle tug. It comes up easily because of the damp soil. Dark, rich earth surrounds the root. He scrapes some off and breaks the root. A vibrant iridescent yellow shouts out against a backdrop of black soil. It looks stunning.

"See, if it's yellow like this"—he gestures the root toward me—"it's yellow root," Eddie instructs. "Then you can taste it if you're not sure. It's kinda bitter." He rinses it off in the pond and breaks a stick off and hands it to me. I put it in my mouth, between my teeth to suck out the juice of the root. To my surprise and delight, it tastes just like the familiar

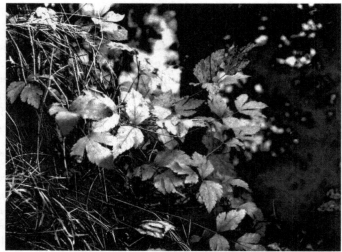

Yellow root growing in the field
Image 1-17

goldenseal extract I've so often purchased and used in my own health and healing regimens. I decide to pull up some yellow root for myself. I dig my hands in the moist soil to get to the root instead of pulling it up by the stem. It's soft and cool and soothing. I keep my hands immersed in the earth for a while before pulling up the root.

Eddie watches me and shakes his head. I can imagine him thinking I'm a crazy city girl, but all he says is "just take what you need. When peoples find a patch they try to take all of it, that's why it's so hard to find."

I nod my head in agreement. I pull a few and break the stem to make sure it's yellow, just like Eddie showed me. I wipe off the soil and rinse them in the pond before putting them in the sack he brought just for the harvest.

I take a moment to exhale and give thanks that we made it safe and that I finally found the yellow root in it's natural environment. I can step back, at last, and appreciate this luscious oasis in the middle of the thorny, mosquito-infested jungle. Vibrant greens decorate the perimeter. The soil is iron-rich, dark, and delicious. Insects hum notes that pulsate high and low pitches, short and long tones. These are syncopated rhythms like the hand claps in the praise houses of the Gullah. Sounds that remind me of fast-moving feet and ankles shackled with those rattling, B.B. shot-filled snuff cans used in the stomp ceremonies of the Yamasee and Tuscarora. Monk, Coltrane and Gillespie—prodigal sons of Carolina soil—must have played unabashedly in these woods when they were children. Carolina fed them her breath and they inhaled. This rhythm permeated their veins, nourished their blood, encoded their DNA and spoke to the ancestors that lived in them. It was an old song, an ancient way of communicating that survived through everything. This was the only music they knew. They had no choice but to try and recreate the sounds in Monkism, Coltranism and Gillespieism.

I now know I understand nothing. I am an infant trying to learn how to speak. My part in this language is listening and feeling the connection in my heart.

Yellow root must be strong medicine if this is what folks have to go through in order to get it.

Oscelena Harris ("Ms. Dot")
"My mother didn't carry us to no doctor"

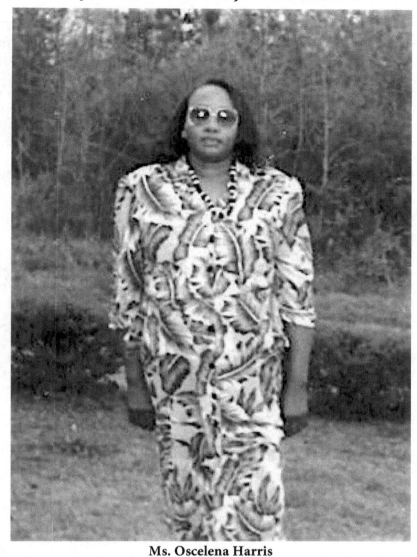

Ms. Oscelena Harris
Photo taken when Ms. Harris was in her 40's or 50's, 20 to 30 years before the time of this interview
Image 1-18

"I come from a little town called Redly and moved to Madison. Madison, Georgia. I'm 73 years old. I just use soap and water on my skin, and I don't wear no makeup. And there's nothin' I do to keep from bein' wrinkled."

Ms. Dot's skin was just like she said, wrinkle free, taut, and even-toned. She was a reddish-brown stocky woman, about 5'6". Her facial features were strong, both African and Native American, but not clearly one or the other. At 73 she still looked physically strong. I can imagine that in her peak, like Harriet Tubman, she was as strong as any man. Except for the tiredness in Ms. Dot's eyes, which gave away her age, she could easily pass for a 50-something.

Madison is in central Georgia roughly midway between Atlanta and Augusta. It took almost five hours of driving from my home in North Carolina, through state highways and back roads, to reach

Ms. Dot's house. Ms. Dot, her grandson, and three of her great-grandchildren greeted us[15] with the warm hospitality that quickly makes you feel like family, as one expects from Southerners. "Ya'll hungry? Can I get you something to eat? I got some soda water. Ya'll must be thirsty after that long drive."

Ms. Dot hosted us in her sparsely decorated living room of one couch and two chairs. She lived in a modest pre-fab home, simple and clean with an air of synthetic modernity. The floors, the walls, everything, looked a generic white/gray and sterile. It was the newest home she had ever lived in. She did not own it, however. The home was owned by the son of the woman who had employed Ms. Dot for most of Ms. Dot's life. The son made good on a promise to his dying mother that he would make sure Ms. Dot would be taken care of for the rest of her living days. But that only gave Ms. Dot the right to live in a home that she will never own, nor be able to pass down to her descendants. Ms. Dot was optimistic, however, that one day the son would sign the papers over to her, making her the sole, legitimate owner.

While we sat in her living room, she told me some of her life's story and her associations with folk medicine.

"All of my family is from Georgia. My mama and grandparents come from down there in Shadydale. My granddaddy was full Indian and my grandmama was Black Indian.

"I was married one time, and that was for four years. He was workin' on the railroad when he died.

"I had four babies at one time. I thinkin' about how I used to pray and ask the Lord to let me live to see my chil'ren get grown. I work hard so they never have to pick any cotton. I thank the Lord I did that. I worked 'til all my chil'ren were grown. When I was a young woman, I used to make my livin' workin' two jobs, in the field and at the cotton mill. I used to get up an go to the field in the mornin' time pickin' 200 pounds of cotton. I get off at 3 and I come home to change clothes and then go on to work at the cotton mill. On Saturday I go to work all day. "When I worked at the White folks house I made $2 a day. When I worked at the cotton mill I made $40 a week. After my day at the mill, I had to go take care of the White folks home and their kids.

"When I had the heart attack, I had worked that Friday, come home, I wash two loads of clothes and fixed supper and that's all I remember. I woke up in the hospital that Wednesday that next week. I didn't know what had happened. The doctor said my heart just stopped.

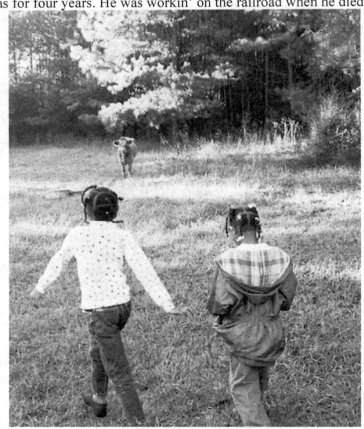

Ms. Dot's grand nieces and her cow
Image 1-19

Ms. Dot pushed herself up from the chair to stretch her body and move around. She moved to the window and said, "See dat cow out there...?"

I followed Ms. Dot to the window.

---

[15] My children and former husband came with me to the visit and interview with Ms. Harris.

"I've had that cow since a baby. I paid $200 for her. I'ma kill it some time in December for Christmas to make beef and stuff like that. I feedin' her dry feeds now, so by the time I kill her, I know she be cleaned out. You can kill a cow by shootin' it and put it somewhere to bleed. I done cleaned plenty cows and hogs by myself. When I was growin' up with my chil'ren, we didn't have nobody to kill our hog. I tell my chil'ren get out there and kill that hog. I got a smoke house back there but we ain't got no time for that now.

"I want me a pig. I got me a cage out there. I'ma get me a pig and watch it eat clean."

Ms. Dot cocked her head toward back-yard-over-yonder and her fattening heifer. She stared out the window. The room fell silent and serene nostalgia permeated the air.

She reminisced the good 'ol days when peach trees were abundant. "Used to be peach trees all up and down here," she said. "I had peach trees in my backyard over yonder. That was before I moved in the city."

These were the same "good 'ol days" of picking 200 pounds of cotton, fatiguing factory work and taking care of White folk's homes. Like the lotus that transcends mud, the human spirit always finds beauty to nourish and sustain the soul in the midst of oppressive situations. The peach trees and their bountiful gifts never did anything bad to Ms. Dot. The leaves gave her medicine, the fruits provided delicious food and the bosom of flourishing peach fields assuaged a "good 'ol days" pain.

Did Ms. Dot know that before her beloved peach trees found their way to Georgia, the Taoist Chinese treasured them just as much? They grew them by the doors of their homes to encourage good luck and believed its medicine carried the elixir of immortality. Peach trees moved from China and lost their supernatural status when they found their way to America but gained a new place of reverence, mostly economic and practical. But for Ms. Dot and others like her, the peach tree retained a semblance of the position it held in China. It gave people hope and solace which is sure to bring good luck and near immortality to any situation.

After a few minutes, Ms. Dot returned to the present reality of our interview and repeatedly apologized for not remembering as much as she once did. She blamed moving to the city as the cause of her not knowing any more. But once moved to the city, Ms. Dot un-remembered some knowledge and gained more.

"Back yonder when we were comin up, my mother didn't carry us to no doctor. We went out there and went in somebody's yard or went in the woods and got sumtin. They [the herbs] cured ya. I learned from my mother.

"For headaches, my mama get out there and get us some jimson weed leaves. She get it, wash the dust off of it with cold water, put it in a poultice and tie it around our head, and it would cure it. It still ground around here. You can find it in the spring in the woods.

"For earaches we warm up some sweet oil and drop a couple of drops in the ear and put cotton in it. We used to blow the smoke from the tobacco in the ear too. It's good for it.

"We used to use them big 'ol wide castor leaves to break fevers, too. We just wrap the leaves around the person until it chases the fever out. You can still find some growin' over here by the school house last year, but they done cut down so much that I don't think you outta find nothin' out there.

"You take the herbs outta them woods down in here. We used to go in them woods and find some scrubby grass when you want your bowels to move. Scrubby grass. It's a green bunch of grass, just like crab grass. You pull it up and the roots are yellow. You bring it to the house and wash it and make a tea with it. It's not yellow root cuz when you pull it out the ground, you can see the roots are yellow, you don't have to break it to see the yellow like yellow root. You make you a tea if you got a cold or somethin' like that. It cleans out your system. The frost kills it. In the spring time of the year, you cain't find it in pine wood, you gotta look for a oak tree and you'll find it. But we done had about three big frosts this year and the frosts kills 'em, you know, and you cain't find 'em out in the woods like we used to."

Ms. Dot paused, sucked on her front teeth and gleaned a wide smile. She rubbed her finger across her top row and proudly declared she's never had any "tooth" problems except for two that were saved by a couple of gold rims. She has all of her teeth, including her wisdom. She pulled her cheek back so I could have a better view of the two salvaged teeth.

"My mama didn't make us go to a dentist to have our tooth fixed. You got some bad teeth, get that little rat-vein. Rat-vein is another weed. It's a scraggly stuff, be 'bout that wide[16], and gets 'bout that high[17], and it have leaves on it, they be green but they have white spots on it. You can still see rat-vein before the frost get it. In the spring time it will all come back up again. You just get it and bring it to the house and dry it and smoke it in a cigarette, just puff on it, and pull on that teeth and it bring that pain out.

"You got a baby that's teething, you give it birdbill. It's a weed made just like a birdbill. Just get you some of that there, bring it in the house and wash it and put it in a jar with some water and we put it in the bottle. We brews it up and when you put it in the jar, you can go ahead and give him some of it. You can keep it for a long time, just keep adding fresh water to it. It will kill that diarrhea too.

"I remember when they took my grandbaby to the hospital and the doctor give out. Her fever so high, they took her home, couldn't break it.

"But I got this young boy, told him to get me all green peach leaves, leaves from the peach tree. I took 'em and dip 'em in dat water, that cold water, wrapped 'em in a towel and put her in it and it wasn't 15 minutes and those leaves dried all out. It took all that fever out.

"They carried her back to the doctor the next morning and the doctor asked 'em, how did they break her fever. She say, she told him, "My grandmother broke it.

"He say, 'Well you tell her I say she come down here and me and her work together.'

"I had a boy, my baby boy, he had sores. Great big husky sores all over him and I thought it was infitaigo.[18] I don't care what I done for him, it wouldn't cure them sores. Every year he break out the same way. So, this lady live next door to us, she was an Indian lady, she say, 'I tell you what you do. You see that pokeberry bush out yonder? You take him out there and let him eat nine poke berries that are ripe. Don't let him eat but nine.'

"I took my baby out there and let him eat nine pokeberries. He lost some scales and then he lost them all. Never found out what it was. I still use all this medicine on my grandkids and children. I brought mines up on medicine like that. They still comes to me first when they get sick. Every year I made my kids go out there and eat nine poke berries. They don't be breakin' out with them sores neither.

"For hives or rash, you use pokeberries, the nine pokeberries. Everybody say the pokeberries is poison but they ain't poison, unless you don't know how to eat them.

"My grandmother used to make pokeberry wine. That's my Indian grandmother. My aunt used to make wine out of it too and sell it to people and folks who come from long way off. She say she had people come from Tennessee to buy her pokeberry wine. She would make it every year. Folks would come and buy it by the gallon.

"There still a lot of pokeberry bushes here in Madison, Georgia. I cook the greens from the poke sallat bush. Cook 'em just like collards and turnips. Wash 'em and put 'em on in your pot. Some folk cook 'em with turnip salad. I cook mine just regular, cuz the doctor told me one time everybody oughta eat overmuch of poke sallat cuz it cleanses out your system. I freeze it. It taste good. When you use it by itself it taste like spinach."

I've seen poke sallat as tall as four feet high with long leaves that resemble spinach. Stalks of deep crimson berries jettied out of the leaves. They looked sensuously sweet and delicious and the birds delighted in their fruits. Most people said the berries were poisonous. Poke sallat grew wild and plentiful in the southern landscape from Appalachia to Florida. If one needed a quick green to cook, poke sallat was the choice because it was free and you usually found it close by.

But I had been over-warned by veteran Southerners not to eat the berries of the poke bush. In making

---

[16]   Sliver of a fingernail

[17]   12 inches

[18]   Impetigo, a highly contagious bacterial skin infection that produces sores and blisters; most common among kids and is treated with antibiotic ointment.

poke sallat, I was also instructed to cook the leaves twice, rinse, throw off the water and then prepare them just like collards. My instructors knew I was green, inquisitive and anxious to claim my Southern roots by doing what Southern folk do, and could possibly get hurt. The plant carries the toxins phytolaccatoxin and phytolaccigenin, which are poisonous to mammals. Cooking the leaves and throwing the water off two to three times reduces the toxins enough to eat without adverse effect. However, eating "overmuch" as Ms. Dot's doctor mentioned above or eating without rinsing off the toxins will give you diarrhea and "cleanse out your system."

The berry is by far the most versatile part of this plant and has been used in many interesting ways over centuries. Ms. Dot and her family, like many others, have used it as medicine and moonshine. The juice yields a rich sanguine dye, and the Native Americans of the Western Continents once used it to decorate their horses, and Civil War soldiers wrote letters to loved ones using pokeberry ink. The Declaration of Independence is often, though incorrectly, stated to have been written in the red ink of fermented pokeberry juice. But, it was Benjamin Lay, the outspoken abolitionist Quaker who came up with the most creative use for pokeberry. He burst into one meeting of Philadelphia's Quaker leaders and plunged a sword into a hollowed-out Bible filled with blood-red pokeberry juice, which he then sprayed in the shocked faces of the slave-owners.[19] From here on, pokeberry juice became a symbol of blood for the anti-slavery movement. One person's poison is another's medicine.

Sharing the merits of poke sallat opened up a flood of memories for Ms. Dot. She continued like a seasoned doctor lecturing to an intern about one remedy to the next, without pause.

"It's another weed called peppergrass. Oh, that's the best stuff. It got a funny leaf on it, and you just go on and pick the top out of it. You use it like turnip greens. They good for you. I used to use that yellow root for high sugar too, but you can't find it like you used to. You can use banana peelings for high sugar. Just peel it off the banana and put it in there and make a tea out of it. But you can use too much of that. If you take too much, it'll get your sugar too low. And for artheritis. . ."

Ms. Dot got up and gestured for me to follow her into the bedroom. It was difficult to see. The room was dark and the curtains were drawn to prevent any of day's light from seeping through. She turned on the bedside lamp. I noticed several bottles on the floor, of varying shapes and sizes, each filled with a liquid and some kind of ingredient: Chopped roots? Banana peel? Kelp? Onion? Root vegetable? Mud? Before I could ask she had already picked up one and was explaining that "This one here is for my artheritis. You get a quart of apple cider vinegar, put nine sewing needles in it, it'll eat those needles up, and just rub the vinegar on you after its eaten up the needles. It works." Ms. Dot put that bottle back and picked up another and another, explaining the purpose of each one in turn.

"This is good for cramps in your muscles. You put a banana in a jar of green alcohol and leave it in there and when it clear up, rub it on the cramp.

"This other bottle is alcohol with lemon juice in it. This for muscle cramps too. I used to get muscle cramps a lot and I just rub this on it.

"I use this bottle, the red clay, for strained muscle or ankle. We get some red clay dirt and make a poultice out of it and put it on the strain.

---

[19]   From the Wikipedia entry on Benjamin Lay (February, 2014): His passionate enmity of slavery fueled by his Quaker beliefs, Lay made several dramatic demonstrations against the practice. He once stood outside a Quaker meeting in winter with no coat and at least one foot bare and in the snow. When passersby expressed concern for his health, he said that slaves were made to work outdoors in winter dressed as he was. On another occasion, he kidnapped the child of slaveholders temporarily, to show them how Africans felt when their relatives were sold overseas.[See: "A Place At The Table: Struggles For Equality In America" edited by Maria Fleming, Oxford University Press, 2001] The most notable act occurred at the 1738 Philadelphia Yearly Meeting of Quakers. Dressed as a soldier, he concluded a diatribe against slavery by plunging a sword into a Bible containing a bladder of blood-red berry juice, which spattered over those nearby. [See: *The Friend* Newspaper (Philadelphia) XXIX (28): 220. March 1856. See also: Jackson, Maurice (2010). *Let This Voice Be Heard: Anthony Benezet, Father of Atlantic Abolitionism.* University of Pennsylvania Press. p. 49. ISBN 0812221265]

"Now for poor blood circulation we go out and find a weed called timtyne weed, but you cain't find it 'til the spring of the year. The timtyne got a white bloom at the top and you take that weed and you kinda crush it up a bit and make you a tea out of it.

"Mullet is good for gout, for when your feet swell up. Get it, mix it, boil it and put your feet in it and bathe your feet in it. Oooh yeah, that works, I done had that, I know. You cain't hardly find it any more. Mullett is a big 'ol beautiful plant. Some people say mullein or mullet, it the same thang 'round here.

"For ringworms, go out there to the fig tree and pull off that green fig and break it open and you will see milk on the inside of the green shell. Then you put the fig juice milk on the ringworm. If you got more than one ringworm, you don't use the same fig for each spot. You get a different fig every time and put that juice on it. You gotta put the fig juice on it every morning. It may take about a week to go away.

"You can also use tobacco for wasp stangs, bee stangs and stuff like that. And ear aches. I didn't chew tobacco, just used it for healin', blow the smoke in the ear and make a poultice to put over the ear.

"Talla[20] is good for colds. If you got a cold, you go get you some talla and get it warm by the fire and you streak your chest and it draws out that cold and then it loosens it up too.

"For upset stomach or stomach ache I'd take caramel[21] root tea. It grows in the yard and you dig up that root. It grow right straight up there like grass, like a bunch of grass. I get me some of it and wash it and chew it. That helps my stomach.

"I like sage bush, too. It's good medicine. I burn it, too. It smell good. I tell you what, you can burn it in your house and you sho' give it a good smell. And then you can take it and make sausage with it. Yeah, it's good. For medicine I make a tea and it cleans out your stomach real good. My mama used to drank it for coffee in the morning."

Listening to Ms. Dot talk about stomach ailments and remedies reminded me of the chronic case of morning sickness I had during the entire term of both of my pregnancies. I'm guilty of holding the stereotype that Southern women can pop out a lot of babies with ease and get back to work within a few days, and also know what to take to curb any discomfort. I asked her if she had any problems during any of her pregnancies.

"When I was pregnant, I didn't have too much trouble; what trouble I did have, we used haasmint[22]. It's down on the river along the creek back here. Make you a tea, and you don't have no pain, no ache or nothin' and when you in labor it come more easier. It helps to get rid of morning sickness, too, and it smell good. It smell like mint.

"And you know that hassmint is a mint weed. You get it and bring it home and wash it and put it on the stove and let it come to a boil and drink the tea. When we was kids, we used to add some lard or vaseline or whatever you want to haasmint and let it cook down, and oooh, it smell good. We used to put it in our hair. It make your hair grow too, we had the softest hair."

The plastic cap covered most of Ms. Dot's hair throughout the interview. Only one lone braid stuck out and fell across her ear to rest on her shoulder. It looked soft, black and silky and gently curled at the end. The "haasmint" hair pomade had served her well throughout the years.

"But we really didn't get sick much, couldn't afford to. For each season we make different teas."

Ms. Dot stopped in mid sentence to get up and turn on the porch light. The sun had set and the last glimmer of that day's light melted into dark right before our eyes. It was mid-October, evenings were cool and nature prepared for her first frost.

"We make teas that we would sip on every day. Like right now, it's getting ready to be winter and you won't be able to find some herbs because of the frost, so I got to go out and get me my teas for the

---

[20] Talla or tallow: fat from cooked beef, warmed and rubbed on chest as a salve.

[21] Chamomile

[22] Horsemint

winter. Rabbit tobacco and pinetop and mullet and horehound is good for the winter season. Mix that together and boil it and make you a tea out of it and sip off of it and you can make cough syrup out of it. Yeah, you can put honey in it and make you some cough syrup. Now honey and whiskey good for colds too, mostly coughs. Get you a pine cone, get you a jar, put that pine cone and some whiskey and some honey in there with it. It good for colds. We give a spoonful to kids and it put 'em right out here. None of my children get their medicine this way anymore. There's a lot. I done forgot what half the stuff I did."

Ms. Dot took a hearty yawn, rubbed her eyes. "I'm sorry," she said, "you got 'ta excuse me, haven't thought about this stuff in a long time and I get tired easy. When I'm tired, I know I just need to rest. Rest would do you more good than any medicine." On that advice, we replaced the interview with cordial chit chat that gradually diminished into silence. Ms. Dot settled her body into the oversized powder blue faux leather chair. It was directly across from where I sat on the matching sofa. Her eyes blinked heavily, her head nodded and finally settled, limp at her chest. I watched until her lids shut and heavy breathing turned to a soft snore. She was secure and safe. We rested together. We had interviewed for almost four hours, and I still had a long drive back to Laurel Hill.

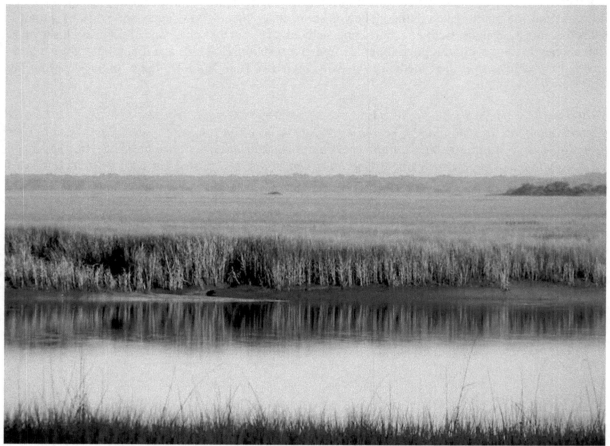

Looking across the marsh to a South Carolina sea island in Gullah-Geechee country
Image 1-20

Description: Greenish yellow sweetgrass used in basketweaving on the perimeter of marsh water

During my early years living in North Carolina I established Wadastick, a non-profit residency for artists and scholars. Wadastick had satellite residency sites at the Tuscarora Indian Nation in Maxton, North Carolina, another on St. Helena Sea Island in South Carolina and a third in El Potrero, Mexico. The goal of the residencies was to offer authentic experiences in traditional cultures. I traveled to St. Helena often while setting up the Sea Island residency and was fortunate to speak with several native Gullah-Geechee and other South Carolinians about their healing tradition. I also visited the Georgia and Florida sea islands just south of St. Helena and experienced more of the rich African traditions that make the sea islands and Gullah-Geechee history so unique.

The Gullah-Geechee[23] people have lived for over 400 years on the coastal Sea Islands that make up

---

[23] A discussion of the origins of the terms "Gullah" and "Geechee"—either in reference to the African continent or to America—is beyond the scope of this book. Historians speculate that the term "Geechee" could have originated from the *Ogeechee River* near Savannah, Georgia. Ogeechee is a Creek Indian word. "Gullah" may have originated from *Guale*, the indigenous American nation whose homeland was along coastal Georgia and South Carolina's low country, or from *Gola* an ethnic group between Sierra Leone and Liberia where many of the Gullah descended. Today we know the terms have overlapping meanings. Traditionally in U.S. history, they both referred to African Americans in South Carolina's low country and Georgia who had preserved a distinctly African culture through the Middle Passage into the modern era. However, "Geechee" was a largely derogatory term that referred to African Americans throughout South Carolina—though more frequently defining those people closer to the coast—while "Gullah" referred largely to people living in the coastal sea islands from Charleston down to northern Florida. African Americans in lower Louisiana also were able to preserve their African traditions through slavery and Emancipation. For the purpose of this chapter, I am

the intra-coastal waterway running through South Carolina, Georgia and North Florida. These people are direct descendants of enslaved Africans who were stolen from the rice growing regions of West Africa.[24] Due to the isolation of these coastal islands, the African people who were settled there beginning in the 17th century had minimal contact with people of other races, particularly Europeans.[25]

Thus, unlike African descendants living in the Deep South and the rest of the country, the Gullah-Geechee people were able to maintain much of their African culture and traditions, in particular retaining a distinct language comprised of over 4000 words from various portions of the African continent. That distinct sub-set of African American culture is what we recognize today as the Gullah and Geechee of the Sea Islands.

A sampling of some of those natural healing practices is outlined below.

Living the Gullah-Geechee Tradition

Many of the herbs and plants used for medicinal purposes and maintaining health are found in the woods and in local gardens. Most medicines were harvested in the winter when the woods were thinner because they were easier to find. But because many plants look alike, people had to be able to identify the top, leaves, and sometimes dig up the roots, break them open and identify the color.

Contrary to Western culture and traditions concerning health remedies, the use of plants and herbs as remedies for specific ailments and/or preventive measures is a way of life for the Gullah-Geechee people.

Preventive Measures

(Cold, flu, cough, ear infections, intestinal worms, etc.)

Garlic is often grown in yards to use as medicine and in food. An effective remedy for cold and cough involved blending chopped garlic with the rosin from the pine tree. It is said that the persons preparing this particular medicine chop the tree until it bleeds. Once the rosin hardens, they collect it and place it in a frying pan along with syrup and stir in the garlic until the flavor is released in the entire pan. When the combined ingredients cool, they harden like a candy bar and are eaten throughout the year. This medicine "cleans you out" and prevents people from contracting such ailments as worms or the common cough. A similar remedy is used among people on the mainland of the Carolinas for colds and worms.

The bay tree grows prolifically on the Sea Islands and the Gullah-Geechee often use the collected leaves to season fish and stews. A tea made out of bay leaf aids in the relief of headaches, congestion, fevers and coughs.

Eucalyptus is also used for its medicinal properties in treating ear infections, chest congestion and the common cold.

Preventive Measures – Winter Months

During the winter months, people make a tea from the plant Life-Everlasting combined with a root referred to as Big Root—named for the size of its root—which bears big leaves and black berries.[26]

---

combining the two terms and using them to mean communities of African descent with distinctive African-identifiable culture living on the South Carolina, Georgia, and Florida sea islands or in the immediate mainland areas some 45 miles or so inland.

[24] The majority of the Gullah-Geechee population are descendants of Africans from the rice coast of Africa— Sierra Leone, Guinea and Liberia. Other countries include Ghana, Republic of Congo, Angola and Nigeria.

[25] The exception to this relative isolation was contact with a few Native American nations like the Cusabo and Yamasee, who occupied a large area from South Carolina through Georgia and into Florida, and the Seminole of Florida.

[26] It may be difficult to ascertain the specific plant referred to as "Big Root." However, "Life-Everlasting" is a commonly-known and recognized plant (Gnaphalium polycephalum), and it is well documented that the Gullah people used it for centuries to relieve cramps, cure colds, combat diseases of the bowel and pulmonary system and relieve foot pain. "Healing and Folk Medicine." Gullah Culture in America, by Wilbur Cross. Westport, CT: Praeger Security International, 2008.

These black berries die off during the winter and are therefore not used to make the tea. Instead, the "Big Root" itself is chopped up and cooked together with Life-Everlasting to make the winter tea. The tea is used to ensure regular bowel movements; similar to the chopped garlic and pine rosin concoction outlined above, it is also said to "clean you out." Most Gullah-Geechee understand that the key to good health is through a clean colon achieved through regular bowel movements.

Specific Remedies

To cure coughs and high fever, people gather mullein, horehound and limbs from the pine tree and cook them down to create a liquid tonic. Mullein is characterized as having large leaves that are whitish-green and fuzzy. Horehound is characterized as a small gray plant and having a bitter taste once it is cooked. Mullein and horehound are commonly found in the gardens of the Gullah-Geechee people. Drinking the mullein, horehound and pine limb tonic causes one to "sweat it out." Within two days, it relieves the fever and cough.

Another remedy to relieve fever is use of the oil bush plant (castor tree/castor oil). People take the leaves from the oil bush plant and wrap them around the feverish body. Once the leaves become dry and parched, the fever is relieved. This same treatment is used in the Creole communities of New Orleans and various Native American tribes in the southeastern United States.

Chest congestion and the common cold is often treated by consuming a cooked tea infusion of eucalyptus leaves. The leaves are boiled and then strained to produce the drinkable medicine. Any unused portion of the eucalyptus drink is then put in the "icebox" (refrigerator) to heat up for later use. Sassafras tea is another common tonic to prevent and relieve colds.[27]

Spider webs are used to close deep cuts and wounds, as well as applied to the skin to alleviate sores and insect bites.

Faith and Spirituality

The cultural traditions of the Gullah-Geechee people and the use of plants and herbs for medicinal purposes cannot be isolated from their faith and spirituality. Traditionally, many of the Gullah-Geechee people participated in small prayer services on Monday, Wednesday and Saturday nights. The opportunity to pray, sing, give testimonials and "thank the Lord" in the "Praise Houses"[28] were an integral component of the Gullah-Geechee way of Life that began during slavery and still exists today. This form of spiritual healing is just as important as the physical healing.[29]

---

[27] An important warning note about sassafras and safrole: Sassafras contains safrole, which is known to have harmful effects if ingested over a period of time in large and concentrated quantities. See warning and instructions in the Sassafras section on pages 319-320 before using.

[28] Praise Houses are small places (average 20'x20') of segregated worship that were established on plantations for enslaved Africans to preach, pray and sing. The Praise Houses soon expanded to be a meeting place that offered support, confidentiality and governance to the increasingly more self-reliant Gullah-Geechee community. Services were held three nights a week on Sunday, Tuesday and Thursday and usually consisted of singing, praise, testimony and the ring shout (people moving around a circle, dancing by shuffling their feet, rhythmic hand clapping and singing a call and response type style). The Praise Houses were considered the heart of the community.

[29] African American people from the Sea Islands to the mainland have always understood that their spiritual and physical health are interrelated. This philosphy was brought from Africa and is recently being accepted by modern medicine. A strong spiritual foundation and the healing and support that is traditionally offered through the Praise Houses and church communities was and still is crucial to African American survival. These are safe places to release frustration, find solidarity, support, strength and hope in overcoming challenges. Today, modern medicine shows a direct correlation between stress and emotional well-being and between chronic diseases like high blood pressure and heart disease and the ability of our bodies to operate optimally. The spiritual and physical mojo worked together makes for a stronger medicine and a stronger people.

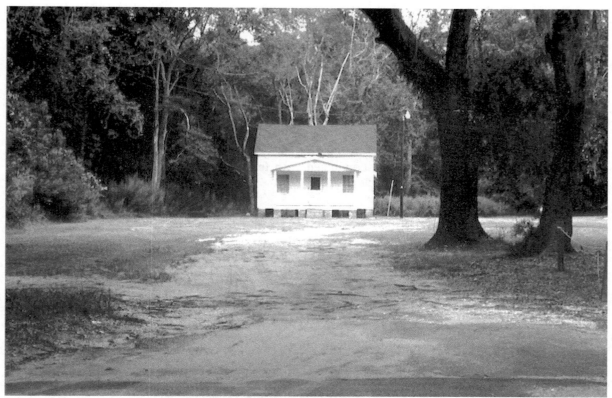

Praise House, St. Helena Island, South Carolina
Image 1-21

The Gullah-Geechee are increasingly isolated into small pockets of their traditional homeland in the sea island area of the southeastern coast. They are losing the ability to practice the fishing, shrimping, crabbing, and farming skills that their ancestors brought with them from Africa, and which formed such an integral part of Gullah-Geechee life and culture until the 1970's.

The Mississippi Valley and West

The Louisiana Purchase and America's victory in the Mexican War in the 19th century opened up vast new territories in the Mississippi River Valley basin and western lands to the rapidly-expanding United States. Down the Mississippi River and into these newly-acquired lands thousands of Africans were shipped and forcibly uprooted from the Southeastern plantations where they had been enslaved. A new American folk saying described these ominous consequences: "sold down the river." These newly-displaced people brought with them their folk medicine traditions and practices originated in Africa and refined in states like the Carolinas, Georgia, and Florida.

The following three narratives were conducted with the descendants of those forced emigrés in Louisiana and Texas.

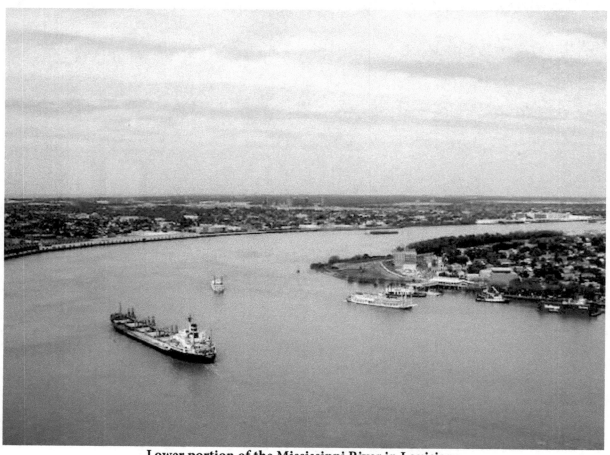

Lower portion of the Mississippi River in Louisiana
Image 1-22

Ms. Levatus Gillory - "We wouldn't get no colds"

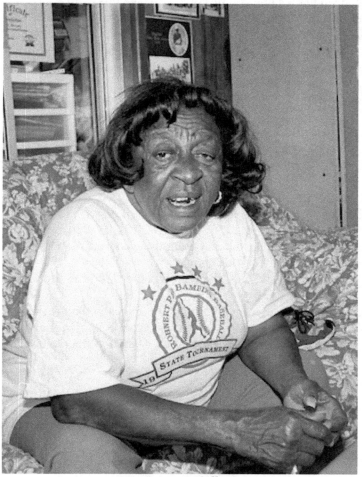

Ms. Levatus Gillory
Image 1-23

People call me Vat or Ms. Vat but my name is Levatus Gillory. I'm from Paris, Texas, not Paris, France. I was born on November 15, 1925. I'm a Scorpio; we are lovers—hahahaha!

I stayed in Paris, Texas until I went into the 5th grade. Then we moved to Oklahoma City and then to Kansas City—my mother, one sister and two brothers. I finished school in Kansas City but I did my 7th grade year in Oklahoma City. But every summer, Mama used to put us on the bus and we went to stay with our grandmother back in Texas.

We didn't go to the doctor or dentist or nothin' like that. I think the first time I went to a doctor, I must have been about twelve. I got all my teeth but a few that been filled.

My mother used a lot of homemade remedies. She was givin us so many different kinds of stuff that we didn't hardly get sick.

I remember Mama used to make flanna, I don't think they have that no more. People go and get black tar and hog grease and turpentine for the winter time. Mama would mix it together and she would put it in a pan and warm it up. Then she would put it on a rag and pin it on us and we slept with that on our chest. Every night she warm it up and pin it on our chest again.

She'd put this on us just before winter, just as winter beginnin', and we couldn't take that off until Easter Sunday. We wore it even to school. And, we really didn't get no colds.

Another thing we had was asfidity. Mama buy that in the store. You can buy it today but it says on the thang that it's not good for internal, but I actually eat it. Mama just put that in a little rag and put it on a string and throw it around our neck. We had to wear that to keep from catchin' colds and germs. We wore that to school even though it stunk.

I use the asfidity on my own children. If somebody drink liquor, put some asfidity in the bottle, you know a little bottle, then when the baby get the colic, you take this asfidity and liquor and put about two drops in it with some milk and give it to em. I put about a whole bag of asfidity in a pint-size liquor bottle and just keep it. I give it to the children to put 'em to sleep. They go straight to sleep.

Mama used to fix a tea with cow manure after she dried it out. We drank it. This helped to clear our chest so we wouldn't get no colds.

I remember Senna leaf tea. It was good too. That was good for your body, it clean you out when you get constipated. I couldn't stand castor oil so Mama give it to us with an orange or lemon cuz that would clean you out too.

We had some kind of wood, it was real red and the tea was red, but it tasted real good. I think it was a cedar. I can see it right now, and it smell good too. Mama used to make it for chest colds and coughs.

When we had earaches, Mama would use sweet oil, put a drop or two in your ear, and that would open it up. And then when we had headaches, she would put vinegar on a brown paper bag and put it across your forehead and we lie down and it would go away.

When the babies be rashed, you brown this flour and put it on with some kind of salve or grease and that clears it up.

We used to boil hogs hoof and make tea and drain the water off. That was the tea. We would drink that hot or cold and it was good too for colds and flu.[30]

Mama would put baking soda on a cut. She would pack it in there and keep it from bleedin and it would boil all those germs out of there.

She would put cold water and butter on a burn and for cuts and thangs she would use iodine.

If you get fever blisters, you take earwax and put it on the fever blister and it would go away.

People nowaday rather carry their kids to the doctor. They don't believe in the old remedies.

---

[30] Hog hoof tea is used to combat such conditions as the flu, whooping cough, congestion, and the common cold.

Ms. Valena Noble - *"People didn't get sick offa pork back then"*

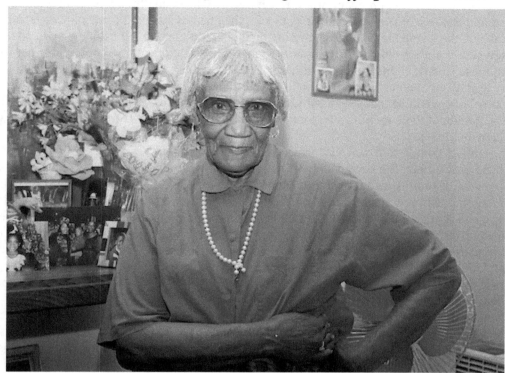

Ms. Valena Noble
Image 1-24

My health is pretty good now. I take a water pill and pressure pill cuz my ankles have got kinda swellin' up. The doctor said it was a lot of fluid. It wasn't natural. That's all he treatin' me for. Other than that, I feel pretty good.

I was born 1909. I was raised in Bonita, Babo Nai Nai. Today that's how we say Bonita. It's between Monroe and Merouets, Louisiana, and Berniece and Oakridge, Louisiana. And then on down from Merouets there's Bonita right there, my little home town. I part-way grew up on a farm. I had seven brothers and three sisters. Some of 'em is half brothers. My Daddy and Mama had seven together including me.

I remember my mother was always out workin' herself with those White people. A lot of people were. She would wash and iron and sometimes she cooked. She was busy.

They would go in buggies then, carry the clothes back up town and come back. She was takin' care of the White family up the street and us too cuz she was gettin' money from workin' round those White people. Mama would work from early in the mornin', 7:00 'til in the evenin' 'bout 4:30 and then she come home. She didn't do much when she got home cuz my grandmother was seein' after us when we was little.

My mother died young. She was about 35. My grandparents raised me after my mother passed.

I never took no tonic 'til I got married. And the tonic I took then I got from the drugstore. I took this cuz they jus' said that would make you stronger and healthy. I couldn't tell if it worked. I was a newlywed.

I married a farmer. My farm was in Babo Nai Nai. I had 20 acres and then another 10 acres. We still have the land. I rent it out. We made cotton and corn, peanuts and beans, tomatoes and all kinds of vegetables, oh, just everythang. We made a lot outta pickin' cotton out there for somebody else that made cotton. After we got that tractor we made fine crops and started with 50 bales of cotton. People went in together helping one another more.

I didn't do nothin' to keep from havin no baby. And I didn't know nothin' then, I don't reckon. I musta didn't. When I was in labor they didn't give me nothin' special. They jus' told me to grease my stomach and work and keep movin', don't lay around. That's all I did and I pushed the babies out.

They told me when I was pregnant not to reach over my head cuz the cord could wrap around the babies neck and choke it. After I pushed the baby out, they had us stay in the bed nine days. You lay up there in that bed, they have the windows, curtain down, wouldn't let the light shine on you and the baby either. They said it ain't good for the baby's eyes and mine neither to have too much light. But now they got all these electric lights on these babies and oh, God, that's tiresome.

I breast feed all my babies 'cept two. I had to ween that baby because he was born with teeth. His teeth was out. Now when dat baby was born he jus' like da rest of us. A li'l ol head jus' like da rest of us. When he got about three months, I be lookin' out at my baby. I say, "Don look like nothin' growin' 'bout dis baby but his head."

Granny said, "I coulda told you that was a waterhead baby, but I wouldn't tell you." Waterhead baby, his head growed big. But he was growin' looong too. We got him a buggy, his face went way out. My husband said, "Nooo! Carry da baby to Monroe." When dey take him to Monroe, x-ray pictures, the doctor say this is not no waterhead baby. Waterhead babies don't last that long. He couldn't hold his head up good, but he could try to talk and play at cha. And he knowed all us. But he just couldn't hold his head up cuz ya see it had boozched-out and got big. He died after he got about 9 years old. We suffered and carried him to different places but he didn't get no better.

I had 10 kids. I guess I'd been dead years ago if my children didn't help me work. They helped me out 'til Uncle Sam got the two oldest. They got drafted in World War II. My oldest son was born 1930 and then next one born 1934. They survived the war.

When I lived on the farm, oh Lawd, I cook all kinds of vegetables and corn and soups and chicken, peas and beans. All fresh out the garden. That work kept me strong and healthy and all my kids.

We didn't go to the store much for anything. We eat the animals on the farm. We had hogs, cows, chickens and geese and guinea. Guinea is a li'l somethin' look like a chicken hen but he walks real fast, fast, fast and look like he ain't gonna ever ever stop layin' eggs. They have their nests on the ground. And they can fly up! I never did have good luck with guineas but I had good luck with chickens and ducks and goose, geeses. I sold some of my hen eggs. Them hens laid some eggs! They lay eggs so much, they lay so many eggs, and then they sit and rest.

Back then, when the grocery truck was runnin' down through there they give us maybe 50 cents for a dozen eggs. Sometimes they go up to a dollar. We get good prices when I was sellin' eggs. We made a lotta money.

We raised a hog long time before we kill it. I had to fool with all this meat, grindin sausage and cuttin' up meat. And, oooh, I would be tastin' them good sausage and love it. They told me, "Onliest way you gonna keep 'Lena from eatin' pork, William have to quit raisin' the hog." My grandmother made hogs head cheese. She put the head in that big pot and find another big pan to put over it. You put your vinegar, sage, and black pepper, steam it down til all the bones off. Oooh, it was good.

People didn't get sick offa pork back then. They show didn't. Today, you don't know what's in it.

Skeeters

The mosquitoes was so bad back then that we have a mosquito ball over the bed. Li'l thin thing you put over the bed to keep the mosquitoes off the babies.

One time they was so bad down at the end of the field. We was pickin' cotton. We had smoke on each end. We made smoke, sulfur smoke, in a bucket or a can and just let it smoke the skeeters away. A bucket down here and a bucket down there. Smoke and smokin'. They go when they smell dat, they gone. Ooooh, it run the skeeters down that way in the woods, a thick place back there. They all go back there. And then you hear 'em jus' singin'. Ooooh, the mosquitoes was singin', they had a hum all back there. I know they was away from me!

No-Shoulders

Oooh, in Babo Nai Nai, my Lawd, my Lawd, they got plenty of no-shoulders out there. My grandmother say they call dem that because dey ain't got no shoulders. She say they enemies. They plagues or somethin'. It was plenty of 'em there. All kinds. Rattlesnakes, water moccassins, copperheads.

When we was workin', we never did get bit. But they was all around there. If you get bit by a no-shoulder, you was supposed to tie sumtin tight around there, and put coal oil on it, until you get to the doctor, quick, cuz dem thangs is poison.

My great uncle say, "Ya'll put a gallon of coal oil right up under the block by the side of your house. That'll keep da no-shoulders away."

Remedies

My grandmother used homemade remedies for colds and made tonics for other sickness. She would go out to the woods and get our medicine when we get sick.

She used to make shuck tea for the measles and chicken pox. Shucks come off of corn, but they be done got dry, and she put em in a pot and steam em, and you drank it.

I had chicken pox once and they would keep some kind of salve rubbed on it and some kind of powder, shakin' powder, to keep the itchin' down. Everybody used those kind of remedies back then.

My grandmother would give us horse milk for the whoopin' cough. She would milk a horse like she do a cow. Milks a horse, a horse! Pull the titty and get the milk. That milk killed the whoopin' cough.

She'd make cough syrup out of onions and sugar. Put tablespoons of sugar and cut up some onions and cook em down to a syrup and that would get rid of the cough. She did all that.

I didn't take my kids to the doctor much. They was pretty healthy but when my kids got sick, I would do the same thang my grandmother did. Give 'em castor oil and rub 'em with it on their chest if they got a fever or a chest cold. And li'l babies, put it in the mole of they head[31] and it bleeds the cold out. I used to hate to take castor oil. They used to have to hold my nose when I was li'l, oooh, but they say it's good.

Then some kind of disease or fever was goin' around. I think it was hay fever. And they say get some astifidisis. We bought it out at the drug store. It would come in a li'l package like chewin' gum and you push the astifist down in this li'l bag, sew it up in a li'l white cheesecloth and wear it around your neck. That keep 'em from catchin' it. When I got out to Oakland, I called for it like I been back home. I say, "Astifist, look like it got a heap'a scent, like a garlic scent. A bunch of herbs in it. And then it got something sticky in it like gum." I called for it but that lady looked at me like I iz crazy. Astifist. These people out there don't know what astifist is.

We would take sumtin in the winter time so they wouldn't get a cold. We'd take teas and cough syrups and totties. It's made out of good whiskey. Put a little water and sugar and let 'em drink it hot. It's good for colds and keepin' 'em away.

We'd take castor oil and blackdrop to keep from getting colds, too. You know, it works you. Keeps your bowels open. Blackdrop is a li'l powder stuff. It's made outta herbs. Different herbs that would grow, we grind it up. Its color is brown. We make a tea from it. You can give 'em a dose or else you could steep it and let 'em drink a li'l bit of it. We would get that at the drugstore. It's in a li'l yellow looking box. They used to give us sumtin else for fever and cough, called Six hundred Sixty Six. It's bitter.

If we get all backed up we take us a dose of Epsom salt and some blackdrop (Black Draught) tea[32]. Drank a big swallow and work myself off. Since I been out here, since I been grown, they told me to take Milk of Magnesia but that stops me up.

---

[31] The mole of the head is the soft spot in a babies head – right on the top in the center—you are supposed to be very careful not to injure or put too much pressure on this area when a baby is young because it could cause brain damage.

[32] Black Draught tea was medicine bought commonly from the apothecary/drugstore and used for many ailments. It is a cathartic medicine composed of a blend of senna and magnesia and acts much like castor oil. It's been sold in the U.S. since the late 19th century.

Ms. Etta Minor-Williams - "We were blessed with so much"

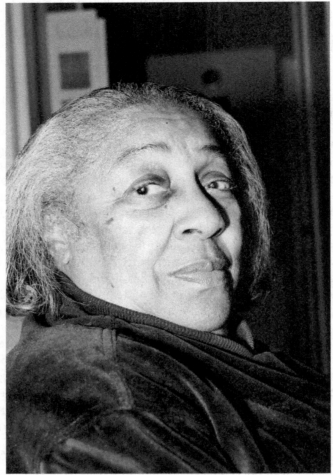

Ms. Etta Minor-Williams
Image 1-25

I grew up in Louisiana 30 miles from Woodville and 12 miles from St. Francisville. We was in between those two little towns.

My family had a 313 acre farm. We raised cotton, sweet potatoes, arch potatoes, string beans, sugar cane, cows, horses, hogs and yardbirds. This was all we raised. We sold gravel and timber off the place. I told my kids if they hadda come up out there like that they would have enjoyed life. I was just raised up with plenty of everythang. Nothin' excite me about what's out there now, because we had plenty to eat and everythang. Every other year my Daddy buy a new car and he couldn't drive.

My Daddy always tell us we was mixed with Indian on both sides. He had 13 brothers and sisters in his family, and then had three sons and it was nine girls – twelve brothers and sisters. I was the eleventh. I was born in the year 19 and 20. I'm 77. I'm blessed. I'm not ashamed to tell my age.

Raising What We Ate

We really had a diet that kept us healthy. We store food durin' the summer time when the okra and beans and corn were plentiful. We'd have to put 'em up for the winter. We had a shelf as long as this kitchen with those quart jars just full of that stuff. They wasn't pickled. You put 'em in a pressure cooker and cook 'em and dey stay there from one end of the year to another. Yeah, you open a jar in winter time when you ain't had nothin' else to cook. You can put sausage in a jar too, fry em and put em in there. Open a jar full of sausage and get some of dat okra and corn and all of that and fix something like a goulash or soup or somethin' and cook rice and put it over that. And, cook that cornbread. You couldn't beat that cornbread. It would be GOOD.

Back then a lot of Black people was so poor. My Daddy had jus' about an acre of garden with everythang in it and the people jus' come to our place and get some crops. They come there with sacks and try to get them somethin for their eat. We raised a lot of sweet potatoes, butter, milk and everythang. We raised all that stuff. We jus' set them out and sell em an there would be a lot lef. Some of them come real poor and didn't have no money and my Mama would jus' go ahead on and give 'em some.

My Daddy would raise corn, too. We had two barns of corn. We would shell that corn and take it to the mill and have it grind and have the barrels of it.

And in the winter time when it start to get cold, those collard greens would be tender and we'd go out there and pick up big ol leaves of collards and put that salt pork in there and get you some cornbread. You cook that cornbread and get you some of that buttermilk. Or smother some potatoes, ash potatoes[33], put some onions in and a piece of salt pork and a biscuit. That's all you wanted. Smothered potatoes and a biscuit and a piece of salt pork. We'd take it to school in those buckets. That would be your lunch. And we could put those buckets on them old heaters, stove heaters, and we set that on there a few minutes and warm dem potatoes, and talk 'bout sumtin good.

We also had pecan trees. Oh they was 'bout three or four big trees. And we would get out there and pick 'em up and sell some and eat some and you ate pecan candy and pecan pie and all of that.

And we used to bake sweet potatoes. And they would be so sweet, you didn't need nothin' but get you some buttermilk and a piece of hogs head cheese and get that sweet potato and sit down there and eat it. That would be like a snack. Some nights when we get hungry, we settin' up there and we go and get some hogs head cheese. Sometimes we had crackers if we thank to get 'em when we go to the store. Crackers with hogs head cheese. Now, I like to cook buttermilk and eat it and drank it with the hogs head cheese, cuz I can eat anything, I liked everythang.

My Daddy had hogs, horses and two or three herds of cows on our farm. We had goats but not lamb.

My Daddy had a cow would give a pail of milk in the evening and a pail of milk in the mornin' and girl, we couldn't keep up wit that milk. Every mornin' I would have to churn. We'd make a whole lot of butter like that so that my Mama had started to make it in a pound and thangs and would sell it. And some would say, "Well save enough butter for we to have to make a cake for Christmas."

We were blessed with so much. If we run out of meat my daddy would kill a cow, kill the hog and we had our meat.

My Daddy would let the hog get about a year old at least before we kill it for food. Today they slaughter pigs only after three months. My Daddy would kill about three hogs, long as this table, and fill three or four barrels with salt pork. We would make sausage, take the lean part of the meat and grind it up in a grinder and season it, stuff it just like you do in the store, and put it up in the smoke house. We would smoke hams, too. We'd smoke the meat and then we'd take it down and wrap it in corn shucks and thangs and put it in a box, just a paper box and keep it like that. It will keep about five or six months when you smoke it. And the ones we don't smoke we put it in salt in a barrel and cure it and top it up in there. It will stay there for about a year. When you ready to use it just take a piece out and cut it. That salt keeps it from spoilin'. Some of that salt pork you buy today ain't got no kind of taste.

We made hogs head cheese too. Souse meat is the same thang. We put the head in a big pressure cooker and cook it real tender and then turn it off. And you pick all them bones out of there and take it and mash it up and then put a couple of hamhocks in there to make it more lean to keep it from being too fat. And you put onions and garlic and bay and peppers and we put it in big pans and we cut it up. And we put it in the refrigerator so it gel good and then we take it and wrap it and freeze it and it will stay there a long time in the freezer.

We raised about 60 turkeys, duck, chickens and ginneys[34]. Well the chickens grow up fast. They just ate corn and we would take 'em and put 'em up in the hen house, about four feet, and keep 'em off the ground so they don't get nothin' but that corn. They would be young chickens around Easter and then about three or four months they be ready before they have to be fryers. When the chicken get around two or three pounds we would kill it then. I used to kill chickens, broke the neck.

---

[33]   A common Southern Black pronunciation of Irish potatoes.

[34]   Guinea, a type of chicken.

They slaughter a chicken from birth to six weeks today. It don't have no kind of taste. When I come to California, I couldn't eat these chickens. And they tell you to wash this and do this to it before you cook it. I say well, why don't they take them off the market if it's that much pollution. Stop raisin' them chickens with all that junk in 'em.

We could gather about four or five dozen eggs a day. We could sell enough eggs to make our little grocery. If we needed sugar or flour we'd take up a thang of eggs and buy sugar and flour.

There was so much there that in turn you didn't want nothin'.

Ailments and Remedies

We really didn't get sick out there in the country, you get out there in that fresh air. We didn't have no sinus and allergies and thangs like the people have now and all that.

I think I gettin' sick today and with all these ailments, it's just somethin' with the food and pollution and thang in the air, I thank. Cuz I ain't never heard of all this cholesterol and we eatin' salt pork and butter and all of that stuff and I ain't never heard of that and no-one ever got sick.

Growin' up we would take sarsaparilla tea, catnip tea. It grew wild out there in the woods. That sarsaparilla, it was a vine. We would pick it and hang it up and then dry it for the winter time. And when we get a cold or we wanted somethin', some kind of tea, we go out there in the barn and get the tea and drink it. It keep you goin' and get the colds outta ya or stopped it from comin'. But we really didn't get no colds.

I never had went to the doctor 'til I got pregnant. I got pregnant right after I got married. 23 years old and had never been to no doctor. I never took a pill until then, neither. The doctor say he wanted me to take vitamins and I didn't know what takin' a pill was. I had a time learnin' how to swallow a pill. I just couldn't swallow. I'd mash them up. Sometimes I let 'em melt in my mouth. I couldn't swallow them whole. But I found a way to take them every time.

I have eight children. I would give my children catnip and sarsaparilla tea for cold and if it get too bad I would give 'em some castor oil. My daughter got a cold now, she been off work all week and I told her she don't need nothin' but a dose of castor oil. It don't taste so bad you just have to make up your mind to take it. My mother used to give it to us all the time. I be in there try to keep from coughin', she say, "Who is that?"

And they say, "That's Ruth," or "That's Etta." And here she come with that castor oil. If I got to take it, I take it plain right out the bottle. She'd give you a big tablespoon and if you waste some of it you got to take a little more. It'll make you well and it cuts the fever too. Vicks salve also helps to draw out fever.

I was visiting my sister and I started to cough, I didn't feel like doin' nothing. Her house is closed up and I can't stand to be fastened up, I need to have my door open, window open and clean out the air. I said, "Girl, let me get home so I can work on this cough, cuz I don't have a cold often but when I get it, it hits me hard." So I got home and take me some hot juice. Didn't have no cough syrup and my son had a li'l whiskey in there and I jus' take 'bout two teaspoons. I wanted it plain. Didn't want nothin' mixed in it and that helped knock that cough out of my throat. Any kind of whiskey a lot of times will do it. But when it first start on you, you got to take that strong, right out the bottle. It really helps. I didn't never give any of my children any whiskey to knock that cold out. I stayed home with my children 18 years 'til the oldest boys got 18 and started to work and go in the service.

If we got bee stings my daddy would say, "Come here baby." He chewed tobacco, he'd spit that tobacco on that wasp stang or whatever stang ya and he say, "Go on back to pickin' cotton." You have to go back to work. It stopped it from swellin' and everythang. The tobacco juice would draw it out.

For cuts, all you had to do is get spider webs, you go to the creek, we had a big crick and go down there and walk in that water 'til it clean out good, then come back and put some of that spider web on there and that was it. That would stop it from bleeding and close up the cut.

Once I stepped on a hoe and cut my feet and it was bleeding, bleeding, bleeding. Today, I'd have to get stitches for it, take a booster shot and everythang. You go to that creek and wade in that 'til it get all that blood stopped and thangs then you put a li'l vaseline on it and then put the spider web on it. If it puffy the next day, you go back to the creek and wade in that water.

I had a friend back in New Orleans, his son-in-law had stuck a nail in his feet and he had to get off from work. I think it was a rusty nail, that foot give him pain. I told him, "You tell your son-in-law to go up there to Bicell Creek and get in there and wade in there so he could get his feet well up." And the doctor had treated him a year or so and he still bothered with his feet. The doctor started to put him in that whirlpool [in doctor's office], in that water, that's the only thang. It was infected. And I say, "I told you that's what you should have done, to go in there and walk in that water, your foot would have been well." After the doctor had tried everythang, he finally put it in that water. Bicell creek. That water was the only clear creek close by and you want the water to be runnin' water, not standing still.

When people would get pregnant, womens would eat red clay, they'd crave for it. When I was pregnant, I jus' wanted to get me some to eat.

For ringworms, a fig tree, it got milk in there. That's what they would use for ringworms, You just put the milk from the leaves on it and it would clear it up. You would never wait 'til it got bad, you catch it right away. My mama would say, "That look like a ringworm comin'. Go bring me a leaf off that fig tree." And she start to puttin' it in there. You didn't have to go to no doctor or nothin'.

To get rid of corns, cut off the bacon. Any kind a piece of salt pork or bacon before it get dried hard. I just put a piece between my toe because if you keep it moister it won't bother you, but if it get hard and dry, it really hurts. So you just take the salt pork and put it on the corn.

We never had teeth aches or cavities because we got our sweets from eatin' apples and plums and berries and all of that. We ain't had no lot of candy, we jus' ate all that fresh fruit. I've never had a toothache or cavities and thangs 'til I was married and had kids and moved to the city.

We never had no earaches or nothin', congestion. I didn't know what an earache was. We had spring water and that probably kept us healthy. Pure olive oil is good for earaches.

We never got constipated because we always ate a lot of greens and fruit. We had a healthy diet. Ain't never been bothered with no diarrhea, no headache. I've never been in the hospital and had no surgery or nothin'.

I heard of pre-menstrual syndrome but we didn't know nothin' about that back then. We didn't have it like it is today. We took catnip tea for cramps and mama make you lay in the bed and stay there and rest the first day. Then after that, you didn't have it any more. When you get cold, that's what makes you start crampin'. When you get warm and take some hot tea and lay there and soon it pass over.

We grew up in the church, you didn't have no place else to go but the church and my Daddy was a bus driver and he had a car, all of 'em couldn't fit in the car. We take the horse and the buggy and the car. My mama and the youngest one would be in the car and he gonna drive the buggy seven miles to the church. But it wouldn't take us no time. Get up, we done prepared that dinner on Saturday evening cuz there's no work on Sunday, just get up and go to church. No ironin' or nothin'.

On Saturday, we'd get up and go out in the garden and pick a big ol' bale of strang beans, butter beans, okra. I used to like to gather that stuff. I sit there and be done shelled a big ol' pan of butter beans and get the okrey for to cook to go in the butter beans. Some gonna want butter beans and some want strang beans. We cook two pots, ol' big iron pots. We use stainless steel now.

But that food in that beef and chicken on the farm is much different than this out here. Even the Louisiana hot sausages taste different out here. They done mixed beef and thangs, they ain't got no kind of good sausage. When I go to New Orleans I always bring me my salt pork and sausage and beef steaks. Oooh, you just get you one of 'em steaks and jus' put in a li'l butter on that stove and cook you some garlic and seasonings on it and turn it over 'bout twice, just as tender, oooh yeah!

I don't really get sick today. Everytime I feel somethin' comin down, I take a little castor oil and it knocks it right out. I hate it too, but once it goes down, I suck a lemon or orange up behind it. The doctor say I got a little artheritis in this knee but it don't hurt or nothin'. The only thang its kinda stiff since it been so cold and rainin'. And, right now, I go to the doctor since I got older, for my blood pressure. I take a little blood pressure medicine and that's all. I go every three months to the doctor. My doctor say at your age you in good health.

I've been blessed all my life. When I came to California in 1952, I had three children. Been married almost 40 years, and have eight children, 12 grandchildren and one great grandchild. We don't have all the acres any more. I sold my part because I wasn't back there and they said you got to keep it up. I had 33 acres when it was divided up. One brother kept most of his and bought some of the other sisters. He got a heck of a lot of land.

But thangs have changed. A lot of Black farmers couldn't get loans to keep their farms goin' and lost their land. There's a big suit against the government.[35] They keep cuttin' the lumber and burning the undergrowth. It burns all the good earth and ecosystem and medicines and other plants that grow there naturally 'til after a while it just don't come back any more. I was just raised up with plenty of everythang. There was so much there that in turn you didn't want nothing.

---

[35] Since the time of the interview with Ms. Williams, African American farmers won a landmark lawsuit in 1999 against the U.S. Department of Agriculture for racist discrimination in loan approval from 1981-1996 in Pigford v. Glickman. In 2010, The House of Representatives approved the decades-old settlement worth $4.6 billion that resolved two class-action suits filed against the federal government by African American and Native American farmers. For more information see Pickford v. Glickman or visit the National Black Farmers Association, www.nationalblackfarmersassociation.org.

Chapter 2 - Strong Medicine
A Blending of Healing Traditions

"If you have one drop of Indian blood in your veins then you are Indian." Black Elk, Lakota

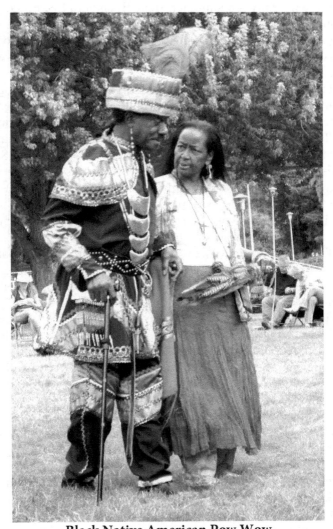

Black Native American Pow Wow
Don Littlecloud Davenport and Bonita Roxie Aleja Sizemore
Pow Wow in Hayward, CA hosted by the Black Native American Association of Oakland, CA
Image 2-1

Introduction

The relationship between African Americans, Native Americans, and European Americans in this country is layered. Our histories and families have been intertwined for over 500 years.

Throughout these narratives, everyone I interviewed proudly claimed bloodline connections to a Native tribe through either a parent or grandparent. How one defined themselves "racially" between Black and Red usually depended on how one was raised culturally. Some said it was easier to just say they were "Black." A few were raised with one foot in the Native world and one foot in the African American world. Despite the fact of having relatives who were staunchly and proudly just one or the other—Native American or African American—many of these Black-and-Red individuals proudly claimed both hertitages and also face internalized racism from both communities because of hair texture, skin color or being accused of "not wanting to be Black."

Growing up, I knew who my ancestors were and exactly where they came from. Yes, I am PROUDLY Colored, Negro, Black, and African American, but I am also Native American as well as Scots-Irish, Creole/French, and Chinese.

My great-grands, the Bowmans and Henrys, were from the Eastern Cherokee and Mississippi Choctaw nations. I can remember my grandmother, Irene Blackburn Lee Ferguson, telling us when she was going to visit an aunt who lived on the reservation.

My mother's people are New Orleans Creole and also claim Louisiana Choctaw heritage. Some of the healing methods passed down to me from my grandmother clearly are Native medicine, specifically Choctaw.

I can trace back seven generations in New Orleans to my great-great-great grandmother Seraphine Tembo. I found her name as the "mother" on the death certificate of my great-great grandmother Elizabeth Augustine. I learned the surname Tembo is possibly of southern African origin. If, however, the surname is actually Timbo, it is of Fulani, West African origin in present-day Guinea.

My paternal great-grandfather, Jem Hing Lee, came from Canton, China to San Francisco at the age of 15 accompanied by his uncle sometime between 1875-1880. It was before the Chinese Exclusion Act of 1882, which were laws passed to prohibit Chinese immigration. In 1890 Great-grandfather Lee moved to Port Gibson, Mississippi. He was part of the largely-forgotten migration of Chinese-Americans into Mississippi from the West Coast during the late 19th century, establishing grocery stores, laundries, farms, and other businesses in that state.

This much-blended family, whose ingredients came from a multitude of nations, resulted in some interesting, cross-cultural pairings. In Port Gibson, Mississippi, for example, my Scots-Irish great-grandfather (I only know that his last name was James), lived down the street from my half-Chinese aunts, who were his grandchildren (they described him as a "mean old bastard").

Today, very few of us are pure-blood. Many Native folks have physical features that are clearly identifiable as African American or European and vice versa. The bloodlines are mixed!

Living in the South, many people did not know how to racially categorize me. When I would go to the heart of Tuscarora-Lumbee region in North Carolina, I saw a lot of folks who looked like my relations. It reminded me of the first time I went to New Orleans as a child and everywhere I went, I saw people who looked similar to me.

Native American and African American bloodlines have a special bond that began during the violent birth of this country. Both peoples were disenfranchised and enslaved side by side. After a slave ship dropped off its African cargo in the New Land, it sometimes replaced that cargo with enslaved Native Americans to sell in another land.

Runaway slaves sought refuge in Native tribes, became a part of the community, had children and fought side-by-side against the colonizers; some tribes adopted the tradition of American slavery and owned African slaves (although they were treated much better).

Because of this close and early kinship, Native Americans and African Americans share similar customs and traditions including traditional medicine, music, food, struggles and survival strategies.[36]

Native American medicinal practices—along with knowledge of the American medicinal plants—crossed over into the African American world at the same time Native Americans on the east coast and in the south were being introduced to African American healing practices brought over on the slave ships. This is one of the reasons why there are many similarities between African American and Native American traditional medicine.

In the spirit of the Lakota belief of *Mitakuye Oyasin*, meaning *We Are All Related*, the following narratives highlight individuals who either completely identified with their Native tribe or who combined the Black and Red folk healing traditions.

---

[36] Professor Jack Forbes' book, *Africans and Native Americans: The Language of Race and the Evolution of Red-Black Peoples* is a groundbreaking work that brings to light this often ignored history.

Hattie Hazel Pegues-Clark

"You used to go out in the field and find all your medicine"

My maiden name is Hattie Hazel Pegues[37]. P-E-G-U-E-S. It's a lot of Pegues in this part of the country.

I was raised in the country, waaay in the country. John Station area in Laurinburg, North Carolina. I was naturally born right here on Sneeds Grove Road. Li'l house still standin' up, bless its heart, you see the chimney part.

My father was born and raised in South Carolina, right near McColl. His mother was Indian, and his father's mother was Indian.

On my mama's side, my grandmother was Indian, too, a Cherokee. Her name was Califia White. She was a pretty brown skinded woman. She had straight hair, reddish. I loved her hair. She taught me a lot. My grandmother taught my mama how to use the medicines and they both taught me.

Rabbits tobacco is the best medicine. I make tea from rabbits tobacco every year, startin' in October. The best time to pick it is the beginning of October thru December, up until February. The brewin' is better during this time of year because the medicine is strongest. You can make as much as you want cuz you keep it all year round.

You don't have to dry it out cuz it already look dry.[38] Then you got some herbs you gotta add in it.

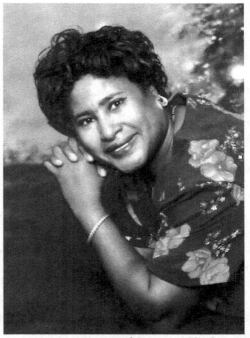

Ms. Hattie Hazel Pegues-Clark
Image 2-2

Some people like lemon in theirs. Others like tar[39]. Whatever you gonna put in it you put that in before it start brewin' so the taste will be in it as it brew. It's accordin' to how you want it. You won't have it too sweet but you add at least two tablespoons of sugar and you drink it while its hot. You keep it in a jar and put it in the frigidaire and heat it up if you want it hot. Or some like to leave theirs sittin' out[40].

Me and my family don't have no problems about runnin' to the doctor cuz I'mma get that rabbit tobacco and say heah, drank this. All of my chil'ren know how to make it. They say "we cain't make it just like yours, but we can try."

It's another tea they call sassafras tea. It's not like rabbits tobacco, it's like a root. I use that to chase the cold away.[41]

Mullet leaf, that's for arther-i-tis and your feet swellin'. You can boil it. It's like a big green flower leaf, but you pull it up from the ground, shake the root off, keep the leaves in all, but you gonna have to cut 'em up. Boil dat in a big pot and soak your whole body or jus' your feet in it. Use dat for artheritis.

---

[37] Pronounced "pah-gheeze."

[38] Some herbs need drying out both for preservation for future use as well as to be able to brew them into teas. But rabbit tobacco, on the other hand, has a dry consistency to it both growing and when harvested, so that it doesn't have to go through the same drying out process before immediate use in teas or for preservation.

[39] Ms. Pegues-Clark explained that the word "tar" in this context meant pine tree sap.

[40] As with other perishable liquids, rabbit tobacco tea kept at room temperature has to be consumed quicker than when refrigerated as it will spoil if it sits out too long uncooled.

[41] An important warning note about sassafras and safrole: Sassafras contains safrole, which is known to have harmful effects if ingested over a period of time in large and concentrated quantities. See warning and instructions in the Sassafras section on pages 319-320 before using.

I see some up there in Paradise[42].

I use yellow root, too. It has a grass leaf on top, not like a flower, but have little egg thangs on the tops of it. My mama used to take yellow root and boil the root, and she put a band in there and soak it, and take it out and wrap it around your head. It was good for headaches. You drink the tea to keep yo blood clean.

People never used to buy yellow root. When we went out to pick it, we picked for other people and store the extra in the freezer. We just pick what we needed. If it was a li'l patch we don' take it all, we jus' pick some and try to find another patch. You couldn't even tell some was picked. It used to stand up out the dirt near the swamps, but you cain't find it no more. It's rare. You used to go out in the field and find all your medicine but you cain't find certain type plants now. They burn the underbrush where they grow the new pine trees fer them to grow up tall. It kills off all the other stuff that gets around it, all the medicine. But you don't wanna get rid of dat pine top cuz dat go wit da rabbit tobacco tea. The needles.

I get my yellow root from that Chinese woman who sells it in her store right there cross from Burger King in Laurinburg. I don't know where she get it from.

* * *

Where I was born and raised over there off of Sneeds Grove Road, it's a walnut tree, and one day I see my grandma getting a walnut from under it and then cutting off the hull, but she put the walnut and the shell away and keep the hull, and I was tryin' to figure out what she was doin'.

I say, "What you fitn'a do wit dat? Eat it?

She say, "No baby. You use it for the ringworm. It's a medicine you put on it. Sit down and watch me. I'mma show you what I'mma do wit it." She had a ringworm patch on her arm. She took the hull and rubbed it on the ringworm. And she say, "That's gonna go away in a few days. You see it won't be there." She say you could boil the green hull and put peroxide wit it and then put it on the ringworm, to make it stronger.

Gwen, my niece, had a bad ringworm on her neck and it was the biggest one we ever dealt with. So me and her and my sistah, Gwen's mama, went out to the walnut tree and got a walnut and cut open the green hull. I told Gwen's mama, "Keep puttin' this on it at least three times a day like a medicine, and it heal up."

"It ain't gonna work. It ain't gonna work. Put calamine lotion on it." That's what my sistah say. That's what she was usin' from the sto.

I say, "Stop usin' that calamine and use this hull." Finally she started puttin' it on Gwen's ringworm and it gettin' smaller and smaller. That tree makes the goodest walnuts. The green ones is da ones you use for medicine. You use the juice.

* * *

We used to get a hornets nest for teethin'. They be an old wooden house, you got to go under there, cuz they grow onto the boards, and you just find one, and you get the whole nest. We let babies teeth on it and they be just as glad.

My Mama would say, "It ain't gonna hurt em it's gonna toughin they gums."

I raised all my nieces and nephews wit dat. I didn't go to no grocery store and get no teethin' rattles.

They was a grass we used to call teethweed, it look jus' like a stalk of grass and babies could chew on that for teethin', too. The medicine from that would toughin they gum.

* * *

We didn't take nothin' for cramps cuz we didn't get 'em. And we wasn't late never neither for our menstruation. One time my niece was pregnant and her baby was two weeks overdue and you know she

---

[42] An all Black settlement in the country part of Laurel Hill.

just got frustrated. I told her, "You know you can't get frustrated cuz you gotta make dat baby come on out." So she was up here one weekend wit me and I said, "Well, I'll see dat baby next weekend." They all looked at me like I was crazy.

They say, "How you know when dat baby gonna come?"

And I say, "It's jus' like I know." She had it dat Saturday mornin. I said, "You weren't overdue you just didn't know your time." Doctors say you two days over due, I say uhuh. I judged all of mines. I hit mines on the head. My oldest one I say Easter, April the 7th. My baby girl I say January the 17th on my sistah birthday. And my son I say December the 7. All of 'em got sevens. And the doctor was tellin' me 28, well, I didn't go by that.

* * *

When mines was comin up and they had colic, my daddy had the ol' cigarettes, not with the menthol on, but they had the cigarettes with no filter. My daddy always smoke Pall Mall. And I looked at my mama and say what you doin'. I see her smokin the baby's head up. She blow that cigarette smoke right in the mole of the baby's head. And I say, "What's that fer?"

She say, "Colic."

I say, "This thang gonna kill that baby."

She say, "No it ain't. It gonna cut dat colic, gonna stop dat hollerin." Da baby stop and she say, "Hold dat teaspoon. " I hold dat teaspoon and she blow in it three times and she put it up in da baby's mouth. Then she give dat baby dat bottle. I was like, dammit it worked on it.

She say, "Don't be goin' to dat doctor for no wind colic."

I say, "What's a wind colic?"

She say, "Dat's when you see dey hold dey li'l mouth out and dey jus' – schwooosh – they suck it all in and dey stomach gonna get hard."

* * *

We didn't get no stomach aches or get backed up. We eats a lot of garden peas, poke sallat, okra, greens. But cabbage give me a stomach ache. Girl I die! Gas! I like cabbage but if I know cabbage gonna give me gas I'mma eat tums befo' den. So I can eat it witout no problem. You can use sugar and a li'l bit of baking soda to cut the gas but da only thang that cut the gas out cabbage is Sprite, Sprite soda. I put the Sprite right in da cabbage, not a lot.

* * *

I got rootworkers in my family, stayin' in Maxton. But I don't believe in dat. I go by the Bible. Daisy[43] had roots worked on her before. She believed in it. She say somebody put some cemetery dirt beside her doors. Somebody been doin' all kinds of thangs to her right before she got saved. I told her it was just the devil. Anythang we need come from God and He put all the medicines right there in the woods.

---

[43] Hazel's first cousin.

Ola B. Hunter-Woods - "Your mind is a muscle"

October 2, 1905 – December 31, 1999

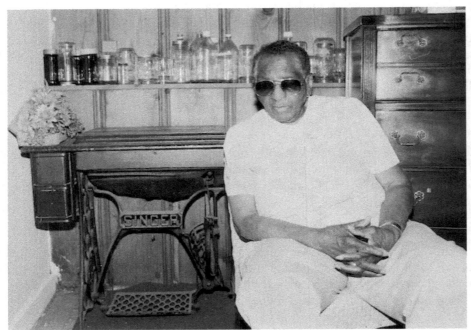

Ms. Ola B. Hunter-Woods
Image 2-3

Ms. Ola B. Hunter-Woods moved to East Oakland in 1962 during a time when the Black community appeared more united and took pride in their neighborhoods. It was the time when the great social changes of our country were occurring and this strong Southern woman from Hope, Arkansas would be in the midst of Oakland and Berkeley's Black Power, Free Speech and Civil Rights movements.

Ms. Hunter-Woods eventually bought a beautiful old two-story home in the middle of East Oakland's Black neighborhood which, at the time, was right down the street from the Black Panther headquarters. Here she set down roots and created and nurtured a southern style vegetable garden in her large backyard that provided her food year round. Her harvest was plentiful and allowed her to can, freeze and share what she could not eat. Downstairs she set up her quilting table and continued to make and sell beautifully decorated quilts. She had a career in teaching, counseling and was a business woman. Ms. Hunter-Woods lived most of her adult life in that East Oakland home, raised children, grandchildren and died there on December 31, 1999, the day before the turn of the new millenium.

I'm 91 now and I'll be 92 in October. I've been in good health all my life and I always get to workin'. I read something all the time. Your mind is a muscle and you got to keep it active. I often tell people you should keep your mind busy cuz when you start talking, your brain stop workin'. I'm reading a book now called *A Conversation With God*.

I got my Masters degree from San Francisco State. When I was there, two young Caucasian men followed me everywhere I went. They wanted me to explain their lessons. Philosophy is a very hard course. The average person can't do it. So then he [one of the men] asked me, "How did you get a Masters in Philosophy?"

We started with Pre-Socratic. That was before Socrates, the very first philosopher. He's on an island that belonged to Greece and the island wasn't far from Egypt. He's on a Greek island. His name is Thales. And he was the first person who had a philosophical mind. You've really got to have a mind for it because it is abstract. You don't have anything tangent. I had two years of law. I had to adjudicate cases to get a Masters in Philosophy. One case I had to adjudicate: Do Trees and Rivers Have Rights? Well I think they do. I don't think rivers should be contaminated with pollution and all this stuff. From the very beginning babies are born in water. You see, this country is so greedy after a dollar that they cut down all the trees. They don't respect the earth. They don't respect that trees have rights. Once we can get to that point, then we'll be alright.

Background

I was born on a saddle ranch in Hope, Arkansas[44]. There was some farmland there also. We used to have all kinds of vegetables and corn and cotton and everythang.

A lot of Indians used to live with us in our community, but they finally run them all out. Now my mother's people were Indian, Quapaw Indian. They a real dark chocolate color and they had straight long hair. My daddy was partly Choctaw. They're from Oklahoma now.

Learning to make money growing up

I learned to pick cotton when I was three years old. I could pick it but I couldn't weigh it 'til I knew how much I weigh. That's the way it work, you could pick it but you couldn't weigh it til you knew your size. I had a bag of cotton ever since I knew my size. My dad used to make big baskets that could hold 100 pounds of cotton. He made them out of hickory stick[45] and he would lace them and sell them. He'd empty that little dab of cotton that I picked out of my bag into the basket until it got enough to weigh.

I didn't learn how to make baskets but I sewed mostly. I pieced a quilt when I was 6 years old. My mother quilted it and sold it.[46] Guess how much she got for it? Two dollars and fifty cents. It fit a double bed size. My mother brought in her money by doing domestic work. After I got older, I was near people who had a lot of peanuts so I used to pick off peanuts on halves. They give me half, I pick 'em off and then I was sellin 'em.

Two nephews came to live with us when I was about eleven or twelve and they and I used to go into the woods and pick up hickory nuts, muscadines and grape and we sell all that stuff. Muscadine is something that look like a grape but it's not as sweet as a grape. We sold all those thangs.

Later on, I started buying war stamps[47], that's what they called 'em. A little snit full of stamps was worth $12.50, so I get it full and put it in my bank account.

When I weren't doin that, I was crochetin'. I'd embroidery, piece another

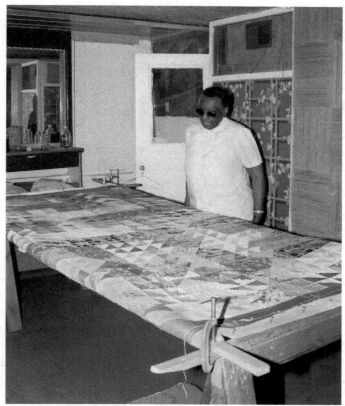

Ms. Hunter-Woods with one of her quilts in progress

Image 2-4

---

[44] A ranch primarily used for raising livestock on large acreage and is maintained by workers on horses.

[45] Flat, thin, flexible slats.

[46] Piecing a quilt is designing, laying out and sewing the pieces/sections/blocks of the quilt together – this is the top layer with the design. Quilting is when you are stitching the top layer (the design), the filling (or batting) and the bottom layer together – the quilting stitch can reflect designs or patterns as well. So the quilt essentially has three layers. The bottom or back of the quilt is usually one solid color.

[47] World War II

quilt and I sell that. Now I jus' finished piecein' a quilt and I jus' finished quiltin' one and I'm startin' another one and I got one in now; that's two quilts. I sell them if anyone wants 'em. I never advertise them. One young man bought six and he bought two later for his mother. He told me, "Mrs. Woods, do you know you sellin' your quilts too cheap?"

I sell 'em for $85.

I says, "John I don't make quilts to sell." I say, "Now if I was makin' 'em for a livin, I would sell it for what the other folks sell theirs." Other people sell them and they don't look like nuthin. One woman charged $300 for hers and another $125.00. I've been quiltin' since I pieced my first quilt at 6 years old and sold it for $2.50.

All my life I been around people who knew how to make money. Nobody ever sat back and waited for someone to give 'em something. If you could make stuff with your hands then you can always make money.

Grandparents

I remember my grandmothers. I don't remember my grandfathers.

I remember both grandmothers because both of them lived with us for a while. I was too little to call them grandmother so I called them Daima. One was named Rachel and the other was named Nancy. I would say Daima Rachel and Daima Nancy and they know who I was talking about. The other kids called them that, too. I know them when I was little and I know them when they died, but I can't remember them dying. I remember them being buried cuz I didn't wanna leave 'em out in the cemetery, cuz I told my dad they be 'fraid to stay out there by themselves. I didn't want them to stay out there. I was 'bout 5 years old when they died. I didn't know they were dead, I jus' didn't wanna leave 'em out there. I say now, "Daima be 'fraid out here at night by herself," and I didn't see nobody else gonna be out there. Uh uh, I didn't wanna leave 'em out there.

Ailments and Remedies

When I was growin' up, I never heard nobody havin' no high sugar or high blood pressure, none of that in those days. People made their own remedies and healed themselves because in those days they didn't see no doctors and they weren't able. They didn't have the money.

The doctors would come if you had the money and send for them, but it depended on how far they were from ya, cuz they drove a horse, didn't have no cars. I remember when Dr. Poole got his first car, I was about eight years old. Most people didn't have no car, they had horses, and they would make those horses go like horses to a firetruck.

They had to call the doctor for me one time and the doctor came. I fell off a banister and knocked my ankle out of place. My foot was standin' straight up like my leg and I wouldn't let nobody touch it. The doctor kept workin' and workin' with my foot 'til he got it down and then he wrapped it with somethin'. I was in a lot of pain but they didn't put nobody to sleep then.

I think people learned what remedies worked from trial and error. And if this one worked, they did this.

The remedies my mother used when we was sick depended on what was wrong with you. Now, in the summer kids used to have a lot of fever because they ate half-green fruit. They come down with flux and fever. Jus' like I got some trees out there now, they be ripe next month but they look like they ripe now. And kids used to eat them, they be so sour they put salt on 'em. It would de-ring their bowels and they'd have fever.

And, a lot of times with a fever, they would take peach leaves, regular peach tree leaves, and put them in a cloth and pour vinegar over 'em and use that as a poultice on their stomach. And if their fever was high, I've seen at times when they take that thang off, the leaves would be dry where the fever had burned them. I had a little niece died with her fever. Her fever was so high until it took her hair. She had beautiful hair. She had the fever for about two weeks. We usually used cold water when the fever got so high and then they used ice mattresses.

We would use sumtin they call buttonwillow. It was good for fever and swelling. It's a bush-like plant. We would boil that and take that water and bathe them in it.

Goldenrod will take the swelling off. It's a pipe-like plant. It's in joints. Golderod would grow about six feet and has a tassle top, and we would boil that, and wherever it was sore, you could have a toothache, and they make a poultice out of goldenrod and put it on it.

Goldenrod with buttonwillow would get that swelling wherever. We just go out into the woods and get them whenever we needed them. Buttonwillow's a bush and goldenrod grows straight up.

If kids had a cold, we used to make muellin tea. It's a little bush-like plant, it looked more like turnips when they growin, but it's a grey plant and it had little fine stickers on those leaves that would hurt you. We used to boil that and put little sprigs off from the pine tree in there and boil it with that muellin because that pine tree has turpentine in it. Kids used to have sore chests and sore throat and we make a tea out of it and give it to them and that would heal their sore throat and sore chest and it would break up the cold.

For chest congestion and cold we used to make something you take from a male calf called talla. We take that suet[48], that fat and stew it down until it was grease. You get it from a male calf when people kill calf for eat. Mostly they took the fat from the testes area and we cook it down 'til it was solid like talla, cold fat from a cow. They call it suet. We used to stew that suet down to talla, and take it and put it in a woolen cloth, some old woolen pants or something, and wrap it real well and warm it, and put it to a child's chest if they had a cold. It would be a poultice and would draw the cold and congestion out. They didn't call that talla, they called it pizzle-grease.

I went to the market not too long ago and I asked for some suet. He didn't know what I was talkin' about. I says, "It's fat from a cow." So he went and got me some of it. He say, "I betcha I know from now on." You can buy a steel skillet if you buy some suet and put it in that skillet it won't stick and it won't turn your food dark. It kind of acts like teflon.

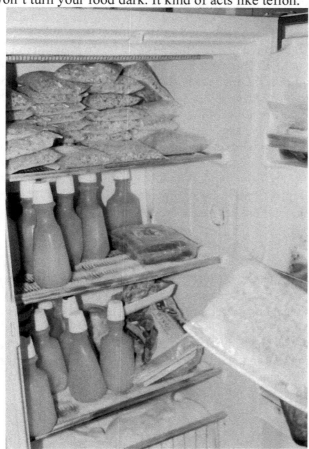

**Refrigerated goods from Ms. Hunter-Woods'
garden**

Image 2-5

I been tryin' to find a steel pot like my mother used to have; you can hang it in a fireplace and cook food in it. So, my friend just gave me a steel pot. She heard me talkin' about it. But it's not like the one my mother had. My mother's pot was tall and had a bell on it, but this one is more less like any pot and has a glass lid on it. She paid twenty dollars for it! But you can put that suet in any pot to keep food from stickin and keep it from turnin' your food dark.

We used to dig blackberry roots and make tea outta that. That's what they used for constipation. Don't take too much of it now. We use it in the spring of the year. And then we would dig Maypock. That's a vine. It runs in the ground. Use that for laxative, too. It has sliver leaves, more than grapevine or muscadine vine, but it looks wild, cuz you see it all in your yard and you dig it up and get it outta the way.

Catnip would grow wild, too, and that's good, cuz I used to drink it. It make tea for the baby to get the hives out. And if babies does get [the hives], they give that catnip tea and those bumps come out. Hives are just something that's endemic to babies. And if they have any kind of stomach trouble, they give them catnip tea. We make that tea and give it to the little babies, even if they are a

---

[48] The fat around the kidney and testicles of cattle and sheep and a common term used to describe most beef fat.

few months old.

You put some catnip in a teaspoon and the mothers would nip some milk from her breasts and give that to the baby. It would regulate them. If you can find catnip in the woods, you know what it is. If you can't find it, your best bet is to go to a nursery and buy the plant and you can grow it in a pot in the house, because if you put it outdoors every cat in the community gonna come over there. Cat's like to smell it. That's where it got its name from.

My dad used to dig sassafras root and that was a tonic for the spring of the year. He make a tea and drink it every morning. You dig the root and let it dry and then you boil that root when you get ready to make some tea and then you throw it away afterward. He just make the tea as he needed it. I used to drink it with him.[49]

Horehound is bitter than bitter. We would go to the woods and get that to make a tea. That used for the whooping cough. I told 'em it oughta cure it, cuz it was so bitter. Horehound look like an ice potato more like. My daddy grew white potatoes, that's ice potatoes.[50] We grew artichokes and ate artichokes too.

We gave hot teas for measles and thangs like that. Mostly it would be sassafras tea and cottonseed tea, from the regular cottonseed. We was separating that core from the hull and you could make tea out of that hull. Most times they would get the hull from factories that separated the cottonseed. It's a core in them and its yellow and we get that core out and make meal out of it and people ate it. We used to make cake from it. Those mills was called oil mills and you pass by that it smell like somethin' you eat. It smell so good!

Hog hoof tea we used for colds. A hog hoof, outta the hog! We'd make that tea and give it to kids. That hog been used a li'l bit for everything.

Back then, all the kids went barefooted. If they stuck a rusty nail in their foot, they didn't see a doctor. They mostly dug a hole, a round hole in the ground and put some bits of woolen material in that fire until it started smokin' and they have that kid hold his foot over that smoke and drawin' the poison out. And what's gonna kill em? They have to hold him there cuz it hurt while it's drawin' the poison out. That's all they did and then, if they happen to have castor oil or turpentine or something like that you could buy over the counter, well, they put some turpentine on it and wrap it and that's all.

If it was bleeding, they got some soot outta the chimney. Now soot doesn't have any grains in it. It's like a powder and they get that black soot and put it on wherever it's bleeding and wrap it. It will stop bleeding. They'd wash it afterward with soap and water. And the funny thing about it, what I remember myself, they had sayman soap. And this you could buy from vendors in a buggy goin around through the community sellin' stuff like that. Sayman soap is some kind of linament. They could buy that linament for sprains or if something hurt like a joint, your ankle or knee or something. They didn't wash their faces with it. They kept it for medicinal use.

For ringworms, they put some of that talla on it. They even put that stuff in your hair because some peoples' hair was dry.

There was a lot of clay, real clay where I lived. It was grey. Most of the people ate it. I had a sister-in-law who used to eat it. That's because it taste good, had a sour taste to it. We would dig it and put it inside the oven and dry it out and eat it. We used to eat cornstarch too. It came in lumps. No medicinal use, just eat it because we liked it.

When women got pregnant they had midwives and midwives would tell them how to treat themselves and not to strain themselves at anythang, but that's all. Now I don't know where midwives got their training. I had an aunt who was a midwife and she was a good one, but she worked with a pediatrican, his name was Dr. Smith. She delivered most of my nephews.

All these things that I have named, that was a remedy, we didn't go to doctors.

---

[49] An important warning note about sassafras and safrole: Sassafras contains safrole, which is known to have harmful effects if ingested over a period of time in large and concentrated quantities. See warning and instructions in the Sassafras section on pages 319-320 before using.

[50] "Ice potato" is a common Southern Black pronunciation for "Irish potato."

Ramona Moore Big Eagle - "That's how smart we were"

Ramona Moore Big Eagle, M.Ed. (Tuscarora/Cherokee[51]), is an oral historian and Legend Keeper of the Tuscarora Nation of Maxton, North Carolina. She was born in Gaffney, South Carolina and currently lives in North Carolina. I met her at the Occaneechi Saponi PowWow in 1997 and we are close friends to this day. Over the years, we've had numerous conversations about many topics. Below, Ramona shares a traditional story about how the people of the First Nations of the Western Continents became known as "Red Men" by using pokeberry medicine, information on health routines she grew up with, and challenges she's faced all her life having "Black looks" while coming from a Native American family and living in Native American territory.

How Native American people became known as "Red Men"

"I was told that in the olden days before Christopher Columbus and genocide contact,

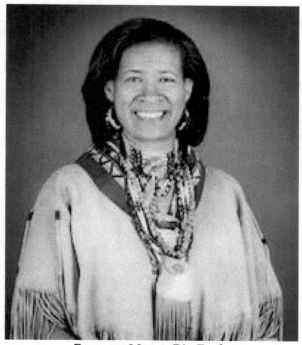

Ramona Moore Big Eagle
Image 2-6

Native American Indian people used poke sallat berry juice to cover their bodies and used that native berry juice as a natural insect repellent and a natural sunscreen, to keep their skin from burning and to ward off insects. As a result, it worked, and this was knowledge that they received from the Creator, possibly through trial and error. That's how smart and innovative Native American Indians were before contact with the Europeans, which changed everything. When the Europeans came here and saw the Natives with red berry juice on their skin, it is said that's why they started calling American Indians the red man, because the brown man had red berry juice on their skin as a natural insect repellent and sunscreen."

On staying healthy

"When I was a child, my mother gave me a tablespoon of cod liver oil every day to keep us healthy, and my grandmother cooked poke sallat. She always made a point of saying you had to know when to pick it and how to cook it. Hence she picked it in the early spring, and when she cooked it, she would boil it about three times and throw the water out each time."[52]

Black looks

Although African American and First Nations natural medicine and culture in the South intersected

---

[51] The Tuscarora Nation's original homeland was in eastern North Carolina. They settled there well before European explorers and settlers came to North America. In the early 18th century, the Tuscarora were fighting the colonists for their homeland in the well-known and historically documented Tuscarora Wars from 1711-1713. The Tuscarora were defeated and most of the surviving Tuscarora left North Carolina and migrated north. They were adopted into the Six Nations of the Iroquois in New York. Today the Tuscarora Nation of New York have their own homeland and is federally recognized. Not all Tuscarora left their homeland in eastern North Carolina and migrated north. Those who remained trace their lineage to those who migrated north. Many have formed Tuscarora Nation tribal bands and are moving to restore federal recognition in eastern North Carolina.

[52] Pick poke sallat leaves when they are young and not larger than a small hand or approximately 6 inches.

and even, in many cases, overlapped, it was not always a smooth blending. Below Ramona talks of the prejudices and racial/cultural challenges she has faced in both her personal and professional life because she identifies as being "Red" with "Black looks."

In Ramona's words:

"Let me give you the story. All my life I have been made fun of because of my hair color and texture, eye color, skin color, and the way I talked. Within my family of Indian people on both sides, no-one, had hair texture like mine. Everyone I ever met in the family had straight hair, wavy hair or frizzy hair BUT no-one, had hair like mine. So I always got the 'where did you get hair like that?' question or look! People would say things like, 'I thought with your light brown hair and eyes you wouldn't have nappy hair like that!!!' I have had hair stylists say 'You may say you are Indian but you have "nappy hair"!'

"When I went off to college in 1972, I started relaxing and blow-drying my hair. Of course, my roots always showed the natural texture of my hair. If you look at the pictures of me on the internet you can see that my roots are not straight. As a result, when I started claiming my Indian heritage and identity in college, people would laugh, make fun, and take it upon themselves to correct me and say 'Oh, you are part Indian?' Out of embarrassment and frustration, I stopped saying I was Indian.

"Then in 1988, as a divorcee with three precious children, I moved back to Charlotte and started aligning myself with the Native community, to again be met with rejection. I was told my children could not be a part of certain Indian programs.

"I started going to the Tuscarora Reservation under Chief Leon Locklear in 1990. We applied for membership and were given Tribal Cards after doing our lineage papers and genealogy. My children and I would dance at the PowWows and attend culture classes in Charlotte, even though some organizations didn't want me to. We were accepted by other people who had mixed Indian heritage who became our friends and supported us and treated us well.

"Now fast forward to 2013. I cut my hair in a short style and went natural, wearing my hair in its natural curliness. I had to come to grips with the texture of my hair. I had to learn to love the real me without the straightening of my hair. I learned to love the look and texture of my hair. I realize that Creator God made me uniquely beautiful, as are all people. I love me and I love every bit of my very thick bushy, frizzy hair.

"Almost everyone had negative words to say about my decision to go natural. The most affirming words I have heard have been from African American friends that have given me so much love, compliments, and acceptance.

"People hire me based on the Bio they see (with a pre-2013 hairstyle) and read on the internet. It is alright for me to come in and erase stereotypes with my words but not by the way I look. They expect to get what they pay for: an Indian that meets their stereotypical "South Western Native look." Corporations, schools, organizations hire me time after time to share Native American Indian Culture programs in which I preserve, promote, and present our culture through drumming, singing, storytelling, and artifact presentation. Their expectations are met as a result of the depth of my knowledge, experiences, communication skills, and transparency, but not necessarily by the way I look."

Beyond The African American

The next two narratives are from two women who are Tuscarora and Lumbee. They are not of African American descent. I included them because they offer additional insight into the challenges of cross-national and cross-cultural identity that is critical to understanding how African Americans and African American cultural traditions—particularly those that involved healing remedies and spirit-work—blended into the American culture as a whole.

These two women were friends of others I interviewed and were excited to offer their knowledge and snippets of their life stories.

Ms. Jacobs is the grandmother of a young lady named Teresa who was my daughter's day care worker in Laurel Hill, North Carolina. I met Ms. Chavis when I interviewed Marjorie Davis in Laurinburg, North Carolina. After Ms. Marjorie's interview, Ms. Chavis was excited to share her knowledge and stories.

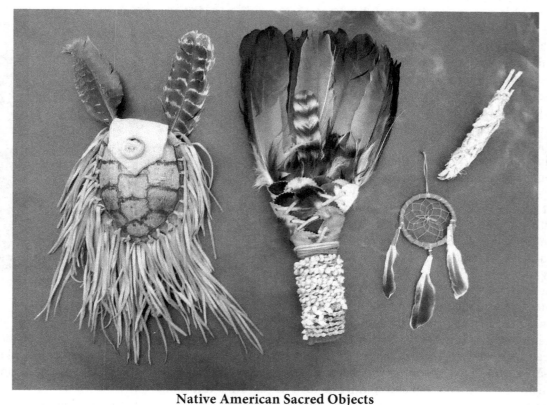

Native American Sacred Objects
(l-r) turtle shell medicine bag, blue heron prayer fan, dream catcher, white sage bundle
Image 2-7

Turtle shell medicine bag: Representing the person wearing it, ceremonial items are put in the bag for protection, guidance, healing, and strength.

Blue heron prayer fan: Ceremonial fan used to sing, pray, and dance.

Dream catcher: Originating with the Ojibwe and Lakota nations, the dream catcher snares bad dreams or spirits and filters threm through its web, protecting the children and families.

White sage bundle: Burning and smudging of sage is used to cleanse any environment and/or person before a traditional ceremony, and is also used personally. Pieces of sage are often put into medicine bags.

Ms. Chavis - "I am Lumbee-Tuscarora"

My name is Ms. Chavis. I am Lumbee-Tuscarora. I was born in Scotland County, North Carolina, in Steel Mills township, but my parents moved to Robeson County. My grandmother went back to her home in Robeson County. That's where I was raised. The town was in-between Red Springs and Pembroke. It was our home. I raised eleven children there.

Bit ya cures from skeeters to snake bites

If anything bit ya, you could put comfrey[53] on there and it would pull it out. Wasp, bee, spider, ant, snake, anythang. We could use some of that now cause the skeeters is so bad. Skeeters didn't used to do people like they do now. And they used to be some of the biggest ol' skeeters, we called 'em yella nippers. They was great big thangs and if one of them bite ya, they would hurt worser than a skeeters. But the skeeters wasn't bad then, they weren't poison like they is now. And the bees, and the wasps'es and thangs weren't as bad as they used to be. But if anyone of 'em bit ya, you gotta beat that comfrey root up 'til it look like jelly. Then when it get real mush and soft, you put you some of that on that bite.

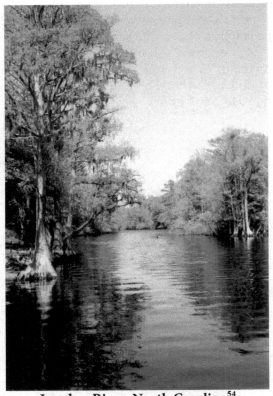

Lumbee River, North Carolina[54]
Image 2-8

One man got bit by a rattlesnake when he was plowin'. So the man killed the snake after he done tied the leg. Then he went home and hitched the mule to his wagon and rode to the doctor. Well, the doctor didn't believe no rattlesnake had bit em cause he was still livin'. Cause he tol' the doctor he didn't do nothin' for the snake bite but wrap it, that's all. He had nothin' there to put on it and then he was getting' the buggy and doin' all that and even kilt the snake. He was supposed to have done been dead by that time.

The doctor made that man take him back to find that snake dat bit 'em cause the doctor jus' wouldn't believe that no rattalesnake bit 'em. They got in the man's buggy and went right back to the field where he kilt the snake and the man gave the doctor the dead snake fer him to believe 'em. The doctor took one look at that snake and knew it jus' like the man say, a rattlesnake. They carried the snake back to the doctor office and that doctor cut that man's leg where that snake bit 'em and split it and then he jus' walk like that.

The man got well, but his leg got an infection in it where the doctor cut it, but that don't mean it was the poison'en from the snake. I believe it was by the doctor cuttin' 'em and probably his systems couldn't take it. And he like to die from that cut.

I don't thank I wanna go to that doctor. Because if I go to the doctor fer sum'tin that bit me and he got to wait fer him to treat me, he got to go way somewhere else and see sum'tin and then come back and treat me and then cut me open. I don' thank he knew what he was doin'. Well, if he had jus' got some kerosene and put on it, that would'a drawed the poison'en out. Or that man might'a been better off had he put some of that comfrey jelly on it.

My cousin John had a dog and that dog would do everythang John told 'em to do. One time they were out and they run on a snake. And John told the dog to get the snake and the snake got the dog on

---

[53] Comfrey root is the root of the comfrey plant which has been used in traditional folk medicine to heal wounds, rashes, burns, broken bones, strains and swelling. The root is often mashed and made into a poultice and then applied to the affected area.

[54] The Lumbee (or Lumber) River, after which the Lumbee people named themselves. The Lumbee are an indigenous people in that region of North Carolina who are a mixture of several related native tribes.

its head. So they come down here after me. Well, that dog was swelt up so big it couldn't hardly get up from the left side. But when they got back home, the dog was layin' in the yard and couldn't get up. His head was swelled that big—[Ms. Chavis gestures the size of a beach ball to demonstrate]— so that dog couldn't pick up his head.

I says, "John, you got any kerosene?"

He say, "Yeah."

"Well, I want ya to get it and wash that dog's head, but don't put it in his ears. If you do, it'll kill 'em." I say, "You don't know whereabout the snake bit the dog, but he had to bite 'em in the face fer it was swellin' so in the head and the face."

John washed him good, all but his hair, washed his whole head good wit that kerosene. And the next mornin' that dog could move his head. And the next day after that the dog could pick his head up. And the next day after that the dog was alright. Kerosene would kill a snake bite.

Grandmothers know best (why ain't no one listnin?)

My grandmother used to go in the woods to get the herbs. She could make a tea and give it to 'em and they would drink it and that would be the end of it. And she could fix a grease.[55] If you had a bad cold and you need to beat it, it would tear you all to pieces. I kept grease made all the time. I kept it in a big jar. I had a bit a everythang in it—quinine, pine tar—a bit a everythang.

Sum'tin bit me one night and my grandmother treated it. She didn't carry me to no doctor. She went in the woods and got a herb and made a tea and I drink that tea and it sweatin' me up. I don't remember what kine'a tea it was. That's where I made the mistake, when I didn't try and learn everythang she knew. After I got married, I jus' wasn't interested in it anymo'. I forgot it all.

When you pregnant and have trouble about carryin' it and about that period, my grandmother had a bush that growed in her yard and she make a tea from that and wouldn't have no mo' trouble.

My grandmother was wit' me wit' one of my chil'ren bein' born, cause the doctor was slow to comin' there, and the baby was born before the doctor got there, and she had everythang fixed up. And he asked her did she have a license. She told him no. He said, "You need it, you need it." But he said, too, "It was nobody could've done no better job than you."

When a baby is born, when it breathes, it breathes the air and it's bound to hurt it. Well that paragart[56] would kill that colic. That's what I gives my chil'ren for colic. When I was tendin' to a baby and my daughter-in-law had some paragart, I reckon the last bottle she could get, well she give my grandson's wife some of it. I give the baby one dose of it for its colic. And do you know, my daughter-in-law, she hid that bottle of paragart[57].

Dr. Purcell dere in Laurinburg was the baby's doctor and my daughter-in-law take that baby 'bout twice a week for dat colic. It was bad about cryin'. It was born six weeks ahead of time, and it would have all kinds of fits and spells. I told her since it been born early, she had to treat it like she been treating it in her womb before it was born. She didn't believe that, so one day, humph, she carry it to the doctor and when she come back, she had 'bout three different kines a medicine. She called me "Grandma" and she say, "Grandma, be sure now that you give Harley this medicine on the right time."

I says, "Ann, when you give Harley to Dr. Purcell and he ask Harley where she was a hurtin…" What I was trying to tell her was she shouldn't be taking that doctor medicine, but she couldn't answer. I says, them youngins, I tell you how to do it and they don't listen, don't believe you know what you talkin' about. Well, when she told her mama what I had said, her mama said she was so glad I told her that cause I stood up to her daughter about that baby.

---

[55] Also known as fixing a talla or tallow: fat from cooked beef, warmed and rubbed on chest as a salve.

[56] Paragart is probably Paregoric, a common household remedy from the 18th to mid 20th century used as an expectorant to treat coughs, diarrhea, and to soothe fretful babies from teething pain and colic and other ailments.

[57] The bottle was hid probably so no one else could use it since it was the last bottle.

Ms. Jacobs - "That's all way back yonder people do"

During my interview with Ms. Jacobs her husband came in and after that her entire posture changed and she wouldn't say more than two words. She looked demure, timid, and knowing her place, almost afraid to speak except when she was allowed. Gone were the stories and long-winded explanations. Perhaps Ms. Jacobs' abrupt change in attitude was because she thought that was naturally a woman's place in the Old South, or because she was of the Lumbee Nation people and her husband was White, or perhaps it was some combination of both. I'm not sure.

But before Mr. Jacobs arrived in the house, Ms. Jacobs talked at length about the healing remedies her mother had passed down to her.

I was born and raised in Roland in Robeson County, North Carolina. I'm a Indian, Lumbee Indian. But when I comin' to Scotland [County] after I married my husband, dey tell me I had to go for White now. That's jus' they sayso. I still say I'm a Indian. Yeah, I know who I is and I act it too.

My husband is White. He come from South Carolina. We been married sixty sumtin years. We met at a church function. Some of my chil'ren favor me some of 'em favor dere daddy. After I got married, I didn't use the teas any more, I was always runnin' to the doctor. The doctor would come out to you then. It got so now that dey won't come out to ya. My husband been to da hospital 'bout six or seven times. He got sugar. I didn' hear tell of no sugar when I was growin' up. I don' know how it happen, but my mother die wit it and I had two sistahs die wit it and now my husban' got it but I didn' hear tell of no sugar den. It's jus' long enough when I hear tell of sugar. I don' know where it come from.

My mama's name was Stroudy Jacobs. Her daddy was a Hunt. My daddy's name was Floyd Jacobs.

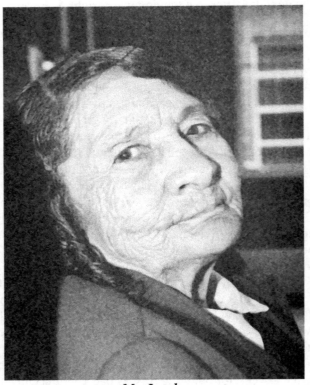

Ms. Jacobs
Image 2-9

I'm da seventh girl in my family. I had three brothers and eight sisters and every one of 'em dead but me. My mama's dead and my papa's dead. I'm da only one livin' and I'm 80 years old. Born in 1918. Count.[58]

The house I grew up in was what you call an ol' timey house. We didn' have no plumin' inside. We had an outhouse. It was a big house made out of good lumber like they did back den. It was worn but it was strong. But you take houses now, it jus' maybe you start on it on da weekend and two weeks you have it built.

I hate to tell you how many chil'ren I had. Nine. And my great-grand chilren, I tell ya I got over 80. I can't count them all, I got so many. All of my chil'rens is grown and my grandchildren, all of dem grown, too, and able to look for dem self. I asked da Lawd to let me live to see 'em all able to get dere own worth. So if dey sufferin' dat be dere fault.

My granddaughter, the one we call Cooter[59], she ain't never give me a sassy word when I raised her.

---

[58] In adding the word "count," Ms. Jacobs was indicating that I could verify her age myself, if I wanted, by counting the years between her year of birth and the year our interview was conducted, either 1999 or 2000.

[59] "Cooter" is the African Americanization of the African word "kuta" (Bambara) meaning "turtle." It is a term

Some of 'em chil'ren did and some of 'em didn'. When I come along my mama would make me go get da switch and I know to go get it. When you say go get a switch now, they go da other way. My mother used to wear a big white apron and would tie dat switch up in her and tote it along wit her. She ain't never had no problems.

It's got so now dat young people don't believe in nothin' now but runnin' to da doctor and taking pills. You don' see any of dem old bushes now that people made they medicine from. Old people is dead and it [folk medicine] died out wit em. But that's all we did in our day.

When I was raised my mama kep' an ol' kettle settin' by da fire. We didn' have no heaters den, we had fireplaces. She made us tea outta everythang and we never did go to da doctor. When we got sick with a cold, she doctor us wit dat medicine.

Now she made shuck tea and run the measles outta me. Shucks out da corn. You know I was breakin' out a li'l bit and she just took dem shucks and made tea and run dem out on me.

Yes ma'am, along den ol' folks made tea out anythang. My mammy would make sassafras tea, and tansy tea, and wormwood tea and mint tea. She growed all dat weed out in da yard. Now dat mint stuff was good but dat wormwood it was bitter as quinine.

Wormwood growed in a bush. My mammy gave us wormwood for medicine, cold and flu, see if she can't break it. It was bitter but you had to take it. But when my mammy say drank, you drank. You take a chile dese days and tell 'em to drink some tea, you can't make 'em drank it.

My mammy used to use a lot of sassafras root. She dig in da ground fer dat, and peel it and cut it up and make tea outta it.[60] It's in da woods. Some people smoke rabbits tobacco but my mammy used to make tea outta it. I hadn't forgot dat. Dat was da first weed dat I knowed of.

Mammy made all da teas for us. She even use da bark from da pine tree and da sap to make a tea outta it. Dats what she tore down da cold and measles and flus and stuff.

Yes Lawd. I thank I cried all night long with a toothache and I had to go to the tooth doctor da next mornin', but he wouldn't pull it. Said he had to wait 'til it quit hurtin'. It didn' never stop hurtin' and I went back and he kept right on 'til he pulled em all. Dis was when I was grown and married. My teeth didn' bother me none when I was home wit my mother. Dat was eight hours wort of hurtin', I was 'bout to have a heart attack but dat tooth was hurtin' and so da denis jus' pull all of 'em. Dat was da first and last time I ever been to da tooth denis.

When we was wit mammy, all dat bother us was worms, and some ol' college doctor tol' her to feed us sum pumkin seeds, and she made us eat 'em all. And you thank I'm tellin' you a story. God knows dat distroyed them worms. Yes sir, and from den on dat woman jus' kep us sum pumkin seeds 'til we lef' home! No sir, never had worms again.

One of my chile got worms when he was small. Well I carry him to da doctor. That was an ol' timey doctor. He said, "You take him some Jerusalem, ain't ya?" Jerusalem is a weed. He tol' me, "Come back and get your seeds (pumkin) and crumble 'em on up in some molasses and let dat boil in." I come back and done what he tol' me, and dat youngin ain't been bodered wit da worm since. And dats da only one I had wit worms. You mix da Jerusalem weed wit pumkin seeds wit da molasses and make 'em eat it. I ain't never hear tell of no worms after dat.

Now the onliest time we had stomach aches was wit worms. You tell me where worms come from, I don' know, unless it come from when you sleepin'.

Mammy give us tea and castor oil for stuffed up nose. Castor oil. We had to take dat stuff! We know not to back from it.

For fevers mammy had carmacrishun. It's a great big ol' bush. You take a leaf and band it to your forehead, and sometimes mama would take alcohol and band it to yo head. You never did hear tell of no aspirin or nothin' like dat. My chil'ren didn' hurt from no headaches, but I had hear tell my mama had one and she band one of dem big leaves to her head. Same thang she used for fever. Carmacrishun

---

commonly used in the southern United States by African Americans, Native Americans, and European Americans as a personal nickname or to refer to a turtle.

[60] An important warning note about sassafras and safrole: Sassafras contains safrole, which is known to have harmful effects if ingested over a period of time in large and concentrated quantities. See warning and instructions in the Sassafras section on pages 319-320 before using.

leaves are green and have seeds on it.

For cuts mama make a salve outta honey and sulfur and put a li'l bit on da cut and give you a li'l bit of it in yo mouth. Sometimes she rub da cut wit Carnation Milk and wrap it up.

For rashes or itches, she mostly put Carnation Milk on it. For ringworms we get a great big patch of black tar soap and scrub it.

If you got chicken pox you ain't gotta thang ta do but go in da chicken coop faurward an come out backwards. Carry em [the one who has it] in da chicken coop faurward an come out backwards and the chicken pox gone. That's all way back yonder people do.

Now, you thank I'm not tellin' you da truth. Come a White woman down heah. Ain't me lyin' none. And she say, "Lady my boy got da chicken pox's, he ain't doin' well."

I say, "You gotta chicken coop?"

She say, "Yes ma'am."

I say, "Carry dat boy in da chicken coop befo da sunrise. And bring 'em out and carry 'em in faurward and bring em out backward again, and the chicken pox be gone."

She come down heah in a day or two, she say, "Lady I don't believe I ever seen dis."

That's all way back yonder people do. Everyone of mine had chicken pox and my mother told me what to do. I carry 'em in da chicken coop faurward and brought 'em back backward. It was gone. Carry 'em in da chicken coop before sunrise at 5:00 and bring 'em out backward. Just one time and dem chicken pox's was gone. That's right.

Chapter 3 - Spirit Work

Introduction

Spirit work in the African American community originated directly from Africa.

Traditional African American healers know there is a healing agent in the medicines they use. They know how to unleash this power—physically through teas, poultices, tinctures and the like—and spiritually by the spoken word, affirmation, or alchemical working of the elements and unseen natural forces.

"Putting roots" on someone, or "goofering," are common southern vernacular used to describe when someone had a spell put on them for good or bad or for love, legal work, negative situations, gossiping, and so forth. Church communities often include intense prayer for the sick to heal by touch and by speaking in tongues. Spreading from east to west and also integrating Native American plant and spirit medicine, New Orleans voodoo, hoodoo, conjuring, hexing, juju, goofering and similar blended practices evolved.

The narratives below are from healers who are also spirit-work practitioners or had close experiences in the world of southern Juju.

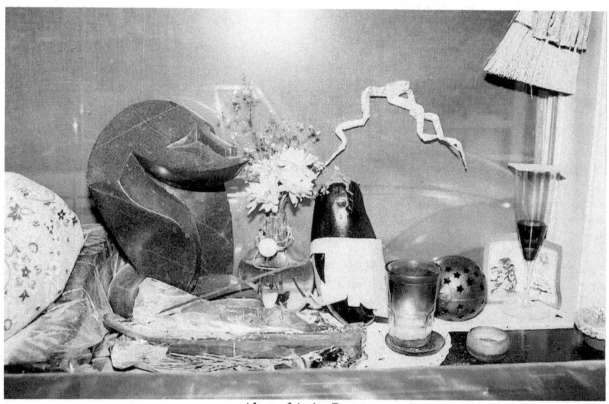

Altar of Anita Poree
Image 3-1

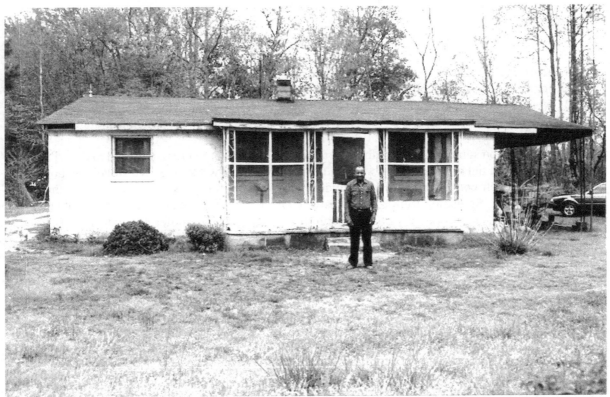

Luther Stelly "Mr. Red" Smith in front of his house
Image 3-2

Luther Stelly Smith—known by friends and family as Mr. Red—built his three bedroom cinder block house with his own hands. The house sat on half an acre of land in Paradise, a Black settlement in Laurel Hill, North Carolina. The Smith family moved to Paradise in the 1960's after a fire destroyed their wooden sharecropper shack where they had first lived, and it was there that Mr. Red and his wife, Annie, raised their five children.

When I first met Mr. Red in 1997, he still lived in that house with his grown daughter Brenda and her two teenage boys, Marvin and Rodriguez. The home was dilapidated by then; it had seen its best years. Some of the boards on the front porch were missing or cracked. The roof sunk in and leaked, and the home inside was dark and dank. The floors were worn down to their dirt foundation. The original paneling was gray with soot.

My visits with Mr. Red would always take place in the front room. He'd get up periodically from the springless couch throughout our conversations and paddle around barefoot while he continued his storytelling. He looked like it hurt to walk, so he kind of shuffled, barely lifting his feet, but sliding them to lessen the impact. "It gets hard around my toe. Gotta soak it and scape it off," is what he said.

His feet were working feet, callused around the toes and edges. They bore testament to the weight they had carried for seventy nine years—their owner plus infinite pounds of pine straw, pulp wood, deer, logs, cinder blocks, children—whatever was necessary to subsist in the rural South.

He worked for himself most of his life and had no retirement to ease him into his golden years. From 1997 to 1999 I had many visits with Mr. Red where he shared his body, mind and soul survival stories.

"I haul pine straw for a livin' now," he tells me. "I'm 79 and can rake 100 pounds of straw a day. I go back in da woods in da sandhills to rake dat straw. Throw it in da back of my truck." He tells me that he puts up plywood on the sides of the truck "so it could hold mo straw and won't fly out. Sometimes I go by myself. Sometime my lady friend hep me to haul straw, but she been sick. I get out dere 'bout 8, cuz when it gets a hotter, you cain't handle a load."

I offer my pine straw raking services to Mr. Red. He laughs and asks, "You like to haul pine straw?"

"Yeah, I like that kind of work." My frame is small by Southern standards, so I showed him my muscles and said, "I'm stronger than I look. And maybe we can pick some medicine along the way too."

Mr. Red's energy perks up when I mention picking the medicine. "Okay. Okay. Yeah, I know where dey at, I know where da medicine at," he says excitedly.

That day never came. A few months later, Mr. Red turned his truck over while driving and rolled it into a ditch. He crawled out through the passenger door, made it to the roadside and rightfully said, "I felt a little shooken up." Eventually, his family convinced him it was time to stop hauling pulp wood and get a doctor's check up. The doctor put him on pills for the first time in his life, and he was never the same. Three years later, his journey here was complete.

And in the year 2000, about two years after the accident, the house where he and his family had lived, and where he had shared so many memories with me, was torn down because it was unfit and dangerous to live in. Mr. Red and his house are gone, but the memories and life story he imparted to me remain.

My Sun-kissed Head

They call me Red since I was 'bout five or six years ol.' My brother say when I was a li'l boy that I go bareheaded out in the hot sun. We didn't have no bicycles and thangs like right now. We jus' be out playin' in the sand, and the sun turn my head red. A lot of people don' even know my name is Stelly. I've been called Red so long, my name is Red.

My sista[61] and I da only ones that are livin' outta nine chil'ren. I'm da knee baby. All the rest of 'em are dead. She live right over yonder 'bout two miles. She take herbs, too, just like me.

My mother's name was Carenna.[62] She was half Indian and half American Black woman. I learned how to use the medicines from her. I reckon she learned from her mother. I never go to no doctor, you doctor yourself. Accordin' to what kind of disease or what was botherin' you, you jus' go out in da woods and find the thangs to cure it.

I take my own medicine for my "sugar."[63] I mix green pine tops, pine straw and peach tree leaves and a li'l thang that grows out in the woods, it's called lion's tongue. I makes me a gallon jug and I put lemon juice in it. I don' take it wit no spoon or nothin', I just take me a jug and shake it up and take me a swallow. A jug will last us 'bout two months. I got to soon make another batch. I don' take nothin' but that for my sugar. I been takin' that for six or seven years.

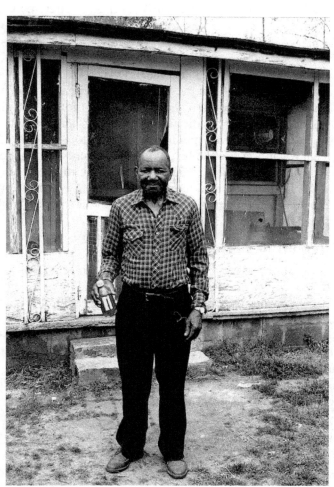

Mr. Red with a bottle of his homemade medicine

Image 3-3

I got five kids by my second wife. None of them use herbs, dey not used to it. They too old for start

---

[61] Ms. Sally Smith McCloud, 84 years old.

[62] Pronounced "Careena"

[63] "Sugar" is a common African American term for diabetes.

them with it now.

When the chil'ren have cold, we go out in da woods and get a herb you call pergiegrass. We get that and drink some rabbit tobacco and horehound, they's a li'l bloomin' weed you can get in da yard. Put all dat in a pot and boil it and make the chil'ren drank it.

My mama used to give us castor oil for colds too. I didn' like it. Dat castor oil, you ever tasted any? I jus' 'bout die when I see her gettin' dat bottle. She had a big ol' bottle, half a pint, set it down in front of da heater in front of da fire, and oh Lawd! She'd get it warm and say, "Come on, chil'ren, ya'll lemme give ya'll some medicine."

"Oh Lawd," I'd say, "I don' want none. I ain't got no cold." She give us all some. My brother next to me could take it jus' like it was syrup. He lick da spoon out. I said if I live to get to be a grown man, I'd never take no castor oil. I ain't took none neither. That stuff is bad.

My father was a good man. He was 'bout twenty-five years older den my mother. He did'n go to church ev'ry Sunday, he would cook. He tell my mother, "You can take da chil'ren an go to church. I'm gonna fix and have dinner done when ya'll come back." There be beans and rice and biscuits. He cook jus' like a woman. He hardly ever go to church, but he take care of dat family.

My father's name was John, John Smith. My father worked in da fields. We didn' have our own farms, we always farmed for the other man, you know, jus' payin' rent for the house we lived in. That's the way we wuz raised up.

We never did own no land when I was comin' up. But after I got grown, I had a farm, 40 acres, when I come down heah from the Sandhills.[64] I had a [cinder] block house and a barn wit' horses and mules. I git somebody who didn' have no chil'ren to hep me plow so I can git thru right quick. I hire some boys to hep me plant cotton, corn, tobacco and peanuts and cucumbers on my 40 acres. Den a man bought that farm from me and turned it into a sandpit. Gettin' rich off dat sand, a sand pit! He gotta bunch of land. It used to be my land. I go across it 'bout every day when I go back in da woods.

I sold it cheap back in dem times. Sold it to him when me and my first wife parted. She wanted her part and I didn' have da money to pay her. I wished I coulda pay her out and kep' da land, but I didn' have da money. Four thousand dollars! Four thousand dollars for da cinda block house, da barn, da 40 acres. Dat was back in da '40's.

Firewater and Bootleg Land

I used to make my own liquor, made it to sell. Dat's da way I bought dat place, dat 40 acres of land, offa liquor. Bought it from a lady for $800.00. An she give me two years to pay for it.

Times were good back den. I paid her $400 dat fall and da next fall I gave her da other $400.00. Land is goin' for thousands of dollars an acre now.

I own dis property heah, it's half an acre. Me and Annie moved heah in da '60's. We wuz livin' right 'cross da road out dere. Dat was da house dat burnt down. We was fixin' to move heah, like tomorrow and dat house burnt down dat day.

Dat ol' house was ol', bout 100 years ol' or more. It did'n take dat thang five minutes to burn down to da dirt. It burnt jus' like paper. Burn up everythang we been buyin' all year for da new house. Furniture and everythang. We got everybody in da house and da next day I went down dere to dat furniture sto and loaded dat truck up on credit. I told da lady dat my house done burn out. She say, "Get anythang I got heah you want an you can pay me later."

Hustlin' out da barrel

I used to haul pulp wood for a livin'. Dat's how I got my foot messed up.

We wuz right back close over yonder, behind dem woods, cuttin' pulp wood. It was windy dat day, Christmas Eve. Da wind began to pick up good and strong, and dat was the last day you could work befo' Christmas. We wuz tryin' to haul two loads.

---

[64]   The Sandhills is a strip of ancient beach dunes in North and South Carolina where the soil is sandy and porous. The region divides the piedmont from the coastal plain and is evidence of a coastline when the ocean level was higher, or the land lower.

Da trees I was cuttin' wuz crooked trees dat bent down in the ice storm the winter befo'. And da wind is gettin' stronger and stronger and pushin' da top of the tree 'round, and when the saw went through, dat tree fell and jumped back on da truck, and hit me and knocked me down. Da tree was on da saw and da saw was on top o' my foot.

I wuz layin' down dere, it mashed it in da mud. I wasn't hurt up dat bad, though.

I worked for a minute at J.P. Steven Mills, made towels and potholders and thangs. I worked dere six years and I didn't like workin' in a mill. Now if I wuz outside, I'd be alright. Da way dey build dese mills 'round heah, you come in dat do, you don' see out any mo, it jus' like you in a barrel. You cain't see nothin' outside for eight hours. I got tired of dat. I make twice da money haulin' pulp wood I wuz makin' on dat job at da mill. I bought two trucks and had a gas tank out dere in da back. I wuz doin' pretty good.

Takin' a heed to it might spare yo life a li'l longer

I ain't took a drop of alcohol, no kind, I say in 25 years. I ain't smoked a cigarette in 'bout 50 years. I was cuttin' pulp wood, me and my cousin. We was cuttin' wit an ol' chain saw, where you need two of 'em, one on one end and one on da other, cuttin' pulp wood.

I had some cigarettes and liquor and listnin' to one of dose ol' battery radios, gotta have a battery, didn' have electricity. Some doctor was talkin', tellin how many peoples died in the United States a year from smokin' cigarettes, lung cancer, how many million people die a year. Listnin' to it dat night and da next night I turn it on, da same thang, tell it again. I took a heed to it. I said dere must be sumtin to dat. I said dat man keep talkin' dat and he's a doctor. I said, "I gonna quit dem cigarettes. So dat day, da next day, me an my cousin was sawin' wood. I said, "Well, when I smoke dis, Im'a smoke at least two or three mo cigarettes den I'ma be through wit 'em."

So dat evenin', I pull out my pack and lit dat cigarette and I balled da pack up and threw it down after. Well dat's it. And I ain't had another cigarette in my mouth since. Dat was back in da '40's. When I got home at night, when I ate, I wanna cigarette, but I didn' do it. I didn' have one and I didn' try and go get none. I said I'ma toughin' it out. I toughed it out dat day and da next mornin' when I went to pick my cousin up to work, he had some. I don' reckon he stopped.

My cousin said, "Wanna cigarette?"

I said, "No, I don' want none. I'm through wit 'em see, and I advise you to do da same thang. You gonna smoke dat and you gonna smoke down to nothin'. Might spare your life a li'l longer."

Epsom salt Chronicles

I don' have high blood pressure. I take Epsom salt for high blood pressure, 'bout every day. I gotta jar and I lay it on tight so it's full strength. I jus' shake a bit a Epsom salt in my hand, not much, throw it in my mouth and take me a swallow a water, three or four times a week. I used to see my mama do dat. I didn' know what she was doin' and I asked her. "Mama what you takin' dat stuff fo?"

She say, "Dat Epsom salt keep yo blood thin down. Son, if you take Epsom salt you'll never die wit a stroke, you never have a stroke." And she didn' either. My mother was almost 80 when she died. Dat will give people stroke, when yo blood get too thick, cain't pass thru dem arteries in yo head. Yo blood get thick and it'll bust tryin' to pass through yo arteries. Be like a pin pop it. Dat's a stroke.

My daddy was 'bout 85 when he died. He took herbs too.

Folks say you betta watch dat ham, it'll run yo blood up. I eat anythang I wanna. I jus' take my Epsom salt 'bout three times a week and keep haulin' my pine straw. I get my blood pressure checked by 'bout every five or six monts at da health department. Don' have to pay for it. Been dere to da health department so much dat da lady knows me. She say, "Mr. Smith, you ready to have yo blood pressure checked?"

I say, "Yessum."

"Well come right on in."

I pull off my jacket an she check it. I say, "Howz it runnin'?"

She say, "Man you got teenage blood pressure and you can haul four loads of straw a day."

Epsom salt would take yo fever down and work for stomach aches too. I take Epsom salt if I get constipated. I make it strong. Take 'bout tablespoon full, put it in a glass, warm water, and stir it up.

You be 'bout ready to go befo five or six minutes. Dat Epsom salt is good for almost anythang, headaches too.

I had a sore on my leg a long time ago when I was livin' in the Sandhills as a farmer. I was gettin' out of my landlord's car and he had a ol' piece o' tin on the runnin' board, been dere for sumtin. That's where you used to step down to get out da car in dem days. That piece of tin, it was dat short [about seven inches]. Dat thang scraped my leg back dere. It got sore and it got sorer and sorer and sorer and 'bout Saturday, my ankle had swolled up yeah 'bout dis large and turnin' blue, dark blue. Couldn' put a shoe on it. Dat Saturday mornin', I said I'm goin to da drug store to see if I could get me sumtin to make my foot better.

So I was goin' down da street to get to Laurinburg, 'bout 8 miles. Cars was runnin' on da left side and I was hoppin' on da right. I met an ol' lady comin' up da street. Ms. Ella Lou. She run a country sto' back then. She dead now. And when she see me walkin' like that she say, "Mister, what you hoppin' fer?"

"I gotta bad sore on my leg Ms. Ella. I gotta get to da drug sto down dere to see if I can get me sumtin fer it."

"You go home and you take you some Epsom salt and you put it in warm water, not have it boilin', jus' good and warm and put yo foot in dere and jus' bathe it good in dat Epsom salt."

That was on a Saturday. I hadn' wore a shoe on it in 'bout two or three days and I could jus kinda tiptoe on it a li'l bit. I couldn' walk on it, dat thang was bad. I went on home and got dat salt and fixed it up and put my foot in it and let it set dere for 'bout twenty minutes. I could feel sumtin ticklin' my foot near'bout. Dat salt was goin' in it.

I had a couch over dere and I got over dere on dat couch. Hadn't slept worth a nothin' in two or three nights. By the time I got on da couch I went to sleep. It was 'bout eleven o'clock when I laid down dere and I slep 'til 'bout five or six o'clock dat next evenin'. When I woke up, dat next evenin' I put my foot on da floor and it did'n hurt none. I said, "Huumph, dat foot ain't hurtin'." Den I stood up and went to walkin'. I was walkin 'round, I walked all 'round dat house. Got up Sunday mornin', put on my Sunday shoes and went to church. Dat Epsom salt is good. I do dat now if I have a sore on me and it don' do right and last too long. Use some Epsom salt. It'll take da fever out. Yeah, dat Epsom salt is some strong medicine.

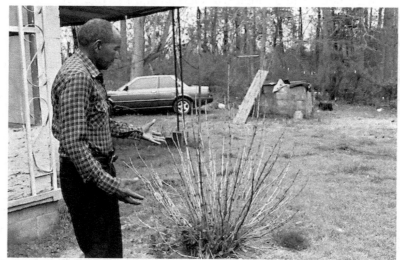

Mr. Red at his house honoring a plant that his sister used to make medicine
Image 3-4

How in da hell can I cure you if I cain't cure myself?

Oak bark is da best for swellin'. Dats good to rub with on my joints and muscles. If yo feet swells or sumtin, rub yo feet wherever yo swellin' is out.

You have to have sumtin like an ax to shave da bark down to get da medicine. Da bark is dry, but you get down next to da wood part, dat's kinda soft. Cut da brown bark off and get down to da wood.

Den you could kinda peel it off jus' like a skin. You boil it down, maybe an hour den rub wit it on da parts dat swolt.

What my sistah made fo me heah in dis jar work good for poor circulation. If yo blood don' circulate good, my feet will get numb and cold. Da next five to ten minutes it gets warm after I put dis on heah. I don know what herbs in it, she jus' give it to me. Dis' don work for ar-ther-ri-tis. Dey say nuthin' work for dat ar-ther-ri-tis. I jus take me some aspirin to ease it off.

Dat ar-ther-ri-tis got to where my Daddy couldn' work. One mornin' my Daddy had to stay in bed when he got thru pickin' cotton. Stayed in da house da whole winter. Ar-ther-ri-tis! He couldn' walk. My mama tried different herbs and thangs to heal it but never did find nothin'.

I was an ol' man befo' I ever went to a doctor but I went to one for this ar-ther-ri-tis 'bout two Saturdays ago, over heah in Laurel Hill.[65] I was hurtin'. What I did dat got me to hurtin' so bad was I went and got a load of straw dat Wednesday and it got to rainin'. It wasn't too cold but I got wet. You cain't get wet wit dat ar-ther-ri-tis. You gotta stay dry and warm. You cain't get cold. And dat night, dat thang tore me up, hurt me so bad. And I come right in da house, pull off all my clothes, top to bottom, put on dry clothes and I thought it would be alright. 'Bout eleven or twelve o'clock dem pains was runnin' up and down from my hip to my toes. When I went to da doctor and he was checkin' me out and thangs, and I tol' him, "There's one thang I want to ask you, have you got anythang that can cure the ar-ther-ri-tis?"

"How in da hell can I hep you and I cain't hep myself? I'm hurtin now!" That's what the doctor said. "If I can cure you, I can cure myself."

I say, "Well can ya give me anythang to hep me or ease da pain?"

The doctor say, "No, no no. I ain't got a thang for dat. I cain't do nothin' for you."

I say what's the matter wit dis doctor, dere outta be sumtin for it but he say, "No we ain't got a thang for ar-ther-ri-tis." As long as you can stay warm, it won't bother you much. But if you get cold, it would tear you up. They had ar-ther-ri-tis back in my Mama's day. I heard her say several times, "Oh my bones hurt, must be getting ol'." Maybe befo' the world comes to an end, somebody will find sumtin for ar-ther-ri-tis.

Make sure da water runnin' when you work wit roots

I known a man near Gibson[66] who is a rootworker. Rootworkers are those who deal wit herbs for tricks. I only deal wit 'em for healin'.

My step daddy John went to a rootworker one time to do sumtin' to my mama. I think he got some of her hair. He got dis woman, another he was goin' wit in Wadesboro[67]. He called and said, "Ya'll come down heah and see 'bout yo mama." We went down dere dat night. She was shoutin' and jumpin' and shoutin' and jumpin' and she had done pulled her hair out on da side of her head.

I said, "What in da world iz wrong mama?" She didn' hardly know us. She looked at us jus' as wild.

My step daddy say, "She been like dat for two days, dis make da third day. Somebody hep me!"

We took her back home to the house. She was jumpin' in da car and we went back home. Den me and my step daddy went and seed dat woman out in Hamlet[68] dat work wit roots. Called her Mum. She give my step daddy John some stuff. It was ground up real fine. It smelt funny and it glitter like gold. He s'posed to give her 'bout a full teaspoon and Mum give him some more stuff.

"You take dis stuff," she say. "Mix dis stuff wit a spoon and give it to yo Mama."

And when we got finished mixin' dat stuff, I dunno what it wuz, and givin' it to her, my mama stopped shoutin' and jumpin' and sat down and looked around. Mama say, "Seem like I been to heaven. Seem like I been in Glory, seem like I been in Glow-ry." Then Mama say, "What I'm doin' heah?"

"You don' even know where you at?" I say.

---

[65] A town in Scotland County, North Carolina.

[66] Gibson, North Carolina, Scotland County, located on the southeastern stateline that separates North and South Carolina.

[67] Wadesboro, North Carolina, located 45 minutes southeast of Charlotte off Hwy 74.

[68] Hamlet, North Carolina, Richmond County, southeastern region, birthplace of John Coltrane.

Her mind jus' kep' comin', and, in I say 'bout thirty minutes, she was back to normal jus' like she always was. After she got better, we took her to another root doctor to get the spell off. The woman tol' us, "Whoever done dis, dey got yo mother's hair. I don' know how or where she live, but look under da north corner down under the pillar, dig down dere and find dat hair and take it and throw it in da runnin' water. Make sure da water runnin' and not no standin' water and get dat hair and throw it." We found dat hair, got it and put it in paper and threw it in this creek over yonder.

It wasn't but a few days after that befo' my step daddy was gone. He was tryin' to git rid of my mama so he could go be wit dis other woman. He didn' say nothin' but he knew that we knew what wuz goin' on. People down heah use root doctors to do devilment. It ain't bad as it used to be years ago. People was bad 'bout dem root workers. I don't hear tell of it too much now.

Ruth Patterson

"I remember workin' cuz I been workin' all my life"

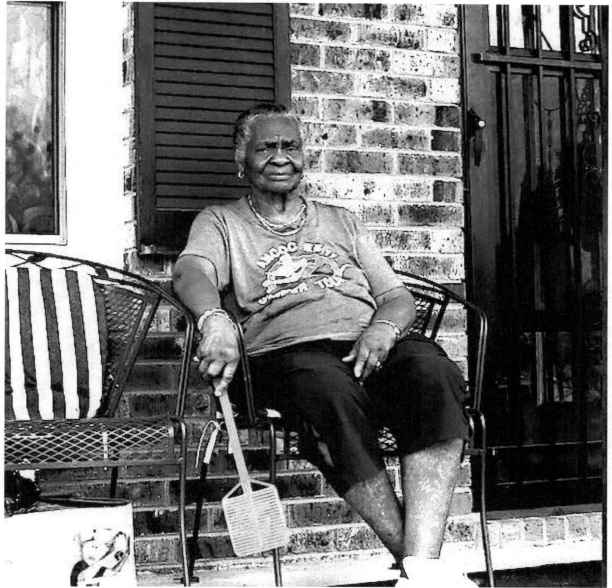

Ruth Patterson on her front porch, circa 1997
Image 3-5

Charlie Patterson used to make liquor in a barrel next to the creek in the woods near the house he shared with his wife, Ruth. Their home was on the outskirts of Rockingham, North Carolina, a few miles away from the birthplace of John Coltrane and Aunt Jemima.

People say Charlie Patterson made the best creek liquor in those parts. Folks would come by to purchase shots or half-a-pints of his "creek liquor" especially after a long work day in the factory, mill or field. They'd stay for a while and drink, talk out their daily exploits and being exploited, dip snuff, chew tobacco, smoke tobacco and then get on home to their families, girlfriends or dogs. To this day, this area of the Carolinas has no bars or other business establishments that sell a little spirits and wind-down for the hard-working Southern folks who choose to partake.

Long after Charlie Patterson's death, the home of his widow Ruth remains the southern version of an underground Irish pub.

I spent a good deal of time with Mother Ruth Patterson over the course of three years, from 1999 until 2001, when I moved back to California. Initially the visits were "interview time," but our fondness and respect grew for each other and my visits became more frequent and longer. I witnessed the daily movement in and around a family that had deep history, rich traditions and a lot of love.

Eventually I became a part of this large blood and extended Patterson clan and Ms. Ruth began introducing me as her niece and Buddy, her son, was like my brother.

Buddy, whose real name is Lacy Patterson, will always have a special place in my heart. Buddy is a Vietnam veteran who was on the front lines of Agent Orange hell for 18 months. His reward for service to his country is an assortment of medications he must take the rest of his life for the trauma he suffered and committed against others, and a modest disability check. Buddy still suffers from hallucinations and nightmares. He, like many others, went to war a whole human being, a teenager at the age of 18 with his entire life ahead of him and few options in Wolf Pick where time moves slow. He came back with his soul broken, fragmented and no prospects of a job. But Buddy comes from strong stock and he is quite brilliant and functional. He is a master builder, farmer and horseman to name a few of his traits.

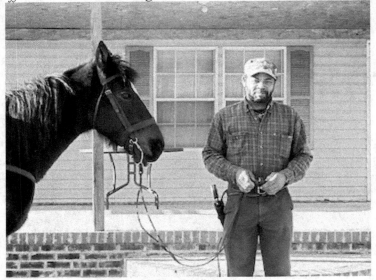

Lacy "Buddy" Patterson

Image 3-6

I asked him why he flies the American flag so prominently in the front of his home. He told me, "I don't fly it for my country, I fly it for the vets who died, still livin', and the POWS. You can tell who a vet is because they fly their flags year round." I have a lot of respect for Buddy and I thank him for introducing me to his family, who is now my family, and especially for introducing me to his mother, Ruth Patterson.

Chewin the fat offa fat back and hog maws

"I go to bed early and I gets up at six every morning," Ms. Ruth tells me one day. "One of the things I do most days is I cooks dinner for Buddy while he's out workin. Buddy like to eat him some fatback; I got to find me some fatback meat so I can season up my cabbage. Yeess, he love fatback. I want you to take dat fatback outta da freezer. You gonna have to cut dat meat too cuz I cain't slice meat. Den you gonna have to fry it up."

I get the meat from the freezer in the shed connected to the side of the house. I bring the meat inside and unwrap the package. A block of frozen white pork fat the size of two bricks sits before me. I have no idea what to do with this.

A few days earlier, Ms. Ruth talked me through cooking and cleaning hog maws and poke sallat.[69] *Now I'll have to do it again, I see.*

"How do you cut this Ma?" I ask Ms. Patterson.

"You ain't never cut fatback either?"

---

[69] Poke sallat is a wild edible green that grows in the south and requires two to three cookings, otherwise eating them will give you stomach cramps and diarrhea. First you parch them, strain them in the sink, wring the leaves like a drenched rag, rinse them with cold water and then put them back in a pot of fresh water (some do this two times instead of one). Then cook the final time, as you would regular greens, with spices and a little meat seasoning.

"Nope, and I've never seen it like this before. If I get it, I get it sliced."

Miss Ruth uses her two fingers like a knife to show me the direction to cut, lengthwise, and the thickness, about one-quarter inch. "And use this knife. It's sharp. Don't cut yo'self Mashell, I ain't got no insurance to cover ya," she warns me jokingly. "You can come on and cut me, but don't cut yoself."

Ms. Ruth never made me feel like I was a "Yankee city-girl" who was deficient in basic Southern cooking. If I didn't know how to do something, she'd show me or talk me through it with a lot of patience.

I cut ten slices from the frozen fatback block, put them in the cast iron skillet on the stove and begin to fry it. The food is now slow-cooking itself. Fatback sizzles, cabbage simmers, and thunder teases about giving some much needed rain.

I join Ms. Ruth at the kitchen table so we can continue our conversations. In Ms. Ruth's house, the kitchen is where everyone congregates. Folks visiting Ms. Ruth knock on the back door that leads right into the kitchen. Few people ever knock on her front door, except for her healing and card-reading clients. A large wooden rectangular table takes up most of the kitchen space. It can sit six comfortably but often holds eight.

The sink, the stove and the refrigerator are in a small open area as you step into the kitchen, fit for only one person to maneuver at a time. We sit for a few moments in silent reflection of our own thoughts, then Ms. Ruth says, "Lemme go see if I can find us some Bailey's." She gets up, goes in her room, and comes out with a bottle of Bailey's Irish Creme. "You make the black tea and I'll pour a li'l of this drink in there." Bailey's Irish Crème and black tea becomes our "special drink" and goes well with our long, intimate afternoon conversations.

We sip and savor our special drink and continue our conversations. A few minutes later, thunder growls and Ms. Ruth stops her words in mid-sentence, gets up and looks outside.

"We got to turn off all this stove and T.V. and cut off all the lights," she forewarns.

I turn off everything and we sit in the dark, speechless, and wait for the downpour. Thunder and lightening storms are always an ominous affair. I want to run to the front porch and watch lightning strike across the sky and the clouds release their bladder. But for Southern folk, it's time to be still and quiet and not call attention to oneself. It's the law of energy attracting energy, and they've seen how one lightning strike can kill or burn your house down.

Ms. Ruth sits patiently and anticipates the downpour. Her head is down and rests in her hands. We hear a knock at the door instead of thunder. "Who can that be?" Ms. Ruth asks with irritation in her voice. I get up to open the back door and three men—all surrogate sons—pile in from their day's labor with gifts for Ms. Ruth.

Surrogate son #1

"How you doin' Mama?"
"Aw right. What is that, a watermelon?" Ms. Ruth asks.
"Yeah. Oranges and everything else," the son answers.
"Put it on the flo over there. Hmmm hmph."

Surrogate son #2

"How you doin' Ma, how you doin'?"
"Jus' fine. What you got dere?"
"Brought you a bucket of small croppies[70]."
"Did ya? Thank you. Do I got to clean 'em?"
"Yeah Ma. Dey ain't been cleaned yet."
"Awright, hmmm hmph."

Surrogate son #3

---

[70] Croppies: a small freshwater fish related to perch or bass.

"How you feelin' today Ma, how you feelin'? I hope you don't feel like I do. Been pickin' in da fields today."

Ms. Ruth answers, "I'm tryin' to get this food cookin'. Didn't know a crowd was comin' up dat fast."

"It pour down, down yonder, we ain't got a drop up heah. Almost had to pull over on da side of da road."

"We gonna get it later," Ms. Ruth advises.

* * *

The three men sit down at the table with us. Now, there's five.

"This my niece, Mashell," Ms. Ruth tells them. "She's from California."

We exchange cordialities while Ms. Ruth gets the bottle of liquor and starts pouring shots. The three men drink their white liquor, Ma Ruth and I sip our Bailey's and tea and we all chew the fat offa the fatback. Eventually the rain drops come down, first slow and intermittent, big hard drops that warn of their presence and then the deluge. In between the raindrops and in the long days before and after, Ms. Ruth tells me her life's story.

Wolf Pick

My name is Ruth Patterson.

I was raised right here in Wolf Pick.[71] Born right yonder where dat house is. Now they jus' change the name, called it Osmond Road, but I guess it'll always be Wolf Pick. When I was growin' up it was my grandmamma, my great granmama and my uncles and all of us, livin' together. We Hintons and Mellons and Elites and Martins and McKeeben's.

* * *

I never seen my mama dat much. She died when I was four years old. The doctor said she had chil'ren too fast. You know, you can get pregnant so fast with chil'ren 'til it wear your kidneys out. My daddy never remarried after Mama died. He raised me. He raised all of us chil'ren along by himself.

There were 16 of us, eight boys and eight girls. Me and my twin sister Ruby was the baby. They called us nicknames but our name was Ruth and Ruby.

* * *

I grew up on nothin' but a farm. I said if I ever got grown I'd never do nothin' else, 'cept farmin. We had fifty acres of cotton fields. Wheat fields. Corn fields. Ten acres of peanuts. Ta'bacca fields. We had our own flour and our own corn meal. Our own beans, pinto, peas. We had butter. We had our own apples, peaches, grapes, cantaloupes. We raised our own hogs, chicken, turkey, cows, and thangs. Everythang we eat, we raised. Didn't have to go to the sto' to buy nothin 'cept sugar and rice and coffee. Now you have to buy most everything from the store, but I still raise a lot of food myself.

* * *

I don't eat pork from the store. When I get ready to get me some pork chops, we kill 5 hogs that we raised. You can kill 'em when they get about five or six months old if you feed 'em right. Feed 'em corn that you raised or go buy corn from other people if your corn give out. Somebody got it for sale, go buy you some corn and then go to the bread place and get you some bread and feed them hogs that.

I don't eat the hog liver and I don't eat no head and I don't eat no foot. If you see the hog graze, you don't want no hog head and no hog feet. They foot nasty walkin' around in hog mud. Well, I make

---

[71]   Wolf Pick is an area in southern Rockingham, North Carolina on the border of South Carolina.

souse meat but I wouldn't eat it for nothin'. Naw, Naw. I gives Buddy, my son, the last souse meat[72] I had.

When we kill our hogs we puts 'em in da freezer and den we make our hogs head cheese. If you get the stuff from the store you don't know what you get. We kill one cow. But one cow don't go far you know. I'll buy steak from the store and beef rib from the store. But I ain't gonna buy no hog and stuff like that.

Two big ol' iron pots, a washboard and lye soap

We had kerosene lamps for light in my time. Had a wood stove and bathrooms on the outside. We had a well and we go there with a bucket to get water. Had wash bowls and a wash tub, show did, two of 'em. If I had a wash bowl now, I'd wash up with 'em. I like to wash up in a wash bowl. You don't waste as much water and it's good exercise for your arms.

There is a lot of lazy people today. A lot of them got washin machines and dryers and thangs now. But I washed all the clothes on a washboard. I had two pots to boil the clothes in, one of 'em big ol' iron pots. I'd boil 'em outside. Put a fire underneath it and water in and stick the clothes in there. I pile a whole lot of wood down dere and lay it next to the wash bottom, so I have some wood to boil the water with and have wood to boil the clothes with.

You tell chilren now to pick up da wood in the yard, they say, "Naw I ain't gonna pick up no wood."

Some folks, after they wash dem clothes they look like collard greens hangin on a line, be so dingy. I'd always wash my clothes in tubs of water with lye soap. Lye soap is better den what dey got today. Makes 'em cleaner and makes 'em smell good.

I made some lye soap last year for a White lady. But I don' have enough grease to make it. You have to have a lot of grease. You buy the talla[73] from the sto' and dry it up. Some folk jus' buy the talla and throw it in da pot and put the lye in and let the lye eat the grease up. But it makes yo soap trashy lookin' ya know. I likes to dry it up.

When I was gettin' da talla I'd dry it up straight. Give da scraps to somebody's dog or throw em away. Take the talla, get you some grease and make you some good lye soap. Used to buy talla in da markets when peoples cuttin' beef and stuff. But they don' keep it no more. Don' save talla no mo. You cain't never find it.

Last year this woman had some lard and it got rank. Everybody don' like rank lard. So, she asked me, "What could I do wit this?"

I tol' her, "Cain't do nuttin wit it unless you give it to somebody's dog or either make up some soap." She said, "If I get some lye will you make me some soap?"

I said, "Yeah."

So she got some lye and I made her some soap.

Anybody can make lye soap but everybody don't make it the right way. I saw a lady one time had some lye soap out in her yard. I asked her if dats lye soap. I asked her how she made it. She tol' how to make it. But I wouldn'a paid two cents for it. She was chargin' fifty cent. A li'l o' block 'bout like dis an 'bout dat big,[74] fifty cents.

I say, "Dat soap stink. Dat grease musta been stinkin' when you made it. I bet it won't even foam when you put it in the water." See, you can tell when dey don' get all da grease outta it cuz it looks kinda greasy lookin' and it was brown, ya know. I say "Isn't nuf lye in it. I know cuz I make it."

We made our own lye soap. You get you some grease. Get you some lye. Put the two together with water in a wash pot. If you got a gallon of grease, you put two gallons and a half of water in the wash pot, then put yo two boxes of lye in it and put that grease in there. Next thang, jus' stir it and stir it and stir it 'til you get dat grease mixed up good in dere. Then you make a slow fire under it, not no big fire

---

[72]   Souse meat (aka hogshead cheese) is a jelly made from the meat in the head of a pig. The meat is cooked out of the head and then marinated in spices and vinegar and refrigerated to turn it into a gel. This is a popular dish in the rural South. It is also processed and then sold by the slice in northern and western state delicatessens that cater to African Americans. Ms. Patterson uses the term "souse meat" interchangeably with fatback.

[73]   Separated fat or grease from cooked beef.

[74] About 2" by 2"

down dere. And then you come and sit down.

After a while you see it come up over dere, like it gonna boil over and then stir it, start stirrin' it. You got to stir it disaway first, and then dataway, back and forth, 'til the water out.

Now put it in a tub, strain it and put yo white satin in it and let it get cold. When it get cold, put it on blocks and lay it on the board in the smokehouse or some li'l place inside so it don' get wet and put it in dere 'til it dry.

When it get dry it's like bar soap. Then when you get ready to wash in two weeks, if you gotta lot a clothes, put two cakes up in dere. If you ain't got many clothes, drop one cake a soap in dere and put yo water in dere, hot water, jus' as hot as you can manage. Den pack yo clothes down in dat water and let 'em set. When it get cool, den wash 'em on dat washboard. I'd be washin' dem clothes and dey be jus' as white. You got to scrub 'em but they'll be white when you wash 'em.

Pinestraw Baskets

I used to make baskets outta pinestraw.[75] You have to get the long pine needles. You can make baskets outta dat green pine straw right out dere, but it's too short.

You can make baskets better outta wiregrass. It's the stuff what you sweep da flo wit it. It's the color of a broom. Some of it git real tall, but it's fine.

My aunt taught me how to make baskets, the woman what raised me. You gotta plait it in separate strips first. When you get a good enough bunch den you start goin' around.

If you got one of dem hooks to put on it then you can do it fast. But if you ain't got no hooks it take you almost six weeks to make a li'l basket. You gotta have patience, time, and you gotta have real good eyes.

The teacher used to have us make baskets in da school. We have a contest to see who could make da best basket. You didn' get no prize but they tell you 'bout the one who made the best basket and everythang. They ain't got time today to teach chil'ren how to make baskets. Dey say, dats ol' time stuff. But it sho iz important.

Before Marriage

I don't remember my childhood much, playin' or nothing like that. I remember workin' cuz I been workin' all my life. Pickin' cotton and pickin' peas. Befo' I got married I was pickin' cotton. Our farm was right there yonder on the hill, right up there. My older sistahs done the cookin'. Everybody worked in the field. We get up 'round 7:00. 'Round then the days wasn't as long as they iz now. We have to hang ta'bacca up in the barn. Have to strang ta'bacca. Have to cure ta'bacca with wood. Get it cured out for market. We worked in ta'bacca when it was cold, too cold to pick cotton. And when it was warm enough to go to the cotton field we quit workin' in ta'bacca and go pick cotton. We done everythang to survive.

* * *

We had to go to school or else we got a whoopin'. We would walk to school, 'bout three or four miles. I never rode a bus in my life. These chil'ren today couldn't deal with that at all. Our school was a one room school house. My first school teacher was Ms. Carrie Wall. My second school teacher was Ms. Lizzie Balwin. She was stayin' wit us. She walk to the school house too. All of us walk to da school together. A road full o' chil'ren and da teacher right along wit us. Didn't have but one teacher for the school house. We get there 'bout 8 o'clock and we get outta there at three.

* * *

On the way to school, we had to pick up cacabugs. Y'all call 'em pine cones. But along den they call 'em cacabugs. Den we go in da woods and break up li'l sticks and bring it to the school house, with the cacabugs, to start the fire in da heater for da school house to get warm. Dey had an ol' long heater

---

[75]   Long-leaf pine needle basket weaving is Native American tradition and craft.

in da school house. Everybody hub-bud up 'round it to stay warm. I remember all dat. Da teacher wouldn't be teachin'. Da teacher be gettin' warm too.

* * *

Everybody's chil'ren 'round here went to dat school. Wasn't but one school house. More den 20 chil'ren. They wasn't cuttin' up back den. Along den, chil'ren knowed how to act. Like I tell dese chil'ren now, "Y'all don' lissen. If y'all was brought up like we wuz, goin to school, you wouldn't do dat." People be talkin' and take da conversation away from you. You cain't even talk about sumtin. Then dey say, "Dat ain't it, Ma, dat ain't it, Ma." And dey cain't say no, you cain't look at 'em to make 'em hush. No, dey gotta get whistled[76]. Cuz da parents don't raise 'em. We wuz raised when we was comin' up, but people don't raise dere chil'ren no more. Chil'ren raise da parents now. That's why I say nobody could adopt me no chil'ren cuz I stay in jail. I beat 'em to death. I sho would!

I ain't never got a whoppin' cuz my daddy would teach us. Didn't know what it was to get a whoopin'. And da chil'ren didn't get no whoopin'. Da teacher would talk to 'em.

Now, da chil'ren tear da books up and you gotta give 'em another one. In my time dey use one book from one year and da next year you had dat same book. Take dem books home and put 'em up when school out. You gotta have dem same books if you go to another grade, and then you pass dem books on to the chil'ren comin' behind you. Wasn't buyin' no books like dey iz now.

All ages be in da same school back then. First grade over on one side. Second grade in another row and on like dat. Didn't know what it was to say high school like it is now.

People oughta be glad to get an education now. They take it for granted. They don't work as hard now as we did back then, neither. We worked all while we wuz goin' to school. It wasn't no stop workin' an go to school. In the evening, you work and go to the ta'bacca fields. After night come, after hangin' ta'bacca in the barn, then you come home and feed up and study the books and get yo lesson done. Yeah, we had to work back then. And it wasn't no goin' to no college.

A child bride

I was 14 when I married my husband Charlie Patterson. He was 55 years old and I was 14. I was finished with school by then.

I cain't tell you how I met my husband cuz he been knowin' me all my life, knew I was born. Along with my Daddy, he helped raise me. Him and my Daddy used to go around together.

My Daddy didn't want me to marry nobody. He didn't want none of us to marry. We jus' married and got out da home. But when my Daddy see I was gonna marry, he say you welcome to marry him and to marry anybody else.

My husband had been married befo. He had 3 girls and one boy befo he got wit me. His daughter was old enuf to be my mama. Sho' was. Everyone of his chil'ren was grown and married when we got married, but they didn't have nothin' to say. Today, kids would have sumtin to say about it. Tell they parents what to do and everythang.

I don't know whether I loved my husband or not before I married him. It was jus', that's a good lookin' man, that's all. He had red curly hair and he had a red mustache and gold teeth. I like-did that gold teeth. I jus' thought he was the prettiest man I ever seen. That's what did it. He was a good lookin' man when he died at ninety years old. Yeah, he didn' look like he was ninety, he look-did 30.

* * *

Charlie Patterson was White. His mama was White and his granmama was Indian but she was White.[77] His Daddy was the doctor, ol' Dr. Patterson. He was Indian though. Dr. Patterson was full

---

[76] Getting sassy, talking back.

[77] In using the term "White" in describing the Patterson family in this passage, Ms. Ruth did not mean that they were full-blooded Caucasian, but that they were light-skinned people of African American or American Indian ancestry mixed with White. This is a common way of describing light-skinned African Americans or Native

blooded Indian. The Pattersons was real bright, got thick skin and they had long black hair, so black it was shiny. My husband had blue eyes. His mama, my chil'rens grandmother, had coal black eyes. She was Indian, had beautiful tan colored skin, not a wrinkle in her face. Her complexion was beautiful. She used white petroleum Vaseline on her complexion and put that on her face once a day and she never had any wrinkles. Didn't use regular soap, used lye soap. She made her own soap. She used lye soap to wash her hair too. To condition her hair, she would use coffee. She would make black coffee and put that as a rinse in her hair to condition it and she wouldn't have to dye it. Her hair was coal black 'til the day she died; didn't have any gray hair.

She had pearly white teeth. Instead of dippin' snuff she dip pepper, black pepper and put it in the back of her mouth. I asked her, "Doesn't that burn your gums?" She said, "No, at first you have to get used to it but then it taste good." It didn't make her teeth black. It made them as white as they could be. She never had any dental problems. She was diagnosed with an illness and only sick for a month before she died. She was 98 years old when she died.

* * *

Everybody like-did Charlie Patterson. I told him they could like him but they ain't gonna get Charlie Patterson. He had a whole lotta women, but as long as I had him here, I didn't care cuz they couldn't get no more than I had got, so I let him go.

Ann, my daughter, would follow him everywhere he go. "Mama, them ol' women were justa lookin' at daddy. They was laughin' and talking 'bout, 'this yo baby.' Ann would say, "I'mma tell my mama. If you buy them anything, I'mma tell. If you buy that I'mma tell my mama."

Ann told me an ol' woman said, "You don' come over here like you used to since you got married." And Charlie Patterson said, "I don' have to come over here, I gotta wife at home."

But I told him, "Well, if they can get any mo from you than I done gotcha, then go'head on and git 'em."

* * *

My husband treat me good and I treat him good, that's why you never see me now married. If I marry somebody he ought to might not do me like Charlie Patterson did. When we been married, shit, I ain't never worked out of a day in my life for nobody else. All the work I done, I done for ourselves. He was a man didn' believe in spendin' a lot of money either. We never did go to da store and buy no meat or stuff like dat. Everythang we need was jus' right here, jus' like when I was raised. When he married me, he know I could work a farm cuz my Daddy raised us like dat.

We was married about 35 years. I had 13 chil'ren by him.

Birthin babies and making yo bones come apart

I had one brother that had 21 chil'ren. I got another brother wit 22 chil'ren who wasn't married but one time. If you take care of yo'self you could have 50 chil'ren and still look good.

All my chil'ren was born at home. A midwife birthed my babies, 'cept for William my youngest. Sally Dawkins and Ms. Ethel Martin; they the only two midwives I had.

If you get out and work it don't bother you when you birth a baby. But if you sit on yo ass when you get pregnant, you know it's gonna bother you. You got to get out and work.

See, I worked when I was pregnant. I picked cotton, two and three hundred pounds of cotton. I pulled ta'baca. Strung ta'bacca. And I walked. Everyday I walk. I cook. Feed a crowd a people. I didn't have to, I wanted to. My husband would go and get a crowd of people and pick cotton or ta'bacca, but I cook. Cook dinner for all dose peoples. And they come to the house and eat and I wash the dishes and I go back to the field and help them work. Work until I had my baby. So it didn' worry me.

The more work you do, the better to have yo chil'ren. If you walk a lot, it will make your bones come apart, it keep yo joints loosen up. But if you sit down, dem bones stay stuck together and

---

American people in some places in the South.

everythang and it's hard havin' a baby. That's what makes you sick. And the doctor tell you when you get pregnant, the more you walk the better you feel. I walk. I lift heavy thangs to make my babies come out fast. I ain't never had no hard time. All my babies were easy, 13 chil'ren, 11 boys and two girls.

When William born, you know what I was doin? Cleanin up my house for Christmas, hangin up my curtains. It took about 30 minutes to push him out. I went out walkin' around and I said I know it's time for my baby to come. I was there by myself. I called Clarence from 'cross the road over dere, I say:

"Clarence come here."

"What is it Mama?"

"Tell yo wife to come here. Cuz this li'l o' baby gonna be born directly."

"Well I'mma go get Ms. Odessa."

"What you gonna get Odessa fer? Shit, dis baby be born 'fo Odessa get here."

But they went up town anyway an told Odessa, "Mama sick, Odessa. She want you to come here."

Odessa went down there to get da doctor. They didn't have but one doctor. All dem chil'ren I had I didn't have but one doctor and dat was doctor McAllister. By the time they got back here that baby and I was sittin' up on the side of the bed. The baby was out. Yeah, looked like it was White, nothing but White. All of my babies looked like White.

With my babies, if it born tonight I have my husband cook me a great big bowl of salad for dinner the next day. Collard green salad, poke sallat or anythang. Anythang green. He would give me some collard greens or either have him go buy a cabbage if wasn't no collards around. He'd cook that cabbage. Cook me some cornbread. Give me some fatback meat. I'd eat me a good ol meal. I put a lot of nutrients in my body. Never had no problems.

* * *

I didn' do nothing to my babies after they come out. The midwife would clean 'em up and grease 'em down good wit castor oil and wrap 'em up and put 'em in da bed. I stay in da bed wit da baby 'bout two days, den I would get up but I wouldn't go out da house for a week. Den when my baby get two weeks old, I go back to doin' my work—my cookin', my cleanin', pickin' my vegetables and stuff. Didn't sit down none, I had to cook. I had all dem chil'ren to feed. Some folks have to go back to the field. But I didn' have to go to the field cuz I had so many chil'ren. When I do my work, da baby would be in da bed sleep. When dey wake up, take 'em and feed 'em good, let 'em nurse your breast, they go right back to sleep. So, there you were.

* * *

All my babies weigh ten pounds. I ain't never had a baby dat weigh jus' a few pounds. They eat everythang they get they hands on. I never had a baby that nursed a bottle. I nursed 'em from my breast.

One of dem, the li'l girl Ann, like to do what her Daddy do. He dipped snuff. He never did put snuff back in his mouth like everybody else. He have a li'l toothbrush, he cut it off bout yeah long and keep it down in da snuff box and make a big ball outta it and take dat tooth brush and put it back in his mouth and put dat big wad of snuff on it. You think he had ta'bacca in his jaw, but he didn't chew ta'bacca.

Ann would jus' beg for it, jus' beg. She wanted dat what he was puttin' in his mouth. He tol' her, You cain't get dis bag, dis is snuff." Oh, she just had a fit on da flo and cried. He said, " I'mma fix her next time, Ruth, I might let her taste this snuff."

I say, "Please, don't."

He say, "Yes I am too."

She got his snuff and started callin' for it, "Snuff, Daddy. Snuff, Daddy."

He said, "I'mma give dis baby some snuff." He got dat li'l snuff wad and stuck it down in dat snuff box and took his finger and stuck it down in dere and wiped it through her mouth and she sit there and smacked it and smacked it and asked him for some more. After then, everytime he would get that snuff box he gotta put a li'l bit in her mouth. And you know when she got big enuf to go to school, she jus' dip in da snuff and hol' it in her mouth jus' like a grown person. Couldn't tell she had it in her mouth. She's in Maryland now. She don't dip snuff no more. She say some time dat snuff taste come to her.

She said one time, whew, she liked to die if she didn't get her a bit of snuff.

* * *

Folks aren't havin' a lot of kids any mo. Too expensive. One cost'es too much. Buyin' all those diapers will make you go broke. All my chil'ren together didn't cost me two hundred dollars. I had to wash my baby diapers, sho did.

When a woman look around nowadays and ain't got but one pamper, you know da baby gonna need more than one pamper at night. So I tell them, "You gotta ol' bedsheet, ain't much good? Take dat bedsheet and tear it up and make you some pampers dat last 'til da next day." That's what we used to do in my time. But dey don't wanna do dat now. Dey say, "Ain't gonna put dat on my baby. I'mma go in dere and buy my baby some pampers."

Healing and taking care of all my chil'rens

My daddy always made tea for us. He didn't take us to no doctor. I used to be scared to death of the doctor cuz I never been to the doctor.

When I been little and people been 'bout to take me to the doctor, I tell them, "You ain't gonna take me to no doctor. You take me down to my daddy."

My daddy would go out in the woods and get me some snakeweed and put it in the bottle. You have to put some whiskey on snakeweed. Let it sit a while an then drank it up. After a while, you gonna be feelin' alright.

Snakeweed is a li'l bitty white weed still over yonder on this hill. It still over there. It lives in the pines, but its hard to find.

I learned my first medicine knowledge from my daddy. Then when I got wit Charlie Patterson, I learned more from Charlie's mama and from Charlie's daddy.

I'm passin my medicine knowledge down to William. He know all dem roots. He can do just what I do. My son Buddy know all dose different roots too.

* * *

People didn't have high blood pressure when we wuz comin' up. They would give you all kinds of herbs and thangs to drink and when you eat stuff it didn't hurt cuz you take herbs on a regular basis. They'd mix it up and keep it in a jar in the house. You be out dere in the cotton field and yo nose be sneekin' and snotty da next mornin', go in dere and get dat jar and get you some of those herbs right now. If they talk about givin' us some castor oil, you go over dere and see us fightin' over dat jar cuz we didn't want no castor oil.

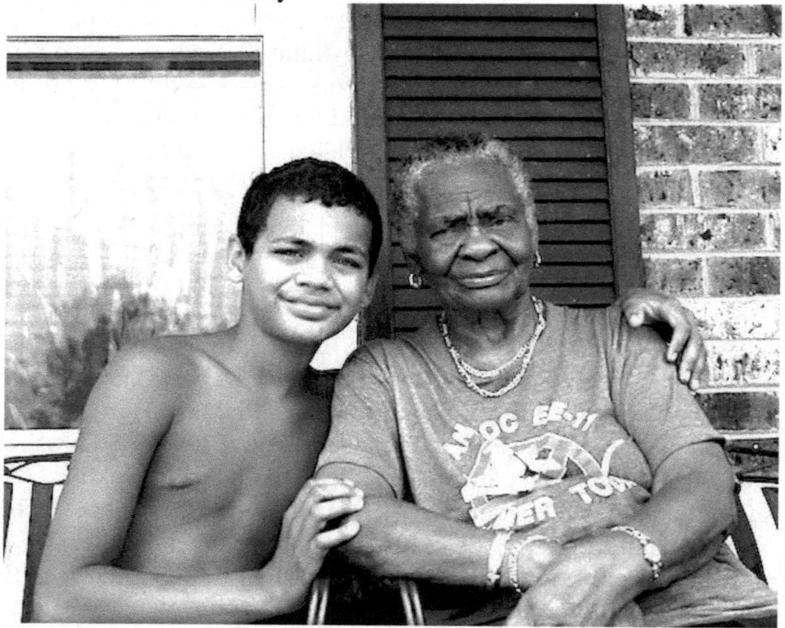

Ruth Patterson (right) with grandson, Bill (William), to whom she has been passing down her medicine knowledge
Image 3-7

* * *

I took care of all of my son William's chil'ren. I even took care of the two chil'ren that Lisa, his second wife, had by her first husband. They was li'l. When they'd get sick I doctor 'em. When they get sick now, they brings 'em to me. They don't carry them to no doctor.

When they get ear infections, I give 'em dat sweet oil. If they get a cold and have a bad cough I get some peppermint candy and get some whiskey and put it in there and make a cough syrup outta it. I give 'em 'bout half a teaspoonful, make 'em go to bed and lay down and be sweatin' and get it on out of 'em. If you go to the doctor and they give you a shot it'll cost you fifty dollars.

If they got a fever, I take that rubbin' alcohol and rub 'em good and make 'em stay in da house and that'll break that fever up.

For congestion, I get me some Vicks salve and mix it up good wit that strong snuff and rub they chest up wit it good, rub it down and it breaks up dat ol' yellow stuff, they cough it up. Sometimes it makes 'em throw-up. They get to coughin' and gaggin', but that stuff will come up outta there. Keep any extra in a jar and when dey get coughin' and dey nose get to runnin' use it again.

* * *

I always raise catnip around my house. If the baby had colic, get dat catnip and boil it. Take a teaspoon full of dat catnip tea and put it in a li'l cup and squeeze some milk out yo breast in dat cup wit dat catnip tea. Den take a li'l bitty spoon and let it drip off of dat spoon in dat baby mouth and won't have no colic.

Catnip grow around a well or a pump. Cat wouldn't bother it 'til it grow right about pretty, but after that, they eat it right up. If people got some cats, wouldn't have no catnip da next mornin'. Funny it ain't got no scent to it. Mus' be sumtin in it dem cats need.

I got some mint out dere right now, but I don't have no catnip because my son got about 25 cats and they ate it up and I cain't grow no more. You can buy it now in da drug store, but you cain't raise it cuz people got cats and dey eat it up. Maybe dats where it got its name from, cats go up and nip it.

Horehound grows around da house, too, in yo yard. It good for colic, too. Make horehound tea. Fix it jus' like you do breas' milk. You boil it and put the li'l tea in it. Then you drank yo tea water and pass it on to yo baby when it take yo breas'. Or you can put a li'l bit of the tea in a spoon wit some breastmilk and give it to da babies.

* * *

Heart leaves is good for swellin'. You gets 'em in the bunch. They leaves is shaped like a heart. You boils 'em and bathes your foot in 'em.

Black clay is good for swellin'. You just take it and pack it on there where it swolt up and wrap it with a bandage. I use mullet for swellin', too. That's all it's good for. And I use Tiger Balm for arthritis.

* * *

When you get a boil, put the skin of the eggshell on top of it to make it go down. If the boil ain't open, get you some fatback and put it on there and it'll jus' open it on up and draw that infection on out.

* * *

Sassafract, you can use that for swellin' and for sores, too. The red leaves, not the white.

The white sassafract, it gotta shiny leaf on it. But the white leaf, it ain't no good. It's pretty much used for the scent, the smell, that's all. You don't use white for cookin', you use red sassafract.

The red sassafract it gotta kinda brown lookin' leaf, a dark leaf, with red streaks in it. It grows out in the old field and peoples ain't tend it in a long time. You can go out into dat field and break a li'l stem offa it and smell it, if it's sassafract, then you cain't tell it's red sassafract now 'til you dig down in dere and pull up a sprig[78] and its white, but if you pop that end loose and it's red, that be the red

_____

[78] Sassafras sprigs are pulled up from the root.

sassafract, and if you pop it loose and it's white, that's the white sassafract. The white will run you blind, stay away from that. You wanna take the red.

You can get them red sassafract leaves and boil 'em and the water be kinda brown lookin'. You can drank the red for coffee or you can take it and make medicine outta it for different thangs. It's good for colds. It's good, too, if you make tea outta that like for a cough and your nose for stuff like that.

A yellow-root cure for a fool and his horse-stick and a dopehead

Them goldenrod is good for colds. It's gotta leaf bought yeah long[79], look like a sage leaf, only it's shiny and it has a heap of leaves grows up on it, and the stem go straight up, jus 'bout dat high[80]. Dat's bitter.[81]

I ain't never had no cold. I drank dat yellow root water twice a day. Also, I makes me some peppermint candy and whiskey. You jus' put the candy in a bottle and pour da liquor on it and dat liquor eat dat candy up and it won't be nothin but a cough syrup den. Den if my nose start drippin' water, I go in dere and I take dat bottle and turn it up and get me 'bout a half of swallow at night.

I don't get sick. Onliest thang bother me is I might get dizzy a li'l bit, sometime I run over dere and get me some yellow root and sit down and in a few minutes I be alright.[82]

* * *

It's a White man down here, he come over here with his liver stickin' out in his shirt like dat. He said the doctor said it's his liver, pushin' out dere. He say his liver is gone. But now, if he hadda been takin' dat yellow root when I told him, wit dat liquor he be alright. He stay close to dis yellow root too. All he gotta do is walk outta his house right on down dere to the branch[83] and get 'em some. Naw, he say, "I want me some liquor, I want me some liquor."

I had my li'l grandson over dere to get him some yellow root brew. I believe he sold it cuz dere ain't no way in da world he drunk all dat yellow root dat quick. He said, "It made me sick, it taste nasty." That's what he said.

I said, "Well, you rather stuff that taste good, and die, than somethin' that taste nasty and let you live?"

"I rather it taste good and die."

I said, "Well go 'head on and die then."

His liver still pokin' out and he still drankin' liquor. He come and got seven bottles of liquor today and seven tomorrow. He got five half-a-pints Saturday night. He got four half-a-pints Saturday evening while Buddy was down there burnin' trash. And he come right back here yesterday and want three more half-a-pints. You know what I tol him, "I ain't got a drop." I wouldn't let him in cuz he jus' killin' himself. I wouldn't let him have a bit. If he didn't wanna die he be takin dat yellow root. So I told him

---

[79]   About two inches

[80]   Two and one-half to three feet

[81]   "Dat's bitter" in this instance refers to the taste of the root or tea as belonging to the bitter family. For example, yellow root is also a bitter. Dandelion root, mustard greens, turnip root and Chinese broccoli greens are also a bitter—similar taste. Often, after someone picks the fresh root or herb with stems, they take a sprig or sliver and put it in their mouth to check the taste and get the medicine directly, right away, as it is most potent. For yellow root harvesting, the root and stems are cleaned of any dirt remaining on them once they are picked from the ground. Then, it's put in a safe place to dry, usually bunched upside down hanging from the ceiling or high point in an outside porch. Once dried, the stems and root are broken up into about 2 to 3 inch pieces and about 1/4 to 1/2 cup is placed in a medium-sized pint to quart-sized jar. Room temperature water is poured over the roots and fills up the jar. The jar with water and roots sits for about 24 hours, then it is sipped on (1 to 3 sips at a time) periodically from 1 to 3 times a day to once a week. As soon as you pour the water over the roots, the water turns yellow, the color of yellow root. Bitters boost the immune system, aid digestion and are good for maintaining and improving kidney and liver health.

[82]   See footnote [13] above for how to prepare yellow root water. EDITOR'S NOTE: This has to be modified so that the referred to footnote reflects the actual final footnote number.

[83]   In this context, branch is another name for a creek or a brook.

I say, "Greg, you know what you otta do.?"

"What Ma?"

All of 'em call me Ma you know.

I say, "You should go home and get you a dose of Epsom salt, get dat liquor outta you or get you some Milk of Magnesia and drank it and don't drank no mo liquor and don't drank no beer, get you some milk and get you some tomato juice and drank it and have somebody cook you a good meal and eat it." I say, "And start eatin' and forget about dat liquor. You live a long time. I ain't gonna say you gonna live forever cuz yo liver gone but you live longer than you gonna live if you keep messin' wit dat liquor."

He say, "Mama, da doctor say I might live six mo months."

"I don't wantcha to die walkin' up in dat road comin' down here walkin'. Stay wit yo chil'ren long as you can. Yo wife done lef ya. Dat boy and girl love ya to death. Try to stay wit 'em if you can."

"Ma, I jus' gotta have me some liquor."

"That's why I'm so glad you ain't got none today."

"Ma, I see ya, I'm goin' to da liquor sto'."

"Lawd half mercy," I say.

Greg is up in his forties. He gonna be dead, I'm tellin' you. His face done turned yellow and it's swollen. He ain't nothin' but a walkin' corpse.

You know how he have to sit down? He gotta sit down easily in da chair, and den when he get ready to lean up he have to lean up sideways, all da way up and then come up holdin' da chair, and when he get straighten up good, he lean over with dat leg stretched out. He say, "I'mma make it now Ma."

He walk straight down in da middle of da road to get down here to get dat liquor. 'Bout a mile and a half. If he give out, he hold on to dat stick. He call dat stick his horse. He talk to it. He say we got to go a li'l further.

Lawd, if he ain't a fool.

* * *

My brother Edgar had four sets of twins. And he got three sets livin'. They in New York.

One twin gotta a sickness dat da doctor say settle in his bone. He say sometime it hurt so bad all over he jus' rather be dead than be layin' there hurtin'. Cain't walk, cain't turn over, cain't do nothing. Then two or three days, he be alright.

You should see the pills that he has when he come here. All dat medication, but you know what he do? He don't take dem pills, he just get him some liquor and jus try to stay drunk all the while he be here.

I gives him some yellow root. He say dat yellow root the only thang helps him. So he come here and he go out in the woods with Buddy and he get him a sack of yellow root and carry it back. He say he can take dat yellow root and he be gettin' on good. He say dem bones and thangs don't hurt him. 'Cept for when he take dem pills, say he nothin' but a dope. Your body cain't get rid of all dat stuff.

Lookin', Readin' and Conjurin'

At Ms. Ruth's house, a steady stream of people come and go throughout the day bearing affection and gifts—children, grandchildren, nieces, nephews, cousins, cousins and more cousins, surrogate sons, daughters and longtime and new friends. And then there are the clients who come for help from everywhere east of the Mississippi.

The entire house could be bustling with cooking, friendly visits and children coming and going, but when the clients come, Ms. Ruth gives them priority. She takes the clients to a private room in the back, closes the door and does her business. When the consultation is finished, the clients leave and Ms. Ruth rejoins her company.

You can look at a person and tell if dey need help. You don' always have to ask 'em if dey need help. And you can look at a person and tell if dey and dey family are gettin' on good. If I can help somebody, I jus' help 'em. I use a regular deck of cards and I use a special deck of cards for nobody else but me. Chil'ren say, "Ma let us play wit yo cards."

I say, "Betta get da hell on outta here. You ain't playin wit my cards."

* * *

When I was a li'l girl 'bout the age of eleven, my daddy was working with the cards, and he said, "Come here, you can do dis fer me."

I say, "What, I dunno how to do dat."

He say, "Do what da cards tell you to do."

I say "Well, I dunno what da cards are sayin'."

He took me to the window to show me the cars that was lined up. He tol' me they was waitin' on him and he wanted me to wait on those people.

I said, "Lawd half mercy."

He brought the people in and said, "This my daughter Ruth. I learnt her to do what I do. She gonna help ya but I'mma be right dere wit her." And nobody had anythang to say. So, we jus' went into the room and my daddy help me wit the first one. Den I start hearin' what da cards were sayin' and I can do it on my own.

* * *

My husband know I can do it when I married him cuz he had brought a lot of people here to my daddy and he know I knew how to do it. So, when I married him, he jus' bring people to me. Sometimes from Monday 'til Thursday, people come to see me. I make about three or four hundred dollars. And the week before last I made $600.

I've been doin' this by myself 'bout 35 years but I been doin' it more than that, 'bout 50 or 60 years, cuz I did it wit my daddy first. My daddy did this and when I got married, my husband, he was doin' the same thang my daddy was doin'. My husband knowed how to do it but I didn't know he knowed how to do it. My daddy learnt my husband how to do this. I don't know how my daddy knowed how to do it. My daddy died when he was 122 years old, so he must've learnt his a long time ago.

* * *

People who believe in it, they come here to me and they tell me they want me to help them. They say, "I gotta problem." And they explain the problem to me.

I tell them, "You cain't brang dat problem to me. You have to let me read it to ya."[84]

So then I read the cards.

If I cain't help people I just tell them to stop cuz I cain't help ya.

I haves peoples from New York. I haves peoples from California. I haves peoples from Detroit, Michigan. Everywhere, they come see me to get a reading.

When you do something for somebody you tell them $30 to start with, cuz that's yo time and that's yo mind. I may be in there with them about five minutes to one hour. Next time you see me go in dat room, don't go in dat room behind me and sit down in dat chair unless you got $30. If you ain't got $30, don't go in there. They know the price.

* * *

I cain't talk about certain thangs cuz you cain't let people know what you use, but you pass that information down. Not everybody can do this even if you show them. It's gotta be in yo family. But a lot of people get they money and they do that anyway. They say, "Oh yeah, I can help ya."

Sometimes I gotta give a person some roots, powder and other thangs and give 'em special

---

[84] Here Ms. Ruth means that a client may tell her what he/she feels the problem is but only through the cards, the truth of the problem will be revealed – the client may or not be correct in defining/understanding what the problem is.

instructions to help them wit they problem. I knows how to talk da fire outta people, but if I tell anybody how to do it den I cain't do it no mo. Certain thangs you cain't tell how to do.

A lot of people think its evil but it's not. But if you use it for evil, it come back on ya. There was a man, a rootworker from Sanford, North Carolina, who did a lot of evil stuff. People would come to him. His wife died, had hair growin outta the palms of her hand and feet. Was as only as big-around as a rail. When this man died, he was as big as a rail too. His roots must have come back on him.

Eveline Elizabeth Prayo-Bernard

"People were real cautious about not leaving their hair around"

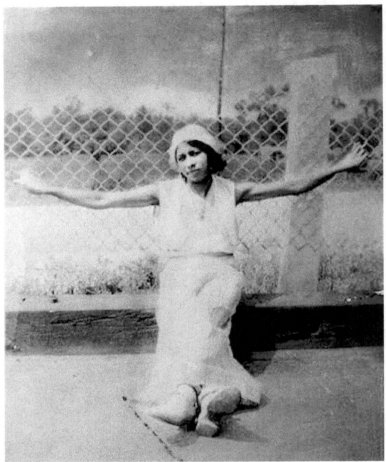

Eveline Elizabeth Prayo-Bernard, circa 1920s, New Orleans, LA
Image 3-8

Don't raise your arms above your head when you're pregnant: 189 years of pregnancy wisdom

I was talking by telephone one day with my Maw-Maw, my grandmother Eveline Prayo-Bernard, while I was hanging up a load of clothes on the line in the backyard. It was 1997, and I was eight months pregnant.

Maw-Maw knew something was happening, and she asked me, "Michele, what are you doing?"

"Hanging up my clothes," I answered.

"You shouldn't be doing that!" she told me. "You're not supposed to lift your arms above your head, the cord could wrap around the baby's neck and it could choke to death."

What a gruesome thought! Of course I didn't believe her and asked for an explanation to justify how on earth raising my arms above my head when I'm pregnant could somehow cause the umbilical cord to choke and kill the baby. She said, "Just don't do it!"

"Okay," I said just to end the discussion and placate her. Maw-Maw knew I had no intention of taking heed to her warning. Ten minutes later, the phone rang again. It was Maw-Maw. Before I had a chance to get the hello out, she frantically said, "I just called Ms. Ethel and I told her what you were doing, lifting your arms above your head, being pregnant and all, and she agreed with me. I don't care what you think, but we've been around a long time and you people do things differently today. We raised our kids right on our own ways and everyone came out all right. You shouldn't be doing that!"

Ms. Ethel was one of Maw-Maw's friends and, at almost one hundred, one of the few persons on

98

earth who were older than her.

The passion in Maw-Maw's words, her deep concern for her yet-to-be-born great-granddaughter's safety and her plea for all of her 89 years of wisdom to be heard softened my stubbornness. This woman graced with sound health, keen sight and good hearing, still lived alone in Oakland, drove, walked unassisted, gambled, danced, went to mass every Sunday, played cards until the wee hours of the morning, caught the bus downtown to shop, volunteered at the hospital and cooked a mean pot of gumbo. This woman and all of her wisdom could be right.

I finally conceded and said, "Maw-Maw, if you and Ms. Ethel say I shouldn't be doing that, I won't raise my arms above my head. I promise." And I honestly didn't for the rest of my pregnancy. My daughter, Nora Irene-Elizabeth Dockery, was born perfect, with no cord wrapped around her neck.

Eveline Elizabeth Prayo-Bernard was born on May 19, 1908 to Fortuna Elizabeth Roussel-Pijeaux and Emile Prayo. She was the second child of this union and the middle child born to Fortuna. Eveline is my Maw-Maw, my Mamere, my Grandmother. On May 19, 2008 she had graced this earth for 100 years. It was only natural that my journey in search of the traditional healing knowledge of my ancestors began with her.

Eveline grew up in the midst of New Orleans' Creole culture and attended Catholic schools all of her life. She developed into a nice, respectable Creole-Catholic woman who worked hard, never missed a mass, and married Creole in order to carry on that bloodline and— most importantly to her and her community—the physical features Creole's coveted: lighter than a paper bag skin tone, sharp features, and hair that didn't need pressing to be straight. (Creoles are a combination of several widely-diffused Old and New World cultures, African mixed with one or more of the Native American tribes of that region[85] and French and/or Spanish, Portuguese, or Italian.)

On the outside Fortuna (my great-grandmother) appeared very much like how she raised her daughter, Eveline. To my knowledge, my great-grandmother was not a full voudoun practitioner, though she did things that would make the Catholic Church cringe and call her a heretic, a pagan, possessed. Fortuna healed people in her community with roots and herbs and energy and other-worldly powers. She believed in spirits on the other side and regularly attended séances with her children, Eveline, Eugene, and Lillian. My grandmother has told me that Fortuna—

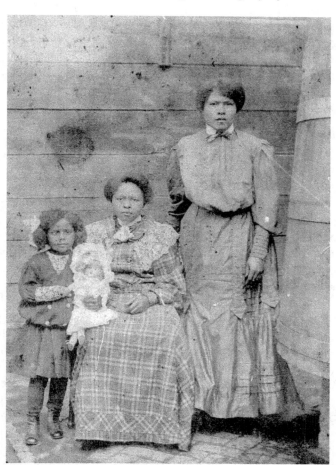

Fortuna Prayo-Pijeaux (Eveline Prayo-Bernard's mother), center, Lillian Prayo (Eveline Prayo-Bernard's sister), left, Josepha Augustine-Borden (Fortuna Prayo-Pijeaux' sister), right, circa 1910
Image 3-9

who spoke the French patois of the Louisiana Creoles—sprinkled salt in the corners of her house to ward off evil and created elaborate novena altars with burning candles and incense to make her prayers more powerful. Fortuna believed in and prayed to Saints who concealed their African origin, much like

---

[85] Alabama/Coushatta, Choctaw, Houma, Natchez, Tunica, Chitmacha, Caddo, Opelousa, Ouachita, Biloxi, or Ofo

people from Puerto Rico and Cuba did in the Santería religion. For most of her life, Fortuna used traditional medicines to heal. Her daily way of life and her healing knowledge was an amalgamation of her African, Native American, and European roots enveloped in Catholicism for purposes of survival.

Where did these teachings and practices come from? "I guess she learned from her mother," my Maw-Maw explained to me. And Fortuna's mother, Elizabeth Augustine, learned from her mother, Seraphine Tembo. And so, the oral tradition survived through the generations, and we can trace it all the way down the line from where it began, back across the Gulf of Mexico to the islands of the Caribbean, and from there traversing the Atlantic to present day Guinea in Africa, (which is the origin of the surname Timbo) or southern Africa which is the origin of the surname Tembo.

Fortuna crossed over at 94 years young. The year was 1980, I was 21 and hadn't even begun to appreciate the knowledge she carried. Eveline, my Maw-Maw, had passionately embraced Catholicism and all of its tenets, and practiced little of what she saw her mother do. Eveline passed her obedience to Catholicism down to her three children—my mother and two aunts —who grew up oblivious to all Fortuna really embodied.

Geneticists say a person carries 14 generations of memory in their genes and certain traits can skip a generation or two. It has been two generations since Fortuna's passing and I have opened this door again to carry on the legacy of my great-grandmother and my mother's people. Fortuna didn't carry the knowledge with her to her grave; it's stored in my genetic memory and like her, I believe in communication with spirits from the other side and the power of root and herb medicines to heal.

But my grandmother also carried the memories of her mother's work, and she shared many of the things with me that she remembered about her mother and the ways of Creole folk.

Marking Your Territory

On the first Friday, early in the morning, some people would get up and scrub their steps off with urine to ward off any devilment or evil or anybody who would try to hurt you. Ms. Coolie, a great big heavy set lady who lived up the street from us, used to do that.

We used to scrub our steps down with red brick dust; we called it brickly powder. Everybody had nice red steps and all around the porch. It was protection. People didn't think you were crazy because people believed in voodoo. They believed you could be hurt by voodoo so they just figured it was something that was being done for your own good. You weren't hurting anybody else; you were just doing it to protect yourself. Most of the voodoo things people did was just taking vent on people that they didn't like for petty things.

If somebody came to your house and you didn't want them back anymore, when they leave, get the broom and sweep them out. Then, take the broom and hang it up behind the door upside down and they never come back. That's right, and throw some salt after them.

I remember this family who lived near us kept on having bad things happen to them. They finally pulled out their mattresses and leaned them against their fence in their yard and cut them open with a sharp knife. They found voodoo potions in their mattresses. You could see through the fence so everyone knew what was going on. This kind of stuff happened a lot. You wouldn't know how the voodoo got there because there would be no cuts in the mattresses to show how the voodoo got there.

There was one family in our neighborhood that didn't like the family who lived next door to them. They wanted to get rid of them so they put some kind of a voodoo potion under the person's front steps to make the person get sick. And by some stroke of luck, the family found this under their step and destroyed it. And whatever voodoo this woman was trying to put on this family backfired and it turned out on her. The family's name was Toumé, and the man, Mr. Toumé got very sick and died. I was very young when this occurred.

People were real cautious about not leaving their hair around. When you would cut your hair, you would burn it. Yeah, you didn't let your hair just loose. They thought maybe somebody could do some harm with your hair, so that was a precaution. You didn't have any toilets to flush your hair down so you had to burn it. I was quite old when we got sanitary toilets, but we had what you called outhouses. That was all over in the South. I've seen a lot of changes and a lot more to come with what's going on today.

There was one woman in our neighborhood who was really involved with voodoo. Her name was

Anne, Miss Anne. People used to go to her house so she could make voodoo packets for them. She made a living doing that. You could say she lived in my neighborhood, on Claiborne Street in New Orleans.

My Louisiana family was part of the wave of Southern folks who migrated west and north in the late 1940's for better jobs and new lives. U.S. Steel, Del Monte, Lays, Mother's Cookies, the Naval Supply Center, the auto plants, and the U.S. Post Office needed reliable, stable workers to fill what seemed to be endless positions with union pay. While the war was still going on, the shipyards were hiring in Oakland and Richmond. These were good longshoreman jobs.

The fresh and eager migrant "Negroes" who came out to Northern California from the South had no problem living in tenement housing, boarding rooms, or shacking up with family until they got on their feet. They survived and lived much like America's new immigrants live today, except without all the social benefits that make transitional life easier such as [welfare], food stamps, medical and other support services.

But there were many benefits in those days for Southern African American migrants that are not always present today. Folks could fulfill the American dream: buy a home, a nice car, and send their kids to a decent school. People also invested their money back into the communities where they lived. The local Black-owned Mom and Pop stores sponsored youth sports teams and contributed to local church and social organization fundraisers. And in turn, those Mom and Pop stores were happily patronized. It was a time of hope, opportunity and progression.

Eveline didn't need to think twice about moving out west to California, where opportunities were plentiful and there were tales that the streets were paved in gold. Her husband of a few years, my grandfather Ernest Bernard II (affectionately called Shine) didn't want to go and didn't want her to go. Eveline left anyway, first for a visit with my grandfather's sister, Mildred Pinion, in 1944. A year later she moved to Oakland, California for good with her two youngest girls, my mother Beverly and my Aunt Joyce. My grandfather, PaPa[86] eventually but reluctantly followed, grumbling.

In New Orleans, Eveline had a lucrative business as a hairdresser and she used those same skills to survive in Oakland until she was told her Louisiana hairdresser's license was not valid in California. Eveline used this as an opportunity to get a stable government job at the Naval Supply Center in Oakland where she worked for 30 years until she retired.

My grandfather, PaPa, worked as a train porter for Southern Pacific and was usually on the "tracks."[87] He gambled and drank his modest earnings away at Golden Gate Fields just north of Oakland, betting on horses and shooting craps with his pals at a nearby pool hall. He never contributed much to the household, though I remember one time, on my 10th birthday, he just reached in his pocket and gave me five dollars. Eventually, my grandmother stopped expecting his help, though being Catholic, she refused to divorce him.

We all were Catholic, even though my mother was ex-communicated from the church for having married my father, a Mississippi Protestant. My grandmother's priest told her that her daughter, Beverly, was going to hell for such sacrilege. Maw-Maw told the priest in her most respectful tone that if her daughter was going to hell then she'd see his mother and him there too. And that was it. We remain ex-communicated Catholics to this day.

Traditional Remedies Spiced with Fortuna's Wit

Visits with my grandmother usually meant eating. And eating in a Creole kitchen meant foods seasoned with a lot of garlic, dashes of cayenne, bay leaf and loads of love. A pot of red beans with rice, chicken fricassee, spaghetti, potato salad, millitont, shrimp Creole and if I timed it right, left over gumbo. This is comfort food. "This is good medicine," Grandma Eveline explained to me during our interview, adding in many other healing practices she had learned from her mother and others and brought with her from Louisiana.

---

[86] The man known as "Shine."

[87] The race tracks.

Mama (Fortuna) used to slice regular beets and put them in a pan and put the pan outdoors overnight. The dew would fall on them, you know, the moisture from the next day, and you would drink it to keep your blood up and keep you healthy.

When you have ringworm, you put a penny in a vinegar solution until it turns green and you rub it on the ringworm until it disappears.

As a child, Mama would take me with her to séances where you talk to spirits. She believed in that kind of stuff. She used to go around and heal different people in the neighborhood, give them baths, herbs, roots, poultices, whatever she could to heal you if you were sick and they called on her. Sometimes she'd stay all night long.

There was one case with a little boy, he was a friend of my brother Eugene. He was sick and had a high, high fever and Mama would go there and put hot compresses on him around the clock. As soon as one would get cool, she'd move it and put another one on. She rubbed him down in that quinine, castor oil mixture and wrapped his body in castor leaves. Once the leaves got parched, she'd put a fresh set on him and make sure his body was still

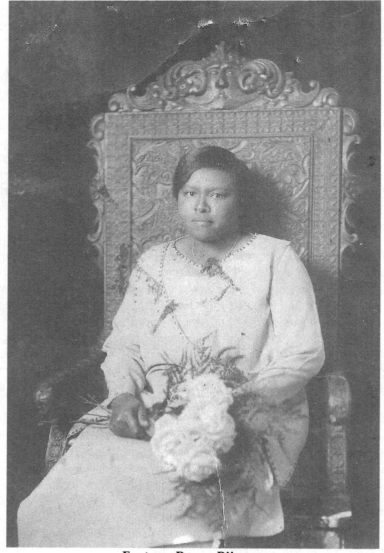

Fortuna Prayo-Pijeaux
Image 3-10

oiled good. She rubbed the oil in all over his body like people give you a massage. She stayed all night. She got tired and she left when he started to get better and told the people to continue doing what she had been doing. But they didn't understand that it had to be a continuous thing and evidently they didn't continue this the next couple of days, and the little boy died.

That was my brother's best friend. I remember he died. Maybe if Mama had the proper schooling, she would have become a nurse or a doctor. She liked dealing with people that were sick. It just come to her naturally.

If babies had an earache, Mama would take a cigarette even though she didn't smoke and she would blow the smoke into the child's ear. I guess the nicotine in the tobacco would ease the pain in the child's ear. She would do this to me when I had an earache. Then she would syringe the ear with a little warm water.

You'd take the temperature or feel the baby's back and hands to tell if they got fevers. If you were hot, then Mama would rub your body down in a mixture of quinine oil and castor oil and wrap your body in the big leaves from the castor tree. You'd stay that way overnight. The next day, the leaves would be dried like they had been in an oven, parched from the fever and the fever would be gone. I did this for my children too. We would also put a flaxseed poultice on your head or chest if you had a fever or headache.

Mama would fill a tub with steaming hot water and put whole bay leaves in it. She'd make you sit in a chair right next to the tub and cover your whole head with a towel. You'd inhale all of that steam and everything and whatever was wrong with you would come out.

I had three children, none with herniated navels. But when a baby's navel did protrude as it sometimes does, you use a dollar or half dollar coin to cause it to be deflated instead of inflated. You tape the coin to the baby's navel. First press the navel down a little bit and put the coin over the baby's navel so that it will push into the belly instead of pushing up and out of the belly. Then take the tape and tape the coin down. That's what you do so you can have a pretty navel and wear a bikini. You leave it on until the navel goes flat. Then you say that person will always have money.

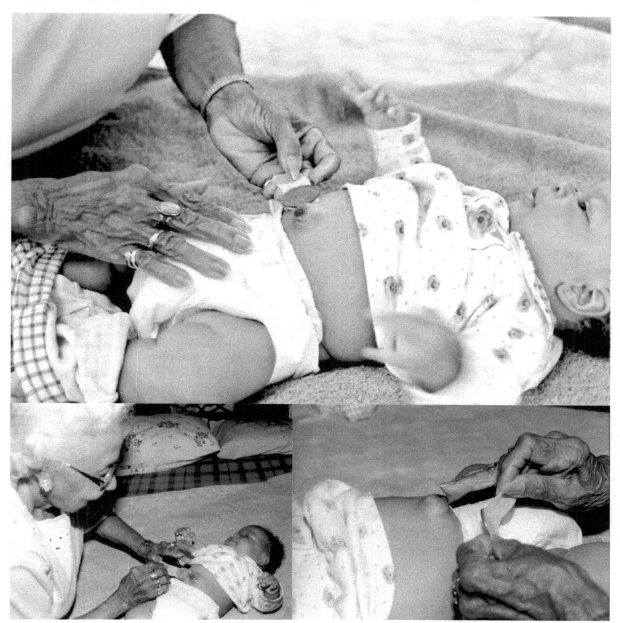

Eveline Prayo-Bernard putting half dollar on her great-grand daughter's "outty" belly button
Images 3-11, 3-12, and 3-13

When I was pregnant, I took castor oil to induce labor, but you never take it if you don't want to induce labor because it will bring it on. It's good for constipation too. Everybody breast fed their babies back then and I breast fed all three of mine.

When children were young and had stuffy noses or congestion and they couldn't blow their nose yet, Mama would use her mouth to suck the mucus from the child's nose and spit it out because the baby would be so stuffy and couldn't breathe. Maybe they didn't have those suctions, but that's what Mama would do.

Mama had such beautiful skin. She used to wash her face and body with watermelon rind. People wash their babies with it too.

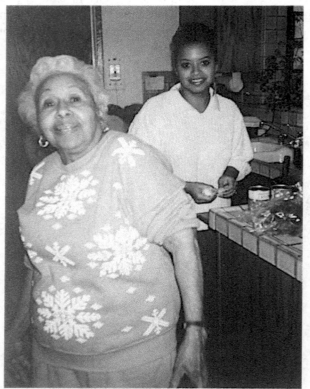

Interviewing my grandmother was a priceless experience. I'm fortunate to have begun talking with her when she was still of sound mind and memory. I learned a lot about her, the Creole culture, my ancestors and those traditions of healing that have been passed down orally for generations. At the end of our conversations, her final words to me were:

There is a book on Marie Laveau who was our voodoo queen and her remains are in the cemetery on Claiborne Street in New Orleans. A lot of times tourists go by and look at her grave and pick up pieces of wood or anything that they think has a connection with her grave, just to take it for good luck. Her grave is still there in St. Louis Cemetery. The people who would be able to tell you a lot of things are long gone. I know that's too bad because a lot of it isn't recorded at all which is really a shame. When you die, you take it with you. That's what they say about our tradition as an oral tradition.

Maw-Maw in her kitchen with future granddaughter-in-law Kimberly Bankston-Lee
circa mid-1980's
Image 3-14

"Now, you got all that on tape?" my grandmother matter-of-factly asked as she let me know this session was over.

"Yes Maw-Maw, I got it all on tape."

"Good. I want to play some of my records." I flip through her albums and call out the names and titles on the cover until she says. "Let's hear that one." While Nat King Cole croons tunes from the 1940's, my grandmother reminisces nights eating out and dancing to live music at Esther's Orbit Room in West Oakland on 7th Street, the hub of Black entertainment during her day. I get great satisfaction just watching Eveline conjure up memories from a past she can relate to.

"I've seen a lot of changes," she concludes, "and there's a lot more to come from what's going on today."

Maw-Maw crossed over at 104 years old in 2012.

Chapter 4 - Coming Full Circle

There is an enduring myth that the moment the African captives stepped off of the jetties into the holds of the slave ships at locations like the Gate Of No Return on Gorée Island, Senegal, they lost all direct contact and connection with their African homeland.

In fact, while contact was unimaginably difficult, it never ceased. As each successive wave of new captives arrived on the North American shores, they brought with them family and village news that was passed along the dark grapevine growing through the plantations and slave farms until it reached the ears of those to whom it was meant.

The spiritual connection between African Americans and Africans was even greater.

While slavery lasted, there was significant sentiment among the African captives to find a way to return to Africa, even by many who had been born in America. That repatriation became possible with Emancipation, and many movements sprang up amongst African Americans to bring it about, reaching their height in Marcus Garvey's United Negro Improvement Association "Back To Africa" campaigns of the 1920's. An unknown number of African Americans made that physical return, adopting African names and building new lives in Ghana, Kenya, Nigeria, and other nations from which their ancestors were taken so many years ago.

In a parallel movement, many African American spirit and folk medicine practitioners have worked to bridge the old Atlantic gap, delving out the roots of their beliefs and practices on the African continent and merging them into a unified whole.

The interviews in the following section reveal the experiences of those who are working to close that broken circle.

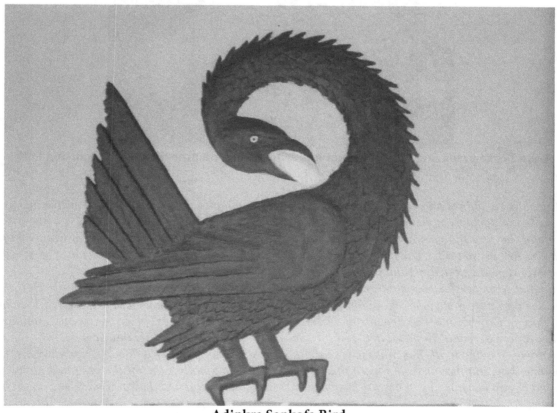

Adinkra Sankofa Bird
Going back to the past to get what you have forgotten
Image 4-1

Anita Poree - "I'm back to drinking pot liquor now"

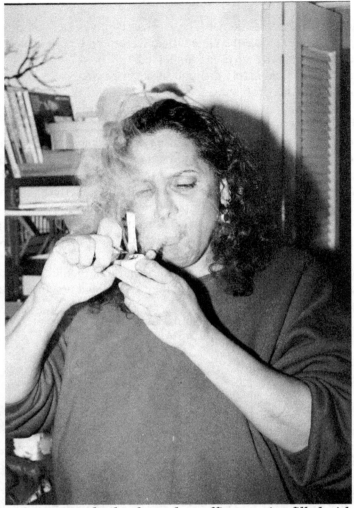

Anita Poree preparing to smudge her home by puffing on pipe filled with cleansing herbs
Image 4-2

Anita Poree defines herself as a Creole/Choctaw woman. She stands about five feet five inches tall and walks comfortably in her dark caramel-colored skin.

One of the first things you notice about Anita is her shiny black hair which hangs wavy and free, much like her personality. The few gray strands are a mark of distinction and experience. And what a life of experience and distinction Anita has lived so far.

She had a successful music career in the 1970's and lived in the center of it all in the Hollywood Hills. She co-wrote many old school hits of the '70's including Eddie Kendricks' "Keep On Trucking" and "Boogie Down" and The Friends of Distinction's "Going in Circles." Her confident, opinionated, and fun-loving personality suited her well for success in Los Angeles' music industry.

To some, she had it all. But Anita was searching for something deeper and more meaningful. "I was going one way, but the ancestors were pulling me another." Finally, she left the glitz and glamour of L.A. and began her journey to the world of her ancestors and reclaimed the knowledge she once called "countrified."

I interviewed Anita two times in a ten year period. The first time, Anita was just opening up to the world of her ancestors and had not yet returned to Oklahoma, Mississippi or Louisiana, the states of her origins.[88] The second interview was conducted in March 2007. By this time, her mother had crossed-

---

[88] Oklahoma and Mississippi are the soil of Anita's maternal lineage. Her mother was born in Waleetka, Oklahoma

over and Anita had the opportunity to return to her ancestral homelands and spend time with her people. Also, a scare with "aggressive" breast cancer really put things in perspective. Her conversation below is an accurate portrayal of her struggles, challenges and epiphanies on the path of her vision quest. It's witty, informative, reflective, insightful and historical. And in the end, she shares her common sense holistic approach to attaining and maintaining her spiritual and physical health.

Survive as strongly as you possibly can without getting sick

I realized after I had the cancer diagnosed that all of those things my mother was raised with that I had looked at as "countrified," or "old hat," were the very things I should be doing. Period! Period!

My parents came from a time when the people from the community they lived in were eating fresh all the time. They were young adults when World War II happened and it was considered affluent if you had canned or glassed goods. But none of my parents and their siblings were raised like that, and my mother, being raised on a farm, felt when she came to the city they got poor. This was before my mother was married and I was born. There was some truth to that economically but they were still shelling their own peas. These folks of the culture knew better in many, many ways, but things like beans and rice was considered a "po folks" food. Well, it's a whole protein and fiber.[89]

They weren't bringing in the higher quality foods in the neighborhoods of color, but even though it was low quality, it was also expensive. So, my Mama said, "Okay, I know what to do." We ate a lot of greens and drank the pot liquor too.[90] Folks would look at it and turn up their nose, but it's extremely healthy.[91] She didn't like to make greens greasy at all and she would overcook them until they were limp as hell and soft. I like leftover greens because they are soft and easier to digest. When I steam vegetables today, I do not throw the water away, I drink the pot liquor.

My mom would make her own clabber. Clabber is sour milk. This is real country, but though people think country ways like making clabber are unsophisticated and backwards, it's actually good for you. She would take the milk and let it sour deliberately in the refrigerator. Our tendency now is to throw it out if you smell something sour, but my mom didn't throw anything away. If she opened up that refrigerator and the milk had turned so sour she could smell, and it had the right consistency, she would get the clabber out of that bottle and pour it into a little bowl. She and my dad would take cornbread, crumble it up in there, and eat it and make it pudding like. It gives you a little more substance so you're not just drinking the clabber straight down. My dad loved it, too.

I would sit there and watch them and my whole left side would start twitching because of the smell and the thought of eating it. My mom would try and make us eat it, but I think for young kids, the taste is just overpowering. As an adult I can probably handle it better. And you know what? Most people on the planet eat some sort of fermented food. Without question, the bacteria are good for you. That's another one of those things that I should be doing now to keep myself healthy, because it is fermented.

My mother didn't use lotion on our skin. She'd use oil, and only then use oil that was edible. If she could eat it, she would use it. So, she used olive oil, coconut oil, anything that you could ingest because

---

in a small area called Clearwater in Okfuskee county. Mississippi and Louisiana are the territories where Choctaws are originally from, before the trail of tears and their forced relocation to Oklahoma. Anita's mother's father was from near Philadelphia, MS, the seat of the Choctaw Nation. Louisiana is the soil of Anita's paternal lineage. Her father's people are from "The House of Poree" in the New Orleans area.

[89] Even though Anita's mother's people were poor and had limited food choices, what they were eating was actually very healthy, beans being a whole protein and rice a fiber—no fat, no sugar, nothing processed.

[90] Anita's mother counters the lack of quality food in their community by not buying canned or prepackaged foods and by cooking fresh beans, rice, and greens. The pot liquor from the greens—which is the liquid that remains after you cook greens in water and then take the greens themselves out—holds a lot of vitamins, minerals and antioxidants.

[91] Anita here is talking about folks in the Los Angeles area where she grew up, and she is referring to the period of the late 40s to the early 60s, the period when a lot of Black folks migrated from the South to the North or West for jobs and a better life. Drinking pot liquor was common in the South, but not as widespread or appreciated up North or out West.

your skin has pores and whatever you put on it goes right into your body. I can't go without oil on my skin because the darker you are, the ashier you gonna look. I don't want any ash on my skin. The only other oil that was used around my house was pure lanolin. Boy, if you could find that now!

Mom didn't use lye or tar soap because she was vain about her skin and she was unwrinkled until the day she died.[92] The Jewish community would sell a lot of chamomile and lanolin soap, so my mom would get it from the Jewish merchants in Chicago, where we had moved after we lost our farm in Clearwater, Oklahoma. Back then chamomile and lanolin soap were considered real basic and what we would call peasant kind of things. I just realized it's good for you, and you know what, I pay more for it now. I learned all this from my mother, saw my mother doing it, saw my father doing it.

My mother used to put straight up oil in my hair. Never petroleum-based products, but olive oil, coconut oil, lanolin. Those were more expensive and my mother and father had a thing about the purer, the better.[93] There was a sulfur product that was on the market that I notice they don't sell anymore. A pure unadulterated sulfur salve is a wonderful healer. I would use this for sores, scratches and scars. Cocoa butter is a miracle as far as I'm concerned.

There was no flaxseed oil back then, but my mom did cods liver oil. She'd make us take it every morning, a little tablespoon and you knock it back with a little orange juice. Nasty!

Now I take cods liver oil daily. Sometimes I take Vitamin E oil too. I find for me, it's better to keep my body guessing a little bit so it doesn't get used to one thing.

And then there was the castor oil routine. If you even looked like you were going to have the sniffles, then we did castor oil. Now that was really bad. There's something about the texture of castor oil that's hard to get down. I don't care what you put in it, it has a gummy quality, a little tackier than the other oils you can ingest. But, it does the job! It cleans you out because it will not digest in your system, so as soon as it goes in one end, it comes out the other and whatever is sitting in there in these little pockets in your intestines will no longer be there. It's wonderful stuff!

My mother had a thing about constipation and about bowel movement. We'd get this question every day, "Did you go to the toilet today?" She'd know if you were lying, and if you were, you'd have to get cleaned out with castor oil.

When I was in my adolescent stage, I didn't go to the toilet at school. It was too nasty. I would hold it until I got home. My mother found out and then scared the "be-Jesus" out of me, telling me "you gonna die," and "it will stop you back up," and "it will go to your brain," and "you gonna fall out," and "we gonna have to put you away for life and you'll get retarded" . . . on and on. She even had the doctor tell me all of that. Now how she pulled that off, I don't know. They realized I was a child that responded very well, not to threats, but to negative possibilities, shall we say. So I figured it out and got used to going to the toilet at school real quick. I put a little stuffed napkin on the seat. I was nine or ten years old at the time. I don't miss a toilet day anymore.

Here again, people isolated out in the country had to stay on top of this and make sure the kids were not constipated, making sure the colon was clean. They knew on a more practical level that if you got backed up, it would cause pain and pain was an indicator that something was going on, and then they would pay attention to where it was. They didn't have all this scientific data that says good health is connected to a clean colon. They knew on a preventive level as opposed to reading it out of a book.

That's where spring tonics came from. And my mother believed in preventive enemas too. Because of that, every once in a while I'll go get a colonic if I feel as though I have too much sitting down in the lower intestine.

You certainly did not want to have an enema when you were a little thing. You know how your little shoes get nailed to the floor...

I've been sorely tempted to take castor oil since I've had my cancer, but I gag every time I think about swallowing it even though it does work. I do other things to keep my colon clean. This is

---

92   Lye and tar are chemicals and very harsh on your skin and irritate and burn your skin. If the lye or tar soap are not made properly, this can happen immediately.

93   Olive, coconut, and lanolin oil were purer than petroleum-based oil in the sense that they are not derived from petrol/oil which is toxic and harmful (not plant based) and you would not put this in your body, so do not use it topically.

knowledge that is passed on down generation after generation.

You can make poultices with castor oil, too. If you have a sore spot or you got something in your muscle that's not quite right, you take a wool rag, fold it over and pour some warm castor oil on it, and take it to the spot. That's why they call it Palma de Crista[94], because it is very healing.

When I was a child, I was the one who was always sick. I had measles and chicken pox back to back. I got through it. I had sprained ankles, hay fever. A lot of people didn't have hay fever back then, but I was so allergic.

My mother would boil things to put up under the bed. It would smell like lavender but it was a little different. You could really smell the oil in it. She'd put it in the room like people use Vicks Vapor to help. It would be her version of aromatherapy to keep the air with something medicinal in it so you could breath, open up your sinuses. We didn't live in an area where there was bay leaves on the trees so she just took whatever she had. Now if we were in Louisiana or something like that, we could easily do that.

She would make poultices out of olive oil and Vicks VapoRub or any other kind of mentholated salve to break up congestion in your chest and bring out the cold. That stuff really worked. She also used something called St. John to clean your chest area out. It was made with pure oil and had a little sweet top to it and was brown. She mix that up, rub on your chest and put a warm wool cloth over it. You could taste the oil up underneath it. I don't even know if they make it anymore. It was very interesting and it worked.

My mother understood about eating clay[95] and what it does, and she considered Milk of Magnesia liquid clay. She gave us Milk of Magnesia before they flavored it. If she could have made her own Milk of Magnesia, she would have.

My mother would also eat a little bar of pure chocolate, dark chocolate, every now and then.[96] It was too chocolate for me. I was being brainwashed that milk chocolate with sugar was better. It was the advertising that was trying to get you to buy a product. The psychology was if you can have it out of the can, instead of shellin' them peas, it was so much easier. Surely you must be tired of shelling! Or Wonder Bread was better than homemade bread. It was not about being healthy at all, but to get people to buy, buy, buy. It's worse today than ever before.

My brother Greg used to have a lot of problems with his ear. My mother would get two teaspoons of water to one of peroxide and heat it up, so it's just warm. She'd tell him to put his head down, and dip cotton in the solution and squeeze it down the ear. You could hear the ear crackling from the peroxide bubbling up. She'd wait a few minutes, then turn him over and do the other side.

If you needed to sweat the cold out, mother would make a mild tottie, and put enough sugar or honey in it so you can drink it down and it would get you to sweating, really strong.

To settle your stomach, she used to make a tea with milk and butter and put honey in it too and it would help you sleep through the night. There's something about it that has a somnic affect.

I had a younger aunt, Aunt Portia, who used to sit in what I now know to be a yoga position. I used to go over to her apartment in Chicago, she and my mother were very flexible. They would sit and do things like that for hours. They would do cobra things, poses where you put the leg on the back of the neck, a lot of torso flexes. They just had a flexibility and innate knowledge especially among the leaner ones. I saw this kind of stuff as a kid and really didn't know what it was and they didn't either.

Rural people have always been stigmatized for being automatically poor. That really is not true, I think they have a good subsistence living and they've never been respected for that. But overall, they did well with what they had because they had real solid principles, solid principles to keep.

It was young and aggressive and had the potential for metastasizing

When I was diagnosed with cancer, it scared me shitless! I was terrified!

Before the cancer I was fit, but clearly not healthy enough for my immune system to ward off the

---

[94] "Hand Of Christ" in Spanish.

[95] Clay: eating it pulls toxins from body and it is rich in minerals.

[96] Dark chocolate: helps lower blood pressure; rich in antioxidants.

little bit of cancer I had. My health slipped by not paying attention, eating bullshit, chewing on plastic, eating styrofoam for breakfast or something like that. We live in a whole other world now. Fortunately, I was born into one that wasn't quite that sophisticated, but it didn't last. I had let something go. I am not going to say that I gave myself cancer, but I contributed to setting my system up to not be able to ward off something that comes in. That's the job of your immune system.

Fortunately they found the cancer way ahead of time, at the early stages. It didn't take any of the terror off of it for me. I had the first stage of breast cancer. They found it with a regular mammogram, then took an ultrasound. When I saw it on the screen, I knew in my soul what it was. That thing looked alive. It was! It was young and aggressive and had the potential for metastasizing.

Fortunately and unfortunately I had a lumpectomy and did the lowest dosage radiation instead of chemo and meds. But before the radiation, I went to a doctor who is a holistic oncologist and we started to prepare my body for the radiation. I was loaded with health building supplements that were all made out of food and other things to make sure my body was prepared for and could tolerate the radiation. And it worked! I still do many of those things today.

Before I even started this process I took my health into my own hands and did a lot of my own research. That's when it all started to come back to me and I realized I needed to do the things my mother did. Everything I turned my nose up as a child I now embrace, except the clabber. But the clabber is creeping up on me slowly. I realize I need something fermented in my diet, so the closest I get to it is goat yogurt, or I'll do raw sauerkraut. That purses your lips and pulls your cheeks up.

I find that the Asian diets, particularly the Japanese, have fermented foods that I can eat. I ate seaweed a lot as a child. We moved to Los Angeles from Chicago right after Martin Luther King's big march in Selma[97]. We had some Japanese neighbors next door who were kind enough to come over and my mother fell in love with seaweed. They showed her how to use it all different types of ways with salad and with fruit and she learned how to make the seaweed rolls with rice. She loved it and I loved it.

I stopped eating seaweed as an adult, but now, I eat it again. I think part of the reason why breast cancer rates in Asian countries are very, very low is because they eat a lot of seaweed.[98]

I'm back to drinking the pot liquor, too. I love it. Tastes good these days. I take a teaspoon of fish oil every day. I can't digest beef or anything outside of a softer meat like fish or certain parts of the chicken, so I eat a little salmon steak or the Rosie chickens which are organic and vegetarian-fed. I'm real picky because everything is over-processed and has so many additives in it. I'm sticking with vegetables mostly and really cooking them down. That works better for my body and digestion.

> **"It's better for me to take some of the wisdom from the ancestors and pay attention to these things that are around you so that I'm not walking around with a case up my ass all the time that just feeds on me."**

My mother's people, Choctaws, originated in Mississippi and part of Louisiana. Her grandmother and mother are from that area. They were people that did not fight back, so what happened was a lot of them were indentured and incorporated into the plantation society in Mississippi. Even on the reservation territories, the designated territory down in Mississippi, they were forced to wear what we would call "mammy" outfits. My great-grandmother's got one of these outfits on[99]. She had hair down to her ankles, but they would make them tie their hair and cover it just like they did with the African women. It was a uniform.

My grandmother was a little bitty Choctaw/White woman, barely five feet. She got married at 14.

---

[97]   The 1965 Selma To Montgomery march that led to the passage of the 1965 Voting Rights Act.

[98]   A recent study indicates that women whose diets include seaweed are may be less likely to develop breast cancer, and that's probably one reason Asian women have a lower overall cancer rate than women in the West. "Anticancer Effects of Different Seaweeds on Human Colon and Breast Cancers." Moussavou G, Kwak DH, Obiang-Obonou BW, Maranguy CAO, Dinzouna-Boutamba S-D, Lee DH, Pissibanganga OGM, Ko K, Seo JI, Choo YK.. *Marine Drugs*. 2014; 12(9):4898-4911.

[99]   Anita is referring to a picture.

My grandfather was Choctaw and Mississippian[100]. He was very tall and handsome and looked more African than Indian. They were truck farmers all of their lives, first in Mississippi and then in Oklahoma. They didn't raise trucks, but the terminology for it back then implied they grew a plethora of things, not just wheat or corn.

At the latter part of the 19th century the KKK was running rampant and everyone was scared. People of color and unassimilated Jews were catching it big-time wherever they were and the Indians were catching it worse than the Black people because at least the Black people had American citizenship, the Indians did not until 1924. My grandfather was very scared about the KKK, and rightfully so, because the Whites wanted the land. So he said, "We got to get out of Mississippi. The KKK gonna end up killing my boys, killing us all." They applied for farmland territory in Oklahoma and were able to get it through my matriarchal side.

My grandparents moved to a reservation area in Oklahoma in-between Weleetka and the Black township, Clearview. That's where my mother grew up. My grandparents started another truck farm and eventually had 13 children. They raised ten to adulthood. With all those mouths to feed, they had to grow as much as they possibly could and raise as much livestock not only to feed the family but to have enough to sell.

In Oklahoma and all throughout the South there was this cross-over thing with Blacks and Indians at the time. They lived together, their bloodlines crossed. The compatibility between Africans and the indigenous was so strong, it scared White folks to death. That's why they had to pass laws to keep them separated. Both people, African and indigenous, kept their traditions secret but you could see some of it at the pow wows or you would never see it. My mother was real privy to all of this as a kid.

They were doing okay in Oklahoma for a long while until a damaging flood hit and wiped out everyone's farmland. There was no crop, no seeds, no equipment. My grandfather applied for a government loan to buy new seeds and new equipment, but he couldn't get refinanced. My family struggled to keep their land and get government help, but the government said, "We can't give you a loan, but we will give you the money to set you up in Chicago and you can get a good job in the stock yards. This is gonna be good for you." Now, there's a place that's a tropical paradise! Can you imagine what this did to my grandfather, a man of the land who had come up indentured, had worked his way to get his own land, raised ten children to adulthood and everybody is doing alright?

They certainly didn't move to Chicago's north shore, but had to live in crowded tenements in Black neighborhoods. And yet they weren't really Africans or African Americans as we know them. They covered up that Indian stuff because it was bad enough if you had Black blood. You didn't want to tell anybody you had Indian blood because Indians were the lowest of the low from where they came from. Plus, if you were trying to pass for White, like my grandmother, in order to get a job and bring in money, you didn't want to tell people you had Indian blood.

My grandfather eventually went to work in the stockyard, slaughtering animals, hitting animals right in the head with a hammer. Get this cow. Pow! On the farm, they did their own doctoring, saving the lives of many animals. He went from life-giving to this deadly piece. He folded right in and never came out. He was a behind-the-closed-door drinker. I personally think he just drank himself to death. I was about 7 or 8 when he died. I'll always remember Granddad. He had this African and this Indian blood, a tall man, handsome man, stoic to the bone.

Some of my family was very successful integrating themselves into Black society. My Aunt Marva modeled for Ebony and married the boxer Joe Louis; she was his first wife. But they really couldn't go back to Indian Territory because the majority of the Indians were too poor. Even the ones that were able to keep some mineral rights and become millionaires were still living in a particular way that was outside of the mainstream society, and the members of my family who had moved out of Indian Territory didn't want that. So, there was all this confusion and this horizontal hostility[101] and hatred

---

[100] By Mississippian Anita means the indigenous people of Mississippi. The Mississippian Native Americans were a mound building culture that flourished in the Southeast, East and Midwest for almost 900 years from 700 to 1600.

[101] "Horizontal hostility," meaning internal hatred, internal racism, jealousy, hostility toward one's own race and culture; adoption of external standards imposed by the colonizing culture resulting in division and jealousy in

among ourselves.

My mom, my Aunt Marva and my Aunt Al were the three that got the most and stayed connected with their Choctaw side. My Aunt Marva is an Owl Woman[102]. My Aunt Al has the gift of sight. And my mother is more of an impath. My mother could hold you in her eyes and immediately see right through you. There used to be a saying in my family, "You don't want Johnnie Iva to dream anything about you because whatever she sees is so."

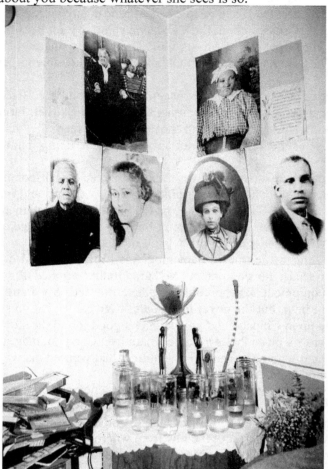

Anita Poree altar with family pictures

Image 4-3

Even though my mother and aunts were secretive and clannish and self-protective around who they were, eventually I started putting two and two together. I used to see my mother and her sisters go in the bathroom and they would do these sweats. It was a part of their little purification stuff. They'd have all these signs for one another.

They had a cousin that used to own a junk shop around where we used to live in Chicago. He was tall and real dark. Talk about a true Black Indian, light eyes, straight black hair, and dark. He spoke Choctaw. I used to think, "Man, he is so cool. Why is he a secret?"[103] You know kids smell things and they don't know the specifics, but they smell things.

That was a man who knew a lot about herbs and stuff. My mother would go and talk to him about stuff and she would come back when I had a cold and she would give me some shit that to this day I don't know what it was. It was just some kind of herbal mixture. I'd ask, "Oh, what is that mama?"

"That's just something. That's just something we do."

That's how I used to get answers. It's hard stuff.

I will never know how much of what my mother knew was passed down to me because they were trying to get away from all of that stuff. They were sooo mixed that they didn't look "real Black" and some of them looked more Indian, a few looked more White.

And the Creole side played a very important part too, because my father's people were more Santería on that side. Creoles are a blend of people that have been that way for a long time. Yes, they are part African, French and Spanish, but it's also the mysticism of the Catholic Church. They were able to hide certain things in it. Some things crossed over and on top of that, they speak patois.

I've been around this stuff all my life even though my family won't admit it. Sometimes I'd find coconuts in the corner of the house. Later I found out they're put there to absorb spirits from the many generations.

---

families; arbitrary decisions in deciding who was more worthy of rights and being "native" such as physical characterists; favoritism toward "Hollywood Indians"—those looking more like what Hollywood portrays as Native Americans. This is as opposed to a heirarchical hostility based on race, culture and economic privilege.

[102] Owl Woman: Choctaw tale of a woman who can transform herself from one body or species to another, a shape-shifter.

[103] The Choctaw-speaking cousin was kept a secret because of the "fear and shame of being both Black and Indian" at the time as she mentioned earlier.

When my Dad's older sister passed, my Aunt Vyv, I couldn't believe all the charms I found in her drawers all throughout the house. I even found her little altar back in her closet. My dad turned white in the face and said, "Don't touch it. Don't touch nothing in here." He loved his sister very much so he was very respectful of her.

It was very interesting, because on the outside to the public Aunt Vyv was proper, educated and cultured. She was very instrumental in my cultural education understanding opera, ballet, theater, the arts. It was a wonderful education. I'm grateful to this day to her for that. But behind closed doors she was a Santería/voudoun practitioner.

I was in my late 20's when I found out that she was a practitioner. I knew a lot about it, but ignored it. I got signals from the ancestors all the time but it didn't register because I was frightened and ignorant and didn't know who to go to, who to talk to. I was busy trying to be in the music business and have material success. My family felt they had to protect their children's psyche from stuff like that. It was common to have that kind of negative beef about oneself because you had to remove whatever society might think is "ignorant." And my family figured this kind of "ignorance" was the kind of thing that would hold you back.

I used to consider all this stuff "country-fied." But when I went to take my mother's ashes back to Oklahoma, I got a whole new respect and understanding for people coming from those areas and the things they practiced. Some of these situations are so tribal, whether you were African or Indian. People would sit down and actually teach you something or just figure out how to do something because of a need to survive.

Healthy living comes from a spiritual base as opposed to just a health base

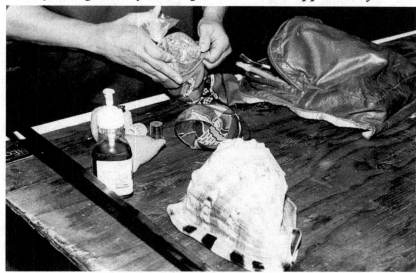

Anita Poree preparing medicine bags

Image 4-4

My spiritual practice is a part of my overall health. I can't really tell you what I got from my mother's side, what I got from my father's side, and what I didn't get from either side but just discovered on my own. I just do it.

My mother's daily spiritual practice was modeled for me and taught me how to have a daily practice. She was very much into prayer. When she passed at 90 years old, I found all her prayer books and spirit-filled literature.

She kept a shit-load of them and would write peoples names in there next to a prayer that would be primarily for their peace and well-being. If some trouble would come up, she'd write your name in the book. She had special intentions for all of us. My mother did this to the very end.

Today, I do daily prayer, light a candle for anything, it doesn't matter as long as the intent is there. I just put gratitude chimes in my house. I am grateful for the little things like waking up in the morning without coughing and the big things like that million dollar check that I'm going to get.

I'm not initiated into any tradition. I'd rather be initiated by a tree than by another human being. That's because of my affinity for being in the woods and a tie that I have with the land will always pull me back to where my ancestors are from. My spirituality is more nature-based. It's a blend of Indigenous beliefs and practices, Creole/voudoun, and Santería.

This stuff that comes from Africa mixed with the indigenous population makes for a very rich combination of things. I switch up my practices and also incorporate other belief systems like

Buddhism, Hinduism and Old World Christianity. In the end, basically, I'm practicing spirituality.

Because my spirituality is nature-based, everything I do for my health is in alignment with natural cycles. I cleanse and purify my system every spring. Country people did this, too, once or twice a year.

I pick weeds that clean me out, eat more fiber and make dandelion tea. If you go to the health food store they charge you more than you want to pay for.

What you eat, how you eat, understanding your body, what it does and does not do are all very important. I try not to eat anything out of season. Don't cut your hair or cut anything off the full moon or new moon. Don't even pick anything or any herbs. If you pick it off the moon cycle, you're not going to get the potency of whatever it is, and I don't give a shit what it is.

I used to think all this was stupid until menopause hit and I suddenly realized that everything my parents and grandparents did was right on. Their whole thing was to survive as strong as you possibly could without getting sick. And they did this by emphasizing what you ate first, taking tonics and cleaning out the colon, so that you didn't have to take any herbs to remedy yourself when you got sick.

Pay attention to the signs

A lot of spirits reside in the woods and visit me there. They feel better in that environment. They follow me everywhere I go. I'm not into different herbs and things for myself, but what I am led to do when I'm in the woods is pick different herbs and things as a remedy or tincture for someone else. I get called for this a lot and I don't even know how I know this stuff, to be perfectly honest with you.

It always starts out when I go to pick sages for cleansing and protecting and knowing that somebody needs this. Then I have a feeling and I say, I better go ahead and pick this or make this remedy or this tincture. I say, who are you and why am I doing this. They[104] say, "Just go do it." They tell me what to do and I just do it. I have no idea where it comes from. At first, it was a little frightening, but you can feel when something is at peace with you, so I just say, it's alright, okay, everything is just fine. I have learned to trust more and I pay attention more so that if something comes up, I know what to do.

I've had a lot of readings and they all come up that I'm a child of Oya.[105] When I walk through the woods on a very calm day (and I am out there a lot), it's very odd when a breeze comes out of nowhere and nothing else is going on. I know configurations of trees and how the breeze sounds. It's Oya coming to say, "Hello, look over there, I'm here."

At first I felt, what the hell is this, why is this blowin' up over here? You could smell things in it and your heart gets to pounding. I now know this is a little signal that's sayin' it's gonna be alright and we don't want you to go over this way, we want you to go on that path over there. I pay attention from now on. If you ever go against it, you will realize why you need to pay attention all the time. I have fucked up royally. You find out quick.

I have altars to my ancestors in my house. Shit moves on my altars constantly. I go through periods where everything is fine and then a picture falls. You really need to pay attention to how a picture falls or how a candle burns. A white candle burning black is a message.

When my ex-boyfriend, Edward, was about ready to die, all them pictures came off the wall in there. I said, "Oh shit, y'all not need do this. What is it that you are trying to say to me?" It was very clear.

I had a candle in here for him and they wanted me to move it and do some things with it because he was having a very hard time. He was tossing over back and forth and back and forth and there were these spirits that were coming to him and he just didn't want to go. He was hanging on to a physical life that was leaving him and he was scared shitless.

The spirits said, "We need to go get him some help." I said, "Lawd I don't want to do this." They said, "Get yo ass outta here and go to work!"

Shit that you've placed on your altar does not move unless someone's trying to tell you something and it depends on how the pictures fall. Ain't nobody in here but me. Cat don't jump up there and the wind doesn't blow anything. It's been happening for a long time.

---

[104] "They" meaning the spirits in the woods and the spirits who speak to her when she is in the woods.

[105] Oya: powerful Yoruba (Nigerian) Goddess of the Wind.

Turning the practical into a sacred experience

About fifteen years ago the ancestors were pulling me and trying to get my attention, trying to get me to open up. I started having these dreams that would wake me up. I would see fingernails peeling the skin off of the dead, which to me signified nightmare!

I went to talk to some Indian friends of mine and they said, "Oh yeah, that's typical Choctaw." The guy with fingernails like a girl, way out and razor sharp, would cut the skin off the bodies, and that was part of what we did as Choctaws.

At the time of this dream, I had never been to my mother's homeland in Mississippi or Oklahoma. I had read some things about the old ways, had done some research and found that this was actually true. But if you stop to think about it, that's just not peculiar with Choctaws. Back in the days, there would always be somebody special who would assist in prepping the body and if their thing was about skinning, then that was their way of doing things. Don't forget they were in a tropical climate, and it was hot all the time. It was my feeling that it was part of a preservation process and you would have to know the subsequent ceremony around that, which I don't know. Any people that live closer to the land, everything they do has a practical reason and they are more in tune to what is going on because it's hands-on. It was their way of turning something that was practical into a sacred experience. I believe had I been living in those times, that would have been my job because I have the stomach for it. To kill something is not my preference, but after something has passed, I'm all over it. That dream was a very poignant piece of information. It helped me understand my mother better.

Bay and Cedar

Bay leaf is a very powerful plant for a lot of things. Not only can you make tincture out of it, you can certainly season gumbo with it, and particularly in this area, you hang it on the door and all over the place. This is not for decoration, it's to keep garbage off of me in here because I have been invaded, though not much, because I keep a pretty safe place.

With bay you have to learn how to read it. It depends on how it dries. I didn't get that outta any book. Nobody passed that down, but suddenly I got this information that said you pay attention to how it dries. It will tell you what's been in here and what hasn't.

I gave a friend of mine some bay because she was having some serious problems in L.A. I went down there not too long ago and I just about freaked when I saw how the shit had dried. I had never seen anything like this. I said, "Child, you burn this and we gonna sage this place and I will send you some more immediately."

It was bizarre how it had dried. It had collected so much malintent that had been focused her way that it was beyond dry. She needed to burn it, not even throw it in the garbage. Burn it!

I'm really big on burning because you need to get rid of some stuff, put it out there and let the ethers take it. In this particular area, Pomo Indians will take the bay leaf off of the stem and line it up around the window sill around all the openings. I thought aah, this is pretty good.

I used to sit in circle with some indigenous women and I have a Pomo friend, and I said that I do the same thing. Except I was taught to put the branch in the center of something because the garbage rises and when it hits the ceiling it catches it right away.

Cedar is another one I collect and harvest and give to some of the indigenous folk around here who do sweats. You take the cedar when they bring the rocks and stuff in for the sweat and you take some of the sprigs and put it on there and it helps to disperse. Cedar is very gentle and penetrates. I always considered it to be for purification.

The Power of Intent

If I need to ask for something, I will do more than what I ordinarily do. One of the things I do is prayers to E-que-co.[106] I did this one of the times I went to Puerto Rico.

E-que-co is a little guy. His mouth is wide open and it's big enough to put a cigar in it. So if something happens that you've been praying for, you give him a cigar and it's really cool. I love my

---

[106] Pronounced a-kay-co

little E-que-co because he looks like my dad's people. And my dad's people used to keep cigars and beer lying around all over the house.

Every Tuesday and Friday, I talk to E-que-co. I put a candle around him and I say, "Where's my studio? You been slackin' off a little bit here." Then every once in a while you hold up a cigar and say, "See this. Wouldn't you like to have this?" You have to learn how to have fun with this stuff too. So E-que-co's message came back and said it's about my intent and the law of attraction, what you're bringing and what you're not bringing. It's an island thing, it's an African thing, it's a Caribbean thing as well as a New Orleans thing.

E-que-co is special. It's a minor entity that is spirit-based for a particular intention or thing that you are asking for. A lot of people are superstitious about this kind of stuff but I think it's the intent behind what you do and they're merely messengers anyway, pure energy.

If you're not about the business of doing your work then your work will do you

If you had been an adolescent 500 years ago, you would go out and get your vision quest and come back and then you know what your life is and you build back[107].

But today, if you're not doing what you were put here to do, the ancestors take your life apart and that is your initiation into modern life. It's like peeling an onion. They take everything off so you can see who you are and then see how you're supposed to operate in this world.

What is happening to me is somebody is rippin' all my doors off the hinges and I am being opened up more and more. So what I find is that I stand out here real vulnerable and naked.

At first, I was keeping a lot of shit secret and it was starting to pound at me from the inside out and I felt, "Lawd, I've got to talk to somebody about this or I'm gonna fuckin' explode!"

My mother and her sisters were never given a safe platform to express this stuff. That's why they were so secretive and clannish. But then the ancestors take you down to your bare essence and then you have your opportunity to pursue freedom and the level of success you actually need.

For me personally, the spirit of my creative art, my creative energy, is where it all emanates from and everything else comes natural to that. I'm a painter, poet and composer. I'm doin' all of it, any kind of ceremony I can find in my art. I stay true to the basics of this as opposed to practicing a contrived ceremony that doesn't mean anything to me.

Right now, my writing is up, my visual arts are up, my music is stewin'. I don't believe in hiding behind my art. I want a full exhibit of my work because I'm a multi-media artist, so I want to show everything!

If you are not about the business of doing your work, what you were called to do, what you were supposed to do, it will do you. I'm a big believer in this and I want to be on the planet a long time. I want to be here healthy. Now I realize that I need to honor myself and take a warrior stance out in the world, which means listening to the ancestors. Once I do that, then I can share this stuff.

---

[107] Meaning to "give back."

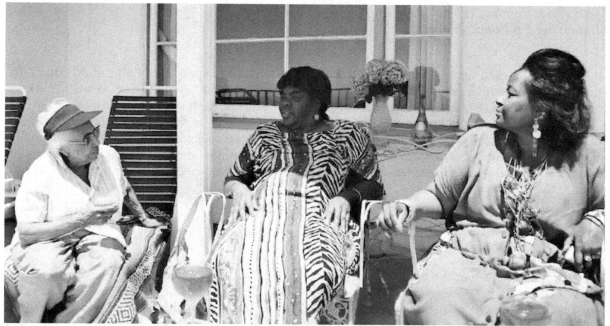

Eveline Prayo-Bernard, Luisah Teish, and Bonita Sizemore (l-r)
gathering at Yacine Bell's home in Oakland, CA to share medicine stories over lunch
Image 4-5

One sunny summer afternoon, I invited Luisah Teish, Bonita Sizemore, Eveline Prayo-Bernard and Yacine Bell-Bayaan to dine and share folk healing remedies from their past.

These women are as diverse in their spiritual paths as they are unified as wise and strong women.

Bonita walks the "Red" and "Black" path and blends the spiritual traditions of her Native and African ancestors. Her early roots are from Ohio and the Carolinas. Luisah Teish, born and raised in New Orleans, is a priestess in the Ifá and Lucumi traditions, which hail from Africa and Cuba. Eveline, also born and raised in New Orleans' Creole community, is a devout Catholic and the elder in the group at 88. And Yacine's spiritual foundation is in the Islamic faith.

The event was hosted at Yacine's home and she graciously prepared a gourmet lunch of Halal[108] cuisine. Feeding the tummy spirit delicious edibles always gets folks sharing and recalling with ease. The entire afternoon was a magical and eloquent call and response that had these elders conjuring up memories eager to burst out. Unfortunately, some of the memories were amputated because so much time had passed since there had been any energy given to their existence and all that would remain would be a name with no connection, like "cow greens." But just knowing and saying the name itself is powerful energy.

Perhaps you, the reader may know the history of "cow greenßs" and share it with us; by doing so part of the reason for this book—to preserve and share the wisdom and to fill in the gaps—would be fulfilled. That would be wonderful! Whenever possible, I include author's comments (in italics) and footnotes as an attempt to fill in those gaps and give more context to the memories and information.

What follows below is that historic and priceless conversation in 1996, held in the comfort and confidentiality of Southern women-folk elders who are long on experience and deep in wisdom. Give thanks for their remedies that heal the whole person, remedies that prevent sickness, remedies that

---

[108] Halal foods are foods that are allowed under Islamic dietary guidelines. According to these guidelines, Muslim followers cannot consume the following: pork or pork by-products; animals that were dead prior to slaughtering; animals not slaughtered properly or not slaughtered in the name of Allah (i.e., limiting the amount of pain the animal will endure by cutting ther jugular vein and allowing the blood to drain from the animal); blood and blood by products. Source: mideastfood.about.com.

protect our spirits, remedies that honor the ancestors, remedies that ensured our survival before, during, and after our time in Amerigo Vespucci's America.

Simmering Up Potent Memories

Luisah

Everybody busted up our families. And they sold the chil'ren apart. We ain't got no papers for knowin'. Just a funny kind of thunk in the heart. Guess the name don' matter none. Whitley, Jackson or Mo'. If the skin is Black and the eyes shine then we be kinfolk, fo sho.

Well, you're not going to find the names they called the herbs in the botanical books. As we're sitting here, species of plants are being destroyed that we'll never get again. What the elders called things is a poetry rather than a botanical genus and species. Sometimes they will incorporate information from the genus and species in the folk name. For example, my mama used to pick what she called "cow greens." Now I have no idea what "cow greens" are.

Eveline

They also have "cow peas." That's what we call black-eye peas.

Luisah

I was lookin' all over the place for somebody who knew "cow greens." And I never could find nothin' called no cow greens. I ran into a woman in North Carolina and I described how mama used to cook 'em and what they taste like and she say, "You talking about poke greens. Poke sallat."

There's an African man named Dr. Anthony K. Andoh. He has a book called *The Science and Romance of Selected Herbs Used in Medicine and Religious Ceremony*. He has done a very good job of cataloging herbs that Black Folks used in Africa, in the Caribbean, and in the United States. It's a very, very good book.

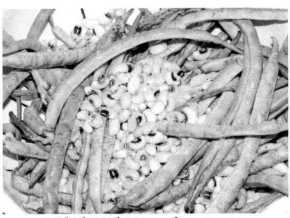

Black eyed-peas and cow peas
Image 4-6

Luisah's voice is a calm, resonating, bass that echoes wisdom from time past. The ancestors are comfortable channeling their message through her. A search on the name and use of "cow greens" has revealed that "cow greens" could be related to the use of "cow peas" as explained in the excerpt below:

"Black-eyed peas, which are actually beans, also were used as food on the slave voyages, and enslaved Africans in the Caribbean thereafter consumed these easily cultivated beans as a basic food. Sources indicate that peas reached Florida around 1700 and then appeared in the fields and on the tables of Whites and Blacks in North Carolina in the 1730s. Although Virginians culti-vated black-eyed peas in the 1600s, they did not become common table food until after the American Revolution.

"George Washington wrote in a 1791 letter that 'pease' (black-eyed peas) were rarely grown in Virginia. He then brought 40 bushels of seeds for planting on his plantation in 1792, referring to them as 'cornfield peas,' planted typically between the rows of field corn. Black-eyed peas were also called 'cowpeas,' because cows were allowed to eat their stems and vines in the fields after the corn crops had been picked. Southerners liked to boil greens and peas of the black-eyed type with strips of salted pork."[109]

---

[109] Source: Joseph E. Holloway, Ph.D, Cal State University Northridge, copied from the site: The Sankoregriot.wordpress.com.

Luisah

I was born in New Orleans and raised mostly in New Orleans. I left New Orleans when I was 14—the way it was with me. We started out in the French Quarters and then we moved to the west bank of the river to a little subdivision to a place called Algiers.

Eveline

I got my marriage license in Algiers.

Bonita

I was raised mostly in Cleveland, Ohio. We did go back and forth to South Carolina and North Carolina.

Luisah

We went to Algiers first and then we were in Gretna for a minute. And then my mama bugged my daddy about getting us some real property. He found a place called Harvey where they had created what they called the Jim Homes (aka Jim Walter Homes), [110] which was a subdivision for colored people.

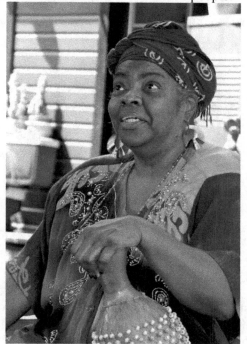

Luisah Teish
Image 4-7

We were one of the first families to move into the Jim Homes. We were across the Mississippi River from New Orleans, way down past Gretna in the Algiers region almost to Marrero, so the Harvey canal was at our back.

What was wonderful about that was when we moved into that subdivision, it was one of those things where everybody got a little two-bedroom house, but you had all this land behind you. They had banana trees and lemon trees and japonica trees and a big willow in the front. The soil was moist and there was a little stream running by the side of the house where the guppies, crawfish and honeysuckle lived. They got wild berries and all kinds of stuff growin', and I go in the backyard and look at all this land, and I thought my mama owned all that land until the day came when a surveyor came with his stuff and drew a line of demarcation. He told me I couldn't go beyond the fence because it belonged to somebody else.

The somebody else that the land belonged to cut all the plants and bushes and trees down, ran shells over the property, and started stacking pipes back there. I was destroyed. That's what comes to my mind. All the things that they killed.

If you didn't study what the original layout was, you don't know what plants were compatible with what other plants, and how those plants were helping each other, and which ones were the most aggressive ones and how they helped keep the balance with the animals and insects in that area.

I was so mad because all of a sudden someone was telling me, "You can't fish over there no more. You can't do this." They came through and rearranged the mussel shells and poured oil on the area and our street became old mussel shells with oil. That's what they did when they decided they were going to get civilized and they shut off the stream, closed it up. They started cutting down the place where my daddy and other neighbor men used to go hunting. Just killin' the stuff that sustained you. The wild herbs, being able to grow your own food, being able to fish, being able to hunt. That all ended. They were steadily making you more dependent on Swagglin's grocery store and supermarkets like A & P, Winn Dixie, and Kroger.

---

[110] Jim Walter Homes are affordable "shell" homes that were water tight on the outside. The customer would finish the inside with their own labor. The only requirement for buying one of these homes was the customer would have to own the land on which the house was placed.

Bonita

I don't remember us ever having to worry about food or having a bad crop. That was one of the things that made me always feel real safe and comfortable. We didn't have to worry about food. I didn't have to worry about a place to stay. I didn't know that we were rich because I would hear them talk about all the land that they had in the South. We didn't have T.V. in those days. So I didn't know that there were really "rich" people.[111]

Luisah

Yes. From one generation after the other. You got a good crop of something and you harvested it, you took the seeds from that and that was what you planted. If something didn't prosper, you didn't use those seeds. Yes, all of that land, the crop, the richness is your inheritance.

Streaming the Medicine Knowledge

Eveline

Do you all remember the castor oil tree? My mother used to rub me down with some oil and she wrapped my body in the castor oil leaves at night and the next morning those leaves would be dry like they were dried in an oven. They took all the fever out of my body. It's a tree with big wide leaves.

My mama[112] used to take fresh beets and spices and put it in the pan and let it out over night and get the dew on it, and they would use that for treatment. Beets and morning mist.

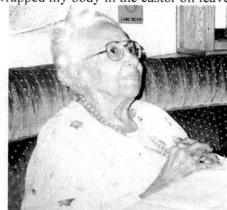

Eveline Prayo-Bernard
Image 4-8

Luisah

Beets and morning mist. That's when it really gets into something that is beyond the medical profession to understand. My mother did onion syrup. Slicin' up them onions and sprinklin' some sugar and she'd always cover it and sit it on the mantlepiece.

We took onion syrup for a whole bunch of things, especially for a general cleanser if she's worried about colds and that kind of stuff.

She'd slice the onions real thin and lay some onions in a bowl, sprinkle sugar, lay some more onions, sprinkle some more sugar. She would cover it with a tea towel and she'd always set it up on the mantlepiece. I guess it had to be in a warm place. She'd leave it there a certain period of time, checking on it until there was this white syrup from the onion juice and the sugar. It was for colds, cleansing and general maintenance.

My memory around that is that I wasn't crazy about the taste of onion syrup. But when she found a substitute for it I wish we had gone back to the onion syrup, because she substituted it with a compound you bought in the store called Three Sixes. 666. It was awful. I wanted the onion syrup because it had a sweet kick to it.

Some people call it evolution but I'm gonna call it devolution, that transfer from the natural concoctions to the concoction that changes the natural product through this now terrible chemical process that we put the natural through. We went from going out into the forest and picking what my mama would call herbs for female trouble and cookin' up stuff for it to takin' "Lydia E. Pinkham."[113] Now if you got some Lydia E. Pinkham and you look on the bottle you'll see Jamaica dogwood root, sassafras, and these kinds of things in the formula. If we wanted to find that stuff around here,[114] we'd

---

[111] "Rich" in the sense of having land.

[112] Fortuna Pijeaux

[113] Lydia E. Pinkham woman's tonic was a popular 19th century medicine. Today it is marketed as Lydia Pinkham Herbal Compound with many of the same ingredients. (See Part II Medicines and Remedies.)

[114] "Here" meaning Oakland, California.

have to go to this drugstore on 62nd and Foothill. These other drugstores don't know nothing about no Lydia E. Pinkham. That compound that my mother used you could find in an old Black drugstore.

We started to lose the identification of the herb and the process for it. While we not lookin', somebody else take Lydia E. Pinkham and put it through a process so that it ain't even what it was no more, and they don't even need the original natural ingredients any more. They can manufacture it and make a synthetic form of it.

Eveline

Cod liver oil was one of the medicines that they gave babies from newborn, so they wouldn't catch a cold or if they had a cold. I could remember how it used to stain up the babies undershirt when it would spill.

Bonita

We took cod liver oil for maintenance and lubrication of the system, but it was also brain food.

Everyone

But they're not the same.
Cod liver oil today is different, castor oil is not the same.
Vicks VapoRub is weaker now.

Eveline

Mama would fill a tub with steaming hot water and put whole bay leaves in it. She'd make you sit in a chair right next to the tub and cover your whole head with a towel. You'd inhale all of that steam and everything and whatever was wrong with you would come out.

Bonita

They used to do that for constipation, too. They'd sit you for a while over hot water. Then you had to get up and walk around and then sit down and then get up and walk around again, while they gave you a drop of turpentine for the stomach. My grandmother said there was one thing that I needed to remember, "If you always want to be healthy, don't be full of shit."

Yacine

My mother used to give us enemas. She was not a gentle woman with this thing. She'd let all that water go and turn this little thing. She was not gentle. She was not kind when she did the enema.

Luisah

Enema is a rude process. It's an invasion. Today we have colonic irrigation which tries to be more gentle but doing the same thing. You gotta fill an enema

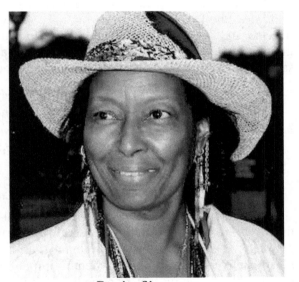

Bonita Sizemore
Image 4-9

bottle four times to get what you get the first 10 minutes of a colonic irrigation. Some people used to do enemas with an infusion of coffee and fennel[115]. It's really quite something.

One of the things that I think about especially for African Americans is that we had our own processes in Africa for things like that and then we had what we learned from our interaction with Native people here. But then the negative part of our inheritance is the attitude that we inherited from the plantation owners' way of dealing with us.

---

[115] The fennel plant is native to the Mediteranean and was introduced to North America by the Spanish missionaries and English settlers, who grew it in their gardens. In the western region, it now grows wild and is known as California Wild Anise. It is generally used as a digestive aid and to relieve stomach problems.

A first generation given an enema and being handled that way knows that it's offensive. A second generation of being handled that way, it's not offensive to them. All they know is that this is the way to handle it. And so it becomes an assumption that a certain amount of brutality is naturally a part of the process. You get a different attitude added to what's being done.

The example that I think about is, I grew up in a huge family, nine children surviving out of twelve. That can work if you got your own garden, your huntin', your own fishin', your own water. But as soon as you move into a situation where mama and daddy gotta work for all of that, then you become what I call the newly poor, no longer self-sufficient. As a child, it becomes tighter, so you start implementing ways that shape the attitudes.

Now in a family like that nobody can be greedy because everybody has to eat. And nobody can be overly-demanding because everybody has to be taken care of. So here I am the oldest girl at home and I'm trying to take care of all the kids and my little brother is waking me up every half hour asking for a drink of water. Now what did I do? I woke him up. I filled four milk bottles full of water and I sat him at the table and I said, "now you drink every last one of 'em right now and don't you bother me for no water no more, at all!" I thought that that was how you solve the problem.

Later on I was reading the life of Frederick Douglass and Frederick Douglass talked about how when he was a child on the plantation, on Sunday they gave them cornbread and molasses for a treat. He asked the master for a little bit more of molasses to go with the last piece of his cornbread and the master brought out a small barrel of molasses and said "niggah drink it all and don't ever ask me for molasses again." And it was like a slap in my face, because essentially I had done the same thing. Now where did I get that idea from? I inherited that.

Bonita

My grandmamma used a lot of camphor from the trees. They have some little fruit on them that you boil. She'd boil it down and and you make a salve, like mentholatum, really potent. She put camphor on cuts and scars and that camphor would pull out the pain and infection. I also remember my grandfather used to give his pigs strychnine for a couple of days before he would slaughter them. He said he would run it through their system to run out all the poison.

Luisah

You can use coal ash to stop the bleeding. And, I'm rememberin' that my mama used to wash her babies in watermelon rind.

Eveline

Yeah, it's good for your skin, wash your face with it.

Luisah

My Aunt Marybelle Reed was the most wrinkle-free woman you ever wanna see. She was one of them red-brown sistahs and she was always glowin'. I remember eavesdropping on a conversation between her and my mama, and Mama was askin' her how she kept her skin so nice. She said she was a baby delivery nurse and that when every baby was born, she would lightly rinse the blood off 'em, and then there's an oil that's on the baby, and when she was cleanin' the baby up, she'd take that and rub it on herself.

We had prickly pear growin' in the yard, and Mama would take the prickly pear, pull the thorns out, skin it, and fry it. She always said it had to be in a cast iron skillet. She would fry the prickly pear in vaseline until it turned green and then she would strain that through three layers of cheese cloth. There'd be this film of very, very fine pricklies left in there. She would pour that in a jar and put it in the refrigerator and leave it there a certain period of time. And that was what she used to oil our scalp with.

Bonita

I used to take sassafras bark and make tea for cramps.[116] I'd boil the bark down with little sticks a

---

[116] An important warning note about sassafras and safrole: Sassafras contains safrole, which is known to have harmful effects if ingested over a period of time in large and concentrated quantities. See warning and instructions in the Sassafras section on pages 319-320 before using.

little bit longer than your finger. You put two or three of them in there and you boil that down. I remember really figuring out that if I got it soon, then I wouldn't have those cramps.

The Art of Being a Trickster

Bonita

They made laws to prohibit us from being able to care for ourselves and to doctor ourselves. "If you practicin' medicine, Ms. Luisah, you violated the code. I heard you gave some cod liver oil to Michele when she had that cold. You ain't licensed to do dat. No you ain't licensed. You violated what we put down. Michele has taken that cod liver oil—we don't know what's gonna happen to that child. You gonna be responsible for her?"

So they put the fear in you and when you might know that the medicine works, no one in the community is gonna say that you're actually practicing medicine. But all they gotta do is ask somebody if Michele is better and they say, "Yeah she real better cuz you know Ms. Luisah gave her that stuff."

"Well what she do?"

They might tell what she did and they might not, because now you know that's against the law. So what we have is not only our own memories of what medicines and potions and what systems work, but we also find ourselves outside of the "law;" a law that really had no consideration about our culture, our heritage or any of that kind of stuff.

With all of this, there are always two or three people in the neighborhood, usually the women, who would continue to work the medicine no matter what.

When I was growin' up, Ms. Gallegos from Cuba, my grandmother, and two or three other people in the area would be the people who would pick potions and do medicine. Of course they did it in secret. They had to. I would be on the walk with her[117] and she'd be pickin' up this, that and the other, and she might tell me, "You don't need to know what that is." And then she might tell me later on, "I want you to remember."

So then your mind is going back and forth.
"Okay, I ain't supposed to remember."
"I'm supposed to remember."
"I ain't supposed to remember."
"I'm supposed to remember."

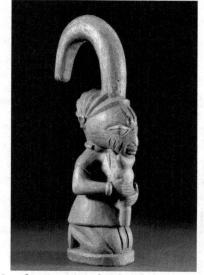

Wooden image of Eshu from Nigeria
Image 4-10

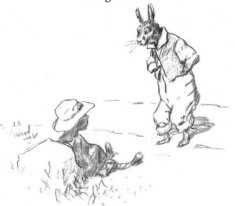

Bre'r Rabbit and the Tar-Baby
Image 4-11

A lot of that is a result of us having to conform and not having clearly accessible the kinds of things that we needed to continue. In order to survive and practice the medicine, you had to know the art of being able to "talk sweet." You had to be able to tell them[118] what they thought they wanted to hear but not tell them nothin'. You had to be a Trickster![119]

---

[117] "Her" meaning her grandmother.

[118] People opposed to traditional healing and conjuring/voodoo.

[119] The trickster is a popular character in African American folktales as well as in many other cultures and mythologies. He appears within many African American stories, story-poems, and songs as extremely intellectual, cunning, and a prankster who relies upon his wits rather than physical strength to protect himself

Luisah

You definitely had to be a Trickster. We were trained about stickin' our nose in other peoples business. We didn't run our mouth about everything because you never knew who you was talking to or what the ramifications was gonna be.

Yacine

Part of survival has been built into us being the Trickster. We do the Trickster without even thinking about it. It's just survival. It's not being the Trickster in the sense of tricking or deceiving someone or lying. It's just a real survival mechanism for us.

African Connections: Animals, Food, Hoodoo and Other Thangs

Luisah

I'm always extrapolating and going back to Africa to understand the meaning behind things we do here. I think that books like Dr. Andoh's *The Science and Romance of Selected Herbs Used in Medicine and Religious Ceremony* helps us to make those connections with what was brought over from Africa and the Caribbean and what we got from the Native Americans.

In terms of healing, there are certain things we can talk about in Ifá[120] and I know where the boundaries are. I think it would be beneficial for African Americans to take initiations and to study Ifá because it helps to fill in the gaps of our inheritance. It's like you don't know why your elders did certain things. It's a revelation to find out that catfish was regarded a certain way here and that it was also regarded that way in Africa. It is stunning to find out that okra is an African thing that we brought here. Okra came from Africa. Words like gumbo means "okra." Peanut is an African thing. And it helps us to understand how much of what is here did come with us. We were not vagabond slaves who brought nothing with us. We brought a lot with us in terms of seeds, in terms of combinations. And looking at that culture helps us to restore the ritual part of the healing that may be missing now.

I left New Orleans in '63. I remember when we went to the west bank of the river, the main issue was which ferry did you take, the Canal Street ferry or the Jackson Street ferry. We went everywhere on boat. We had to get around on boat. We had to relate to the water. We ate a lot of catfish. I found out that the oil of the freshwater catfish is now being used to heal cancer. That's the steak of fish. I've eaten armadillo, eel, possum. Mama wouldn't let us eat coon for some reason.

And the other thing I found out is the catfish, with its distinctive black skin and its whiskers—in Africa they call that mudfish and it's highly popular and considered to be highly sacred there.[121]

Now they got guinea hen in Africa, which is a bird that is eaten. There's a lot of folklore and stuff

---

or "play games" on other creatures. These trickster character depictions were notably represented in the Signifying Monkey rhymes popular in African American culture as late as the mid-20th century, in which the monkey traditionally escapes the jaws of the lion by turning the lion's wrath on made-up disrespect by the elephant. Another popular African American take on the trickster meme were the folk tales surrounding Br'er Rabbit (Brother Rabbit), a clever character who overcomes oppressive situations through his wits and trickery. These were told and retold in the cabins in the slave quarters long before they were collected in book form by the white writer Joel Chandler Harris in the 19th century and thereafter entered into general American life. Many historians believe that the Br'er Rabbit stories may have evolved from an integration of the African-Ghanaian folk tales of Anansi the Spider and Native American folk lore, specifically the rabbit in Cherokee folklore. Eshu-Elegba, the orisha of the Yoruba people of Nigeria, is also considered a trickster and may have also been transformed into the Br'er Rabbit folktales and Signifying Monkey prose-poems.

[120] A relgion and system of divination from West Africa, primarily Nigeria.

[121] From the Akan peoples to the Yoruba to the Benin kingdom, there is a fish— commonly called the mudfish — that is both mythical and real. In art and oral literature, the mudfish combines the traits of several species of fish and is an icon of wealth and the divine powers of rulers. The real fish lives when others would die—either by crawling on land or burying itself in the mud of the streambed. Some of the fish also have a dangerous electric charge, which one might equate with the ruler's power as a judge. Picture a combination of a catfish and an electric eel. Often smoked on sticks, the fish can be purchased in the market to be eaten or used as a sacrificial offering. [Source: Africa.si.edu]

about the guinea hen down South. They call that a frizzy hen.[122] It was a special thing if you had a frizzy hen. Now, frizzy hen was a magical thing actually. You let a frizzy hen move in the yard to scratch up conjure. Pay somebody to throw something at you. You let a frizzy hen loose in the yard and the frizzy hen would find it. That's right. I knew people who kept a frizzy hen on a leash at the front door. Now where did that come from? It was a tradition that came from Africa.[123]

It helps to reconstruct the folklore around the medicine so you can fully appreciate its use and power. A lot of the things have folkloric connections and ritual connections we may not think about because in this culture, you only look at the medicinal properties. Going into Yoruba or Akan tradition or Congo tradition will help fill in the gaps in there.

Most people associate the peony flower with China. Around here in the Bay Area, if you try to get a peony, what you gonna get is the plant and that is going to be expensive.

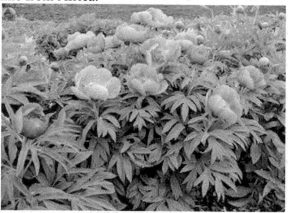

Peony flowers
Image 4-12

Description: magenta colored flowers, yellow stamens in center, green leaves

However, there are Cuban and Puerto Rican shops in the Bay Area where you can go in and get a string of peony seeds with a hole bore in 'em and strung to make a necklace or eleke.[124] That string is only gonna cost you $15.

I have a Goddaughter who's from Trinidad who sent me a whole jar of peony seeds. It's a red seed with a black dot on it. Now we may look at it and see a pretty seed that you can plant and will grow a flower, but there is folklore that talks about how when the Creator was giving everything it's property, the Creator asked the peony, "What color do you wanna be?"

And the peony said, "I wanna be a black seed." But then it changed it's mind and said, "Oh no, I wanna be a red seed."

And so Creator made it black and then threw red paint on it and most of it is red and only the tip of it is black. So, it's not just the flower that you grow, it's a seed that you give to somebody when they're suffering of indecision.

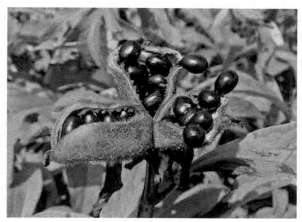

Peony seeds
Image 4-13

Description: shiny black seeds bursting out of a tawny colored pod, green leaves in background

Okra is a natural cleanser. The only time I use okra is as medicine. I don't eat it. I leave it out of my gumbo. When I was a kid my mama would make a pot of gumbo and she'd a make a pot of okra and tomatoes and stuff on the side, and those of us who wanted the okra would scoop it up and put it in our gumbo. I wouldn't, because I can't stand the texture that okra makes.

What's interesting is when I got initiated into Ifá and Lucumi, they give you your taboo foods.

---

[122] Most often spelled "frizzle hen" or "frizzled hen."

[123] In African American spirit medicine, black hens or frizzie hens are used to scratch up conjure and hoodoo in yards where an enemy may have laid down an evil charm. The scratching footwork is a protection from evil and ensures uncrossing of a spell for the restoration of good luck. One can also clean sweep an area or wash areas of foot travel by sprinkling protection herbs and minerals and sweeping briskly. Chicken foot charms are also made for protection.

[124] Elekes are bead necklaces or bracelets worn by an initiate of Santería or Ifá. The color and shape of each eleke represents a certain Orisha (spirit).

Watermelon is a taboo of mine. Pumpkin is a taboo of mine, as well as yellow squash, eggplant, and okra. But they're all things that I use as medicine. So for me to sit down and eat a plate of okra would be like drinking a glass of penicillin.

We always think of tea as boiling the herb and drinking it. But you can go to Africa and you'll find women sittin' with a bucket of water and they are rubbing and rubbing the herbs in the water. Then they pull the crushed leaves out and that water has just the pure chlorophyll property in it. So there's more than one way to use the herbs.

Also, there are songs that go with that medicine and special times that you prepare it and take it. You have a relationship to the herb that ranges from what phase of the moon you planted in to what kind of offerings you make to the earth before you plant it – what kind of prayers you do before you harvest it, what the process is for preparing it, when you take it, and the folklore that embodies it. The relationship gives you the whole thing. You're not a lone somebody somewhere swallowing a pill made out of something you don't know nothing about.

The timing for everything is important. We say, always cut your hair on a new moon. People used to cut their hair on Good Friday. Never pierce ears on a full moon because the ears would bubble up. I've seen that.

We were told that doing things by the time of the month was not respectable, or it was born out of ignorance so we let a lot of the tradition go. Once you find out that there's a whole continent of people who also practice and believe in that tradition you don't think that anymore. Then that whole notion that culture is something that trickled down to us from the Europeans becomes the exact opposite.

European indentured servants were also land-based people and there were times and places when the African people and Native American people converged along with the Europeans, and all three cultures exchanged knowledge and learned from each other. There were many places where one culture didn't know nothing about something that was grounded in that environment and so we learned it from the indigenous people. As people on this continent, we all got a job of restoring an ecological balance.

Red Brick Dust

Eveline

I remember something else that folks used to do. If somebody came to your house and you didn't want them to come back anymore, when they leave, get the broom, sweep them out, take the broom and hang it up behind the door upside down, and they never come back. That's right. And throw some salt after them.

Another lady lived up the street from us on St. Phillip Street, Ms. Coolie, great big heavy-set lady. She get up on the first Friday, early in the mornin'. She had the house with the li'l bit a li'l step,[125] she brush it down with urine.

Luisah

That's right. Establish their territory. And my grandmother's thing—which is something they did at the church, at the cathedral too—is to scrub the steps down with red brick dust.

Eveline

Oh, yeah I used to go and grind that brickly powder 'til it was fine and scrub the steps. Everybody had nice red steps and all around the porch.

Luisah

It was a protection!

Bonita

That's why people paint their steps red. A lot of people paint their driveways and their steps red nowadays. It's transitioned from actually havin' the herb to havin' it refined, to now using the chemical product, from painting it with brick to painting it with red paint.

---

[125] Meaning narrow steps

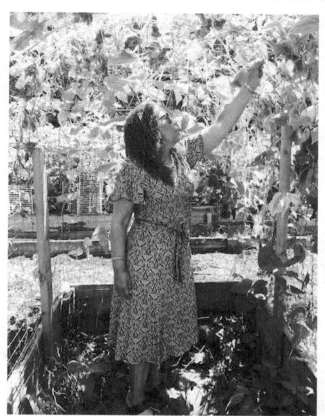

Yacine Bell

Image 4-14

Yacine

But the power is not in the red paint. The power is in the belief, the grinding down of the brick, because as you're grinding it down you're putting it in there, you're putting your protection in there, and you're grinding and putting that energy there, and then as you move it around and sweep it around and pat it, you make it powerful.

Bonita

My grandfather was a brick-maker and so he would take me with him on jobs so I would know how to make mortar. We'd bring some red dust —that mortar dust— home and he would have red brick dust in his pocket.

Luisah

They say as a child I used to eat red brick dust. That's what scared my father about me.[126]

You know, Mississippi clay dirt is medicine when you pregnant. We used to feed women Mississippi clay dirt and I remember folks sendin' for dirt from Mississippi and eating starch until they got it.

I remember my Aunt Marybelle Reed, bless her heart. She was in that in-between place because she knows all this root stuff and she'd also gone to nursing school so she had a foot in both worlds. Aunt Marybelle Reed would send for Mississippi clay dirt. And she would put it on a cookie sheet and run it in a slow oven sumtin like 250 degrees. She would leave it in overnight, pull it out and pound it, and give pregnant women Mississippi clay dirt. For the mineral content.

Now you can go to the health food store and buy something they call Vanity Cleanse. You get this green French clay drink as a cleanser. It's the same thing. The mineral content. It's really something. The trick that gets played on the people is we get told that what our elders knew is inaccurate or even evil, and they steady stealin' it and then putting it through some other process where they then gotta go sell it back to us. That's what pisses me off. And the rhetoric undermines the confidence in the elder.

Inheritance

Luisah

One of the famous stories in my family is the one I always come to when I talk about missin' my grandmother.

My grandfather was a big Black man of Haitian extraction. They say Papa[127] got sick and they took him to a place where colored people were treated. Someplace in Slidell, but it wasn't no hospital in Slidell.

They tell me that the man in Slidell told Big Mama,[128] "Take this niggah home and build a pine box because he gonna die."

And the way the family story go, Big Mama opened the trunk in the bedroom and she took a comb

---

[126] Red brick dust is a component used in spirit work.

[127] Luisah's grandfather

[128] Luisah's grandmother

and bust her hair down into two braids. Then she put on a grey tan hide dress with fringe on it and picked up a medicine bag and started singing and went in the woods. She was gone for three days and three nights. She come back with a pouch full of green berries that she boiled up, boiled up several times, puttin' it aside and boilin' it some more in the morning. They said she fed Papa a fusion of that tea. The man got up and lived another 30 years. Outlived her. And when he died it was because he got hit by a car. So there.

Now, I wanna know what them berries were. I wanna know what songs did she sing when she went in the forest. I wanna know why she put her hair in two braids. You see what I'm sayin'? And I wish I had that dress. Now there's a piece of information that at this point all you can do is pray that one day somebody who knows it will lead me to it, cuz I ain't got no other description other than that it was some li'l green berries.

Bonita

You start thinking about who your mama is and who your mama's mama and your daddy and all them kinda things, you know that's a whole lot of people. People would ask me, "How did you learn to do this? How did you learn to do that?" I would say my grandparents taught me. I realized that the vastness of what our knowledge was and is, is just indescribable, and now a lot of it is lost.

Luisah

What you learn from your people, that's your inheritance. All of it! It's a shame to have inherited all of that and then to have a culture twist itself so that it's not possible to really know, appreciate, and pass on the value because it's not honored. It's up to us to make sure its passed down and honored.

At this time Yacine tells us lunch is ready to be served! We are ready to eat! She places in the center of the table a plethora of Halal cuisine that includes lamb ribs and chicken, an okra corn and tomato casserole, rice, cabbage and pasta salad. Luisah asks Eveline to lead the grace because she is the elder, but Eveline says to her and us all, "No I'm not, I'm gonna listen to you pray." And, Luisah graciously accepts the honor that has been passed to her.

Luisah

I want to take this moment to give thanks to Almighty God, to the Unity of the One, to the All That Is.

I want to give thanks to the power of the Heavens of the Sun and to the power of the Earth and the Rain which took these seeds and produced this food so that we might take it into our bodies and sustain our lives. I want to give thanks to the knowledge of our ancestors, the ones who came before us, who taught us the art of cooking so that we might put this gift together in a way that nourishes us.

I want to recognize the work of the people who harvested this, who brought it to market so that we might have it to nourish ourselves, and to give thanks to our parents for bringing us here, and to acknowledge that we are wise enough to be here together for this purpose today.

ASÉ

Imani Ajaniku (aka Ochunnike) - "From Cherokee to Geechee"

This narrative is from the words and experiences of Imani Ajaniku, aka Ochunnike. A priestess in the Lucumi and Voudoun religions, Imani also holds a Doctorate in Biblical Studies and a Master's Degree in Science, both from the Universal Life Church in Modesto, California.

I had the pleasure of meeting Imani in early 2008 through her sister and my dear friend, Dr. Sala Ajaniku, who lived in the apartment directly above mine in Oakland, CA.

Imani has chosen a life path that she's been endowed with since birth. She was fortunate to be raised in a family that nurtured her gifts, which in turn gave her the courage to become her destiny. Like Anita Poree, Imani was raised by parents from the South who migrated north for a better life. They brought their medicines and culture with them and made sure that Imani and her two older sisters would be molded by that magic. As a young woman, Imani searched for truth in spirituality and was faced with many more questions than answers. Eventually, her sojourn led her to the religions and medicines of her African ancestors.

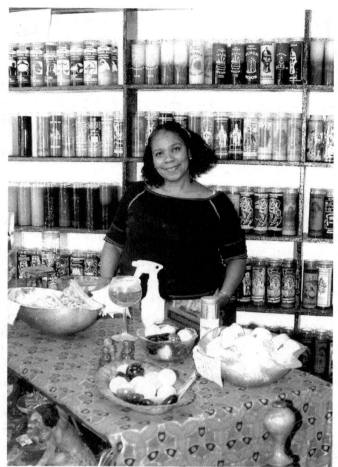

Imani Ajaniku in her Oakland, CA botanica
Image 4-15

In August of 1994, when it was really taboo, Imani became initiated into the religion Lucumi, which simply means "Friend." Lucumi was brought to Cuba by enslaved Africans determined to continue their faith by blending it with Catholicism. Three years later, in the spring of 1997, she became initiated in Voudoun in Haiti. It is in both of these religions, which have their roots in West African traditions, where Imani finds a connection and compatibility with her Southern lineage and the possibilities for infinite spiritual expansion.

Her journey is a testament that celebrates how she's woven together the early influences from her Eastern Cherokee and Southern African American roots with the religions of the African Diaspora. Imani Ajaniku, aka Priestess Ochunnike, has made it her life mission to help people lead spiritually full, physically healthy and balanced lives. Priestess Ochunnike has over one hundred Godchildren whom she has initiated into both Lucumi and Voudoun, and she continues to counsel and guide many of them.

From 1996 to 2008, she was owner and guardian of Botanica Ellegua located in the heart of East Oakland. During those years, Botanica Ellegua served the needs of the greater African Diasporic religious community in California and beyond, and of people of all backgrounds seeking guidance. It was in the perfect location in the heart of the East Oakland community, on the corner of 42nd Avenue and Foothill Boulevard.

East Oakland is a vibrant community full of life and a gumbo of cultures predominantly from Meso America, the African Diaspora, Asia and Polynesia. That area also boasts one of the largest American Indian populations in the country, with the Intertribal Friendship House located a couple of miles away.

Botanica Ellegua was one of the epicenters of the community that welcomed everyone of all faiths, *and tended to the spiritual and medicinal needs of the community and practitioners. People obtained their medicines, recipes and sought guidance through Diloggun consultations at Botanica Ellegua. Priestess Ochunnike cultivated an organic herb garden in the back of the Botanica so her medicines would be potent and truly come from the environment.*

Botancia Ellegua was a gathering place that celebrated, supported and preserved Lucumi and related traditions. Its doors were open to educate as well.

In this interview, Imani also speaks about the misinformation and misperceptions surrounding the religions from the African Diaspora. She also shows how they are just another way of honoring all life and praising the infinite power or state of being that Lucumi practitioners call "Oludumare."

Below is the fascinating and insightful interview with Imani Ajaniku conducted on August 15, 2008 in her Botanica Ellegua in Oakland. It is filled with terms and a vernacular that many are unfamiliar with so there is a glossary at the end of this chapter to help you reference any word you do not know. Sit back, read and enjoy.

Bloodlines: From Cherokee to Geechee

I refer to myself as a Native African American. My mom is Cherokee, from the Eastern Cherokee Nation, and my dad is Geechee.[129] His mother's father was from the Carolina Sea Islands. My father was very dark and mom was fair. Together they were a very striking couple. Up until the time my mom

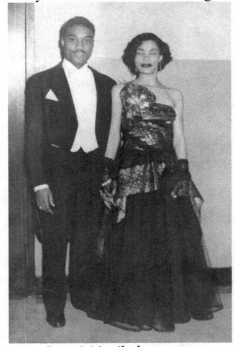

passed away, I thought of myself as Black. African American. I learned early that when I attempted to identify or include my Native roots, what I got back was, "You just don't want to be Black," so that didn't work for me either. When I got older, I was able to find out more about where I came from and now I claim my Native roots and I don't have anything to prove to anybody. I have the blood that runs through my veins, I know who I am, I know what I am, and that is really what is good enough for me.

I was born in New York, but we took regular trips to the South every summer until my Grandmom, my mom's mom, passed away in the 1950's. We simply called it going-down-South. The most vivid memory I have about being in the South is my grandfather going outside in the backyard, grabbing a chicken, wringing its neck, plucking it, and serving it for dinner. The other thing I remember is the dirt. It is very red, and it's very rich, and my mom used to eat it. Later in life, she would eat Argo Starch. I know there's definitely a correlation between eating the dirt and eating the starch.

Imani Ajaniku's parents
James Albert Hadden
and Cora Helen Smith-Hadden
(circa late 1950's to early 1960's)
Image 4-16

When we'd go down South, we'd stay near the Cherokee reservation in North Carolina. My mom used to tell us stories about her dad, my grandfather Joe Parker. After he passed, my mother's immediate family moved from North Carolina into South Carolina, mingled among the African Americans there, and really went forth as coloreds. It's a very common story. Mom would tell us how the kids would throw stones and sticks at them and call them "dirty reds" and "injuns." It was bad—very, very bad—and so painful to hear those stories.

---

[129] "Geechee" is a term used interchangeably with "Gullah" to refer to a group of people living along the southeastern Atlantic coast from Jacksonville, NC to Jacksonville, FL, taking in all of the Sea Islands and 35 miles inland to St. John's River. Here people from numerous African ethnic groups linked with indigenous Americans and created the unique Gullah language and traditions from which later came the term "Geechee."

When my mom passed, I was having such a hard time dealing with her transition. Aunt Millie taught me whenever I wanted to talk to my mom, just take a stick, pound it three times and call her name three times saying, "Corrie Helen. Corrie Helen. Corrie Helen. Mommy wake up. It's your daughter." Just call her three times and pound the stick three times and she would hear me. So that's what I would do. Later I learned that in Ifá, and Voudoun, we have an Egun (ancestor) stick, and we pound it on the ground and say, "Wake up, hear me, hear me, hear me" three times, when we want to talk to the ancestors. It's just like what Aunt Millie taught me. The Black American community and the African community have so many similarities in their spiritual traditions. They both have a strong belief in God and a reverence for our ancestors.

After my mom passed, we wanted to know more about our family, so we started tracing our lineage. That's what led me to the Cherokee reservation. It was in the early 1980s when that happened. I was 31 then. Going to Cherokee was a hard trip and a very beautiful trip.

Although I looked a lot like the people, the people knew I wasn't from there. I met a woman there named Bea who took a liking to me. She took me in and had a traditional sweat for me.

The next day, her daughter gave me a tour of Cherokee. It is very beautiful! Leading up to the reservation you can see the Smokey Mountains. As you get closer you start to see the trading posts, big headdresses made of feathers, hides, and a lot of stereotypes about what the eastern branch of Cherokee Indians look like.[130] I found it really insulting.

I learned a lot and experienced a lot on this trip. It was the first time I had a traditional sweat. I learned that to the Cherokee, bear and snake are two very important symbols which mean strength and luck. In the culture, every piece of the bear is used and all parts of the snake are used as well.

As for my father's people in South Carolina, my father was the eldest of nine children. His mom passed when he was very young and his Aunt Millie raised him. My youngest sister Millie is named after her. I don't know much about my dad's mom, but I was told that she had long black hair and spoke Spanish and Gullah.

Gullah/Geechee people speak so fast. When I was young I used to understand them and speak Gullah too. Geechee [Gullah] is a combination of a lot of different dialects. It was a language that they [Africans who were brought to the Sea Islands] created over time for survival and it's something to be proud of.

The Expanding Branch

I definitely feel that the ways and traditions of your parents and grandparents shape and form you to do what you are doing now and the life path you take. My mom shaped me to respect all life and everybody. When I was young, my mother didn't allow us to kill bugs. She would say, "That bug is just as important as you." Spiders were a definite no. We could not kill spiders, so I didn't grow up afraid of bugs.

When it would storm, my mother would line up my two older sisters and me (we were two years apart) at the foot of her bed and tell us to listen to the storms. These were terrible storms. Thunderstorms where the sky would get black and I wouldn't hear anything but thunder. Mom would turn off all the lights and we had to be still and be quiet and let it pass. It used to scare me. We had to stay away from the window because electrical storms would go through the house and find energy. We were fresh energy and energy finds energy! Mom never talked about God being angry or anything like that. I understand now that my mom was really attempting to teach us that if you're quiet long enough you could learn something, and you could hear something, and know that even Spirit moves on the wind. It was a valuable lesson.

When I was young girl, a woman would visit me at night dressed in white and would cover my feet. This happened often. I talked to my mom about it and she acted like it was very normal. When I got older, and expanded my search beyond Christianity, I realized that my visitor was a spirit or a guardian angel that came to watch over me.

---

[130] Imani relates that she saw this on billboards, wooden carved statues, and in pictures. She was referring to what are called the "Hollywood"-looking Indian people and not Native Americans who have any Black or African American physical features, and who fulfilled the stereotype of what we see on television projected by Hollywood.

My mom never made me feel self-conscious about seeing spirits so I never said anything about that until I started studying more about spirit and manifestations. And then when I was in college, for a period of six months on a regular basis I had dreams where I was dressed in white and I was speaking French. At the time, I didn't know what that was. Years later I found out it could have been Egun ("ancestor" in Ifá). So, it's not an accident that I am on this path and got initiated in Voudoun and Lucumi. These values are completely compatible with my upbringing. That is why I feel great about what I am doing.

Sound Remedies

We were pretty healthy kids growing up. We didn't get a lot of colds, infections or flus and I didn't go to a dentist until I was in junior high school. Once a week, every week, when we were young, my parents would line us up and we would have cod liver oil and castor oil together. It cleaned us out and we did not get sick when we were little. This went on until some time in junior high school. But every once in a while we would get a cold and Mom would do mustard rolls. She'd actually get the mustard seed and she would pound it and then mix it with some oil, I think talla or pig fat. She'd rub that on our chest and on our back and cover it with a piece of cloth for warmth.

No matter what was going on with us, my mom would mix raw egg and milk together and make us drink that. That was her thing, raw eggs and milk; her cure-all along with cod liver oil and castor oil once a week. And in the wintertime, she would just reach outside the window and get snow and add the snow to the egg and milk and put some sugar in it, and then we'd have ice cream.

Naked Mud Baby

When I was little, my family called me little naked mud baby because I would take off my clothes and play in the dirt naked and rub it all over my body. My mom had to put a rope on me—I had enough room to move —because I would take off my clothes and run up and down the street naked. My daddy would come home from work and I would say, "Hi daddy," and run up to him butt naked. So, I feel very comfortable in nature and I've felt that way since I was a child.

The earth means something to me. I like the way it smells. I can tell different kinds of soils. There's a fertile red soil, there's a fertile black soil, there's brown, there's sand, there's the soil that nothing grows in, and all of them have properties.

There's something we do in Lucumi that really shows this understanding. If someone has something they need to get rid of, like a bad thought, a memory, an illness or a growth, you take a cloth or a fruit and rub it on your body and then go bury it in some soil that is barren, because nothing grows there. I find this practice universal in some Native traditions such as with the Lakota and Cherokee and some different African traditions as well. In Christianity, it would be the same as saying, take your burdens to Jesus and lay all your problems down. The main intention is for you to take whatever you have that you don't want, give it to something else (such as the fruit or cloth) and then let it go.

Knowing and understanding soils is very, very helpful. If we need something to grow then we use fertile soil. I also learned that voice is important when doing this or anything. The power of our word means something. And when our words are combined with the words of our ancestors, saying the same prayers just makes that voice stronger. That's why it's really important to say what you mean and mean what you say. That is the oral tradition!

I know I come from a people who worked with the earth and were definitely at one with nature. As long as I can remember, I've always been in the earth. I ate it, I played in it, and I dug in it to plant seeds.

Some of my earliest memories are of the garden we had growing up in New York. Mom loved to grow pansies and potatoes and roses and tulips all together in our yard. Those were her favorite flowers. She had corn, string beans, collard greens, and kale, and there was a grape farm in the back of where we lived. We had our own seeds and we planted and we burrowed in the earth. To this day, I like to grow all my herbs and vegetables together.

I decided to study health in college because of my affinity for working with herbs and medicine from the earth. It's as natural to me as breathing. I received a Master's Degree in Science and a Ph.D. in Biblical Studies. I also studied Buddhism and African religions because I really love God. I wanted to know how people all over the world worked with the earth and healed themselves. I even made an herbal first aid kit for one of my final projects in college. I made tinctures, extracts, balms, put together teas, got into massage therapy and polarity. I wanted to understand the healing power of touch and the laying of hands. I was on this quest to know how the spiritual side really worked and how the theoretical side really worked and to put this expansive belief into some kind of formula.

The last 32 years of my life have been in pursuit of more knowledge about spirit, about healing and how that relates to me, how that relates to other people.

Ochunnike

This section is Imani's narrative about her path in the Ifá, Lucumi and Voudoun religions.

I am initiated into two religions, Lucumi[131] from Cuba and Voudoun from Haiti. These religions are very different than the mainstream religions in the United States. Unfortunately, everything that is a little bit different than Christianity gets lumped into something that is against God or against Christ. It can appear that these religions are going against the mainstream but they aren't because they are good and they are beautiful and they have integrity.

I've found that most religions from people of color around the

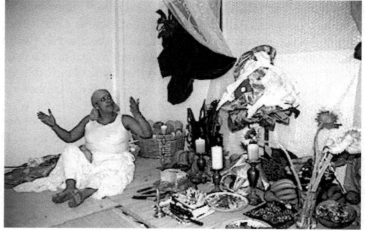

Imani Ajaniku in her altar room
Image 4-17

world have the same basic philosophy and respect for nature. There's the belief that everything is alive and everything has purpose from the tiniest insect to the largest, and that we need to leave the Earth better than we found it. I feel Lucumi and Voudoun are more encompassing of these ideals than Christianity.

Africans brought their belief in God with them during the slave trade, and then they were stripped of their humanity. Everything that they did that was African was forbidden. When you take away someone's belief in God then you reduce them to an "it." Then folks can justify treating "it" any way.

Africans are strong and very spiritual and they found a way to continue their beliefs and their religions took on different forms, usually mixed with Christianity.

In Voudoun and in Santería, for example, you will find a lot of pictures of Catholic saints. Africans believe that more is better and that is why they were able to accept the saints that the Spanish and French conquerors carried with them. They felt that if the Catholic saints made their conquerors so strong and magnificent, then it could also work just as well for the Haitians and Cubans.

In Voudoun they have their own saints, too, which they call Loas. In Lucumi, Santería, and Candomble they call them Orishas. Lucumi is just one branch of the religions that were brought over from Africa during the slave trade. It means "Friend."

I first got initiated into Lucumi here in Oakland in August of 1994 and not in Cuba because I didn't want to jump over all of my native ancestors and dishonor them. I walk on their graves everyday.

Lucumi is a religion that is based in Ifá, which is from the Yoruba region of West Africa in Nigeria. The belief is that with the advice of God—whom we call Oludumare—our ancestors, and the Orishas, we can build a good life and have good character. We don't have to do it all and figure everything out by ourselves because we have the advice of God, the different Orishas and also our ancestors to help us.

---

[131] Continue to use the glossary of terms at the end of this chapter to look up words you don't know. It will help you to really appreciate this section "Ochunnike" which bears the title of her initiated name.

For any situation, we can call on an Orisha and use their particular property of nature to aid us. For example, we may need to call on Oshún, who is fresh water and embodies the courage and determination of the river. We can't hold back the river. Or we could use the power of the wind, who we call Oya. Because we are a part of nature, we could use whatever property to help us to be better human beings and assist the world that we live in.

I didn't know Lucumi when I was a young woman living in New York. I was searching spiritually and my studies eventually led me to Voudoun, but back there it was called Voodoo. Voodoo didn't resonate with me so much because it seemed to be a practice of revenge. I can imagine in the course of history that desperate people do desperate things. So there was a time and a place for revenge, particularly during colonization and slavery. I also came across Wicca and kept searching until I finally found Voudoun and read *The Divine Horsemen*.[132] Shortly after that, I moved out here to Oakland and met Luisah Teish, who took me to my first Bembe almost forty years ago. Luisah was at one point a mentor and when Luisah and I met she hadn't become a priestess yet.

A Bembe is a celebration with drums and music and it's usually in honor of a particular aspect of an Orisha. The first time I went and heard the drum I knew this was what I had been searching for all my life and I didn't even know it. I wanted to take off my clothes and run right in. Since then I never looked back. Today I am a full time Madrina[133] and a servant of spirit. They work through me and it's wonderful. It's also very, very tough because I don't have my own life. I have over 70 godchildren that I baptized in Lucumi. Two have their crowns. And in Voudoun I have over 20 godchildren with different levels of initiation.

I went to Haiti to get initiated into Voudoun during the spring of 1997. What really struck me is that Haitian values are the same as mine. If somebody is hungry you feed him or her. If there is a little, everybody gets something. If someone is cold, you share what you have. If people come to my house, I offer them food and something to drink. These are values I learned from my parents.

In Haiti, everybody in the family root[134] worked to make sure people were taken care of. And it was the same way when I travelled to Senegal, Mali and in Gambia.

I was in Senegal the longest. There's no infrastructure in the smaller towns. There are no faucets. You have to go to the river and get your water and your fish. Everybody participated to make sure that the people ate and drank. Rice is the staple and for a meal, they make rice balls and eat fish and a green that is very similar to our collard greens. Everyone eats out of a central pot and they eat with their left hand. There is a lot of spiritual significance eating with the left hand. Everything good passes through the left. That's the receptive side. The right hand is used to wash the body.

The homeless people in Senegal are treated very different than the homeless in the United States. Many homeless in Senegal had leprosy, but they didn't leave home because they were kicked out or shunned by the family, they left because they did not want to inflict the illness on the other family members. People give them food and clothing and money willingly because they were all kin. It was really very beautiful the way the community looked after everyone. It's very different here in the United States.

Lucumi

Lucumi is one of the fastest growing religions in the United States. Lucumi came to the United States in 1957 through a man whose name is Eshu B. It was in Cuba that Eshu B. initiated the first Americans into the Lucumi religion, Oba Seijeman Adefunmi I and Obayalomi (Chris Orleando). That was in the 1950's. Today we have practitioners in the millions.

Adefunmi came back to the United States and bought some property deep in Gullah/Geechee country about a half-hour drive from the Atlantic coastline in the lower end of South Carolina and founded the Oyotunji African Village.[135]

---

[132] By Maya Deren. Originally published by Vanguard Press in 1953, it is still available for purchase as of the publication of this book. Deren also produced a companion movie by the same name.

[133] Godmother/sponsor of intitiates in Ifá, Santería, Voudoun and other African diasporic religions.

[134] "Root" in this instance means initiates in Voudoun and the extended family.

[135] Oyotunji means "rises again" and Oba means "King" in Yoruba which is both the name and the language of a

Chris Orleando, a well-known drummer, was Eshu B's other initiate. His Eju name is Obyalomi and he is with Chango.[136]

Power of Prayer

In Lucumi and Voudoun we have certain prayers called Moyuba that we say to honor our ancestors. We say Moyubas to honor ancestors connected by blood or ancestors who may be in our spiritual lineage but not connected by blood. These can be living elders, priests, medicine men and women, healers, folks who have walked the road of truth all over.

We start the Moyuba by calling out the ancestor's name. This is another way for us to call on the four directions, using our bodies and voice to get that unseen but felt support that we look for in our prayers.

A prayer is a statement that facilitates life on some level because there is no room for any other kind of prayer. So when those words come out, I know the ancestors are elevated and are there to help too. I strongly believe that everybody has a way to identify him or herself through language, movement and sound. When we mimic those movements we attract the same energy from generations on back. Whatever we do taps into that power. It's like having a posse that's not seen but felt.

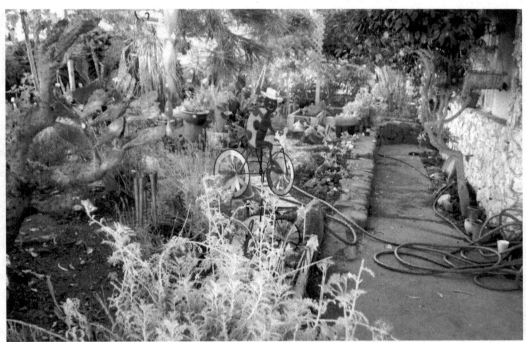

Medicinal and ceremonial plants in Imani Ajaniku's garden
Image 4-18

Holistic Wisdom for Spiritual Health

A lot of the medicines I have in the garden and in my store are used in particular ceremonies. We refer to them as Ashé's because they have certain powers. All of them are from Nigeria. They are all authentic.

---

distinct Nigerian tribe. Founded in the early 1970's, the Oyotunji Village is a product of the sixties' struggle for Black liberation and the growing Yoruba religious and cultural movement in New York. After the establishment of several temples in Harlem in the mid-sixties, the movement relocated to a rural setting near the town of Sheldon in Beaufort County, South Carolina, to continue its cultural development there. According to its founder, the Oyotunji Village quickly became "a place of rehabilitation for African Americans in search of their spiritual and cultural identity."

[136] Obyalomi was intitiated under the protection of the Orisha Chango, who is his primary Orisha. During inititation, a reading is done to determine "who owns your head," that is, which Orisha has claimed you.

Strong Medicines

Obi Kola

This is Obi Kola. It is used with Oya or Chango or given as food or nutrition.[137] The purpose of this medicine is to make the words that come out of our mouths stronger. It has to do with being successful. One of the attributes given to that divine infinite Voudoun Orisha we call Chango is success, and the power of our word helps us to achieve success.

Efun/Cascarilla

Efun is powdered snail shell and lime chalk. It comes from Nigeria. You can put this in a bath or put Efun directly on your body. It is believed that this is a medicine of good. You put it on your body just like baby powder to hold in the goodness so that anything that conflicts with that will be repelled. It's not poisonous. You can even use it on babies.

There is an American counterpart to Efun we call Cascarilla. It's made of powdered egg whites and eggshell in the United States, not the powdered snail shell and lime chalk that is Efun from Nigeria. You can really feel the spirit in both Efun and in Cascarilla. Some people say that Cascarilla is American Efun but it is not. Cascarilla has the same principal as Efun, but Efun is stronger. People use them interchangeably.

The Parable of Human Desires

Many people are bred to believe that White is better and that people of African descent were there to serve the Whites. It's not a matter of better, it's just different, and together we can really change this notion of horizontal prejudice, the skin prejudice, the language prejudice.

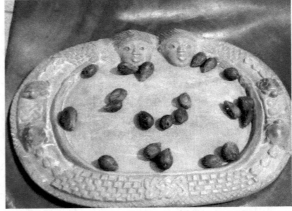

Obi kola nuts used in a divination tray
Image 4-19

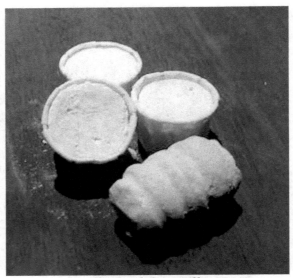

Efun and Cascarilla
Image 4-20

Description: Efun is the white colored snail shell shape in the foreground and cascarilla is the white chalk in the 3 cup-shaped containers

In Lucumi there is a parable that says it is a crime committed against the Gods to have prejudice. This story tells of a time when the Orishas were walking the Earth doing good deeds among the humans. One day, the humans told the Orishas that they wanted to be different. So the Orishas appealed to the highest in the pantheon, Oludumare, who is the deity of all the Orishas and humankind. Oludumare knew it would be disastrous to give the people what they want, but knew if he did, they would learn this to be true. So Oludumare told the people and the Orishas to meet him in the town square at a certain time.

When all the people got there, Oludumare threw out some palm nuts into the air and when they came down, they came down into the desires that people wanted. Some wanted to live on the water, some on land, some wanted straight hair, others curly hair; some wanted to be light skin, some dark skin, and the people wanted to speak in different languages. Oludumare gave the people their desires and they were

---

[137] The nut is often chewed.

all happy and satisfied.

A while later, however, the light people began to come together and began to dislike the ones who were different. That's when the wars started and the land stopped producing.

The youngest Orisha, Oshun, was very upset over all the misery the people caused themselves. So when everyone went to sleep, she assumed the form of a bird and flew up to the heavens into the clouds and went to Oludumare, and said, "You lied to me. Look down on earth, your people are suffering."

Oludumare looked out and saw what was going on and said, "Because you alone came to me and are telling the truth, I will always listen to you."

And for that reason, anytime something important happens and you need good advice, everybody visits their local river to talk to Oshun. She always speaks truth.

Diloggun Divination

The system of divination we use in Lucumi is with the cowrie shells. In Africa they use the sacred chain or Epele and palm nuts for divination. I use the sacred sixteen cowrie shells in my divination along with a lot of prayers and Obi's. The shells are prayed over and bond to a ceremony that makes them sacred and gives them the ability to talk. They are no longer just cowrie shells. They are referred to as Diloggun. It's very similar to what a priest may do when blessing something sacred. After we pray over the shells, we cast them in a form of a pattern that we call Odu.

The Odu is very similar to a parable from the Bible or ancient wisdom from an Asian saying. It's usually applicable to what's going on with that person. The magic comes in when the problem is stated and the recipe is given to restore the balance. When that advice is followed, the balance is restored in that person. That's the defining moment. We have free will to accept the advice or not. If the advice is to make a cake with special ingredients then you put it together, bake it, and you have your cake. You have your medicine and it works! It's really beautiful. I've witnessed this time and time again. Lucumi is as old as time.

Voodoo, Juju, Hoodoo, Misconceptions

There's a big difference between Voodoo in New Orleans and Voudoun, the religion that comes from Haiti.[138] In Voudoun the religion, they refer to their deities as Loa or Lwa, which means the law. Practitioners of hoodoo or voodoo do not call on the deities. They don't call on the divine, and that's the difference.

In Voudoun we say prayers that actually call on God. In Lucumi we have prayers that call on God. If you have something that goes against life, it's not of God. The misconception comes when people lump all of these religions from Africa together without even knowing what they actually are.

Juju is a spiritual practice where people can decide to make things happen in a good way or not, but it does not call in the divine. To me, if something goes against a life force, whether it's a person's life or an intent, it goes against God.

The origin of the Voodoo doll is from an Nkisi. An Nkisi is a figure from the Congo (Zaire) that represents a community. It's a human figure that has no gender because it represents the entire community.

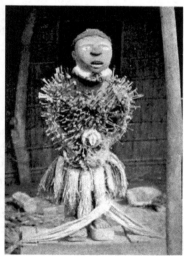

Nkisi from Zaire (Congo)
Image 4-21

Description: Nkisi with nails, cloth and other ceremonial accessories

---

[138] Enslaved Africans brought Voudoun to Haiti from Dahomey, which is located in West Africa.

Whenever there was a dispute among the community members they would go to the Oba, who was the king at the time, to settle the dispute. And when it was settled, the king then would take a piece of iron or a nail and hammer it into the doll to seal it, to give the agreement a seal of approval.

So the Nkisi was a public agreement for all to see and acted as a reminder of the intent of absolving the problem and honoring the settlement reached. Imagine Westerners and other outsiders coming to Africa and seeing all these Nkisis with these nails hammered into them. Westerners automatically said, "Aaaaaaahhhh, that's evil." But its completely opposite from what people imagine the voodoo doll to be. And that's the origin of the voodoo doll, not with intent to harm someone but to do good and restore balance to a community.

I'm over 60 now and realize that I'm at the point where we are getting to be our own elders. I'm closing the botanica and will continue my work from home. I'll do consultations there and grow my herbs in my garden. I don't want all that I've learned and have become to be hidden away in some room. Before I leave this planet, I am determined to document more of what I do, more of what we do in Lucumi and Voudoun and share it with the world. There are so many unheard voices that really contribute to our humanity and to our survival, across racial lines and across cultural lines. I'm honored and proud that mine is one of them.

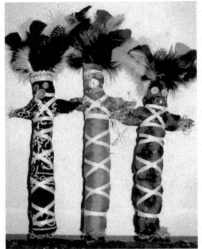

New Orleans Voodoo Dolls
Image 4-22

Description: Contemporary New Orleans-style voodoo dolls made with cloth, feathers, and buttons and bound with ribbons. The color of the dolls' cloth from left to right is black, lavender, and red. All dolls are bound with white ribbon and multicolored feathers top the crown. The interior of authentic voodoo dolls were made with Spanish moss and other roots. The dolls have more power when made by the person who wants to direct the intention and energy embodied in the doll. Using the ribbons to bind helps to secure the intention. Sticking colored straight pins in the doll and other embellishments (that may include personal effects such as hair, nails, or clothing) intensifies the affirmation for the desired outcome.

Botanica Ellegua

Before Priestess Ochunnike established Botanica Ellegua in 1996, the location operated as another Botanica under the guardianship of a Preistess from Puerto Rico named Rosa. I went to Rosa to get a reading at the Botanica right before my journey to North Carolina and the beginnings of my research for "Working The Roots: Over 400 years of Traditional African American Healing." *At the time of that reading with Rosa, I had no idea that I would return to 4212 Foothill Boulevard in Oakland twelve years later (July 2008) to interview Priestess Ochunnike, the last person I would include in* Working The Roots. *This serendipitous chain of events was affirmation that I had come full circle on a journey that is cosmically led by higher powers and our ancestors. I am so grateful and honored to be a constant witness of this.*

Live Healthy,
Michele Elizabeth Lee

PART II - THE AILMENTS AND MEDICINES

"My chil'ren, dey know when I was givin' dem dat same thang my mama and granma give me. I gives it to my chil'ren and I told dem what I was givin' 'em and what it was for and what dey had. My Uncle Red should have passed it on to Bobby [Red's oldest son] cuz he know. And den Bobby should have passed it on down to his chil'ren. It's got to be handed right on down through the generations in da family. So Red would have passed what he know on down to Bobby, and Annie [Bobby's mother] should know somthin' 'bout dat stuff by her mama and pass it on down to Bobby too. 'Bout all parents were dealin' wit some kind of herbs and stuff."

Pete Smith

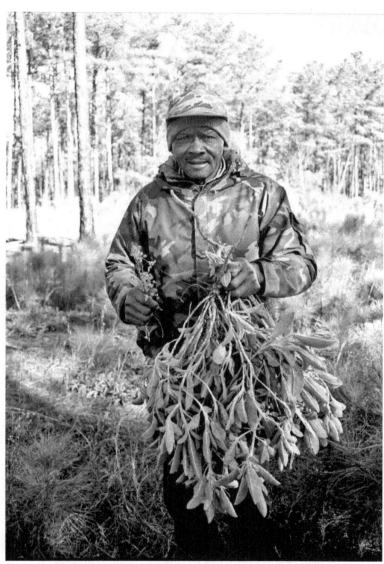

Mr. Pete with lion's tongue and rabbit tobacco
Image II-1

Traditional Healers

Imani Ajaniku: North Carolina, Georgia, New York, California
Yacine Bell-Bayaan: Mississippi, California
Ramona Moore Big Eagle: North Carolina, South Carolina
Irene Blackburn Lee-Ferguson: Mississippi
Eveline Elizabeth Prayo-Bernard: New Orleans, LA
Joanne Carol: South Carolina
Ms. Chavis: North Carolina
Marjorie Davis: North Carolina
Nora Lee Dockery: North Carolina
Ms. Ethel: Donaldsonville, LA
Levatus Guillory: Texas
Myrtle Harris: Florida
Ms. "Dot" Oscelena Harris: Georgia
JoeHayes: North Carolina
Opensanwo Ifakorade: Georgia, California
Ms. Jacobs: North Carolina
Sally McCloud: North Carolina
Eddie Nelson: North Carolina, South Carolina
Valena Noble: Louisiana
Hattie Hazel Clark-Pegues: North Carolina
Ruth Patterson: North Carolina
Anita Poree: Mississippi, Louisiana, California
Pete Smith: North Carolina
Mr. "Red" (Luther Stelly Smith): North Carolina
Ron Smith: Alabama
Luisah Teish: New Orleans, LA and California
Etta Williams: Texas
Ola B Hunter-Woods: Arkansas

Prescriptions for Healthy Living

Medicines, Ailments and their Remedies, and Hoodoo

The foundation of most traditional or folk healing is to stay healthy so you don't get sick and, if you do, to have the knowledge to heal oneself with natural medicines. Ever wonder why people took a spoonful of cod liver oil daily or weekly? Or castor oil at the first onset of a cold, or right before each season? How about sipping on herbal teas to "cleanse your blood," or taking a shot of apple cider vinegar to "cut the mucous," or drinking the "pot licker"[139] from a pot of greens? These were some of the preventive health routines used in African American healing traditions that kept the immune system strong and sickness at bay. In addition to sound preventive health routines, moving the body was and still is essential to good health.

If someone did get sick, there were natural medicines and remedies used to treat the ailment or ease the difficulty. Natural medicines and remedies came from all parts of plants, minerals, and animal by-products. Moving energy to heal with hands or massage and the power of affirmation, meditation, and prayer were used in the past and are still used today as a treatment for a number of ailments. Life challenges relating to relationships, emotions, health, money, court cases and other situations were often dealt with through the ancient wisdom of working the unseen natural forces such as rootworking or conjuring. These practices may also have been complemented with plant, mineral or animal medicines.

This section presents and categorizes into four chapters and two glossaries the healing information collected from the interviews and narratives in Part I and other interviews I conducted with healers over the course of 15 years.

Chapter 5: PREVENTIVE HEALTH CARE
    Routine health maintenance and seasonal tonics used.

Chapter 6: THE AILMENTS AND THEIR REMEDIES—TREATMENT OF AILMENTS
    An overview of several medicines in various forms that were used to prevent and treat many ailments. The information in this section is alphabetized by ailment.

Chapter 7: ANIMAL CARE
    Specific treatments for a few animal ailments.

Chapter 8: THE MEDICINES
    Lists and describes natural medicines commonly used in African American healing traditions derived from plants (roots, herb, bark, stem, berries/fruit), minerals and animal medicines (such as spider webs!). In this alphabetized section you'll find the alternative names, health benefits, and how the medicines were prepared and applied.

Chapter 9: WORKING THE POWERS: CONJURIN' AND HOODOO REMEDIES
    Several spiritually-based wellness practices are explained.

GLOSSARY Of CULTURAL TERMS
    You'll find the meanings and significance of several cultural terms such as *Ashe*, *Egun*, *gooferdust*, and *juju*.

GLOSSARY Of MEDICINAL PROPERTIES
    Definitions of *antioxidant*, *cathartic*, and many other curative properties are provided.

---

[139] The liquid left over after the cooked vegetable has been removed.

As you review the two chapters dedicated to general health care and the treatment of specific ailments ("Preventive Health Care" Chapter 5 and "The Ailments And Their Remedies" Chapter 6), you may want to refer often to Chapter 8, "The Medicines," which provides a summary of the healing properties of each medicine, health benefits, and how they were prepared and applied in African American healing. The medicinal properties information may explain why some of these "old timey" remedies actually worked.

Some natural medicines in Part II were not used in African American healing traditions (to my knowledge) but are medicines that are currently incorporated into healing practices from healers I interviewed in the "Coming Full Circle" section in the narratives of Part I. These natural medicines have been used for thousands of years in older healing traditions (such as Chinese and Ayurvedic) to prevent and treat certain chronic ailments. I have noted in the text where any such medicines are part of contemporary, but not traditional, African American use.

Today, many people are returning to the healing and health maintenance traditions of their ancestors or complementing modern Western medicine with those traditions.

I hope you find this section useful on your path to remembering the healthy living practices of your ancestors.

To Your Health
Michele Elizabeth Lee

A Precautionary Note on Self-Treating, Recommended Dosages, and Regimens

Today, like our ancestors did in the past, it is popular to self-treat or use alternative and complementary medicine treatments along with conventional treatment. If one is already taking conventional medicine for ailments, natural medicines may pose a serious contraindication to the conventional regimen. It is best that any treatment of self care be done under the advice of a health care professional.

The medicines listed in this section contain suggested dosages and regimens based on information provided from natural healers who self-treated. *They are not intended to treat, diagnose. or prescribe, and are presented for educational purposes only.*

There may not be a generic dosage or regimen that fits all bodies, health conditions, and/or treatment for a particular ailment. It is best for anyone taking natural medicines and/or self treating to be in tune with their own body, to have some knowledge of the ailment being treated, and to pay particular attention to how the body responds to suggested treatments.

Until one is familiar with the effects of a particular medicine, it is best to start off with the lowest recommended dose, working the way up to the larger recommended dosage if needed, while continuing to check on both the positive and negative effects on one's body.

Special attention should be paid to any side effects while taking any self-treated medicine, such as headaches, diarrhea, upset stomach, vomiting, or similar conditions. If such conditions occur, one should discontinue use of medication or treatment and contact a health care professional. In some cases, reducing the dosage of medicine may eliminate the side-effects or a possible cause may be an allergic reaction.

Chapter 5 - Preventive Health Care

"Clean and purify your system every spring, and then in the fall, right before winter..."

Author unknown

General Health Maintenance

"We got a cleansing every spring and reinforcing every winter. We all had to line up and drink cod liver oil and castor oil while it was foaming. Every spring and every fall we would take this elixir and it would foam up. It was ugly, it would make you want to gag, but you had to line up and take it in a spoon. I think they put sulfur and honey and something else in it too." Author unknown

IMPORTANT: Before taking any of these medications, you should consult the "Precautionary Note On Self-Treating, Recommended Dosages, and Regimens" at the beginning of Section II.

Apple Cider Vinegar (ACV)

Medicinal properties

antibacterial, antibiotic, antiseptic, anti-inflammatory, prevents indigestion, reduces mucous and sinus congestion, assists with sinus drainage

Health benefits

Before the days of natural food and health stores, people used to make their own apple cider vinegar (ACV). [140] ACV is a potent healing agent when it is raw, unpasteurized, unfiltered, and contains the "mother," the ball of living enzymes and nutrients in the ACV that makes it an active healing medicine.

Southerners often add ACV as a flavor to their collard greens and then drink the pot liquor, which is very nutritious and full of all the ACV benefits. Some folks even drink a shot glass of ACV to "cut the mucous" build-up in their body.

Adding ACV to your diet makes the body pH more alkaline, which helps the body prevent and fight off sickness. ACV is high in acetic acid, which can help our bodies absorb minerals from the various foods we eat. ACV may lower glucose levels, cholesterol levels, and blood pressure, thus helping prevent and treat chronic health diseases like diabetes, high blood pressure, and heart disease.

People have also used ACV to assist with weight loss, reduce nighttime leg cramps, combat body fatigue, provide sore throat relief, relieve achy joints due to arthritis and rheumatism, and treat gout, as well as to boost immunity so the body can fend off colds and flu. ACV provides calcium, phosphorus, magnesium, copper, iron and potassium.

Preparation and application – Dosage used for Prevention

Take 2 tablespoons of ACV in four ounces of warm water or juice, once per day. Add honey to sweeten.

Add 2 or more teaspoons of ACV to your greens during the last 10 minutes of cooking.

(See Chapter 6 "The Ailments And Their Remedies" for specific ailments that have been treated with apple cider vinegar.)

---

[140] Use raw apple cider vinegar that contains "the mother," the tiny, web-like ball of living enzymes and nutrients in unpasteurized, unfiltered ACV that makes this liquid an active healing agent.

Castor Oil

More than just a "nasty tasting" medicine and purgative

During our grandparents' generation and for generations before them, castor oil was a staple in every Southern person's medicine cabinet. It was usually administered at the onset of a cold or flu, as a seasonal purgative, or given at the beginning of winter to build up one's immunity.

Medicinal properties

analgesic, antifungal, anti-inflammatory, antiviral

Health benefits

Castor oil has been used since ancient times to cure a wide range of diseases and to boost immunity by increasing lymphocytes, the white blood cells that fight disease, colds, flu, and infection. Castor oil's purging effects cleanse and remove parasites from the body. Castor oil is rich in ricinoleic acid, which inhibits the growth of numerous species of bacteria, viruses, molds, fungus, and yeasts. When rubbed into the skin, castor oil penetrates deeper than any other essential plant oil. Castor oil packs have been used externally to relieve pain, reduce inflammation, reduce fever, detoxify the body, and boost lymphatic circulation.

Preparation and application – Dosage for Prevention

At the start of each season: 1 tablespoon of castor oil to detoxify the system, clean bowels, and strengthen immunity. (See Chapter 6 "The Ailments And Their Remedies" for specific ailments that may be treated with
castor oil.)

Castor oil was also used in the treatment of the following ailments:

External

arthritis and other aches and pains, boils (skin), cysts, fever, hemorrohoids, lymphatic congestion, respiratory ailments, skin conditions

Internal

colds and flu, colic, constipation, fever, hemorrhoids, intestinal worms, respiratory ailments

Clay/Chalk/Bentonite

Red or White
(Ingested and used as a poultice and salve)

Scientific name

Phyllosilicate

Also known as

dirt, kaolin clay (kaopectate), Mississippi Mud

Medicinal properties

absorption of toxins and heavy metals, antibiotic, anticarcinogenic, antidiarrheal, anti-inflammatory, antimicrobial, antiseptic, detoxifier, emollient (softener), refrigerant (cools body), provides trace minerals

Health benefits

Clay/chalk has been used internally and externally as a healing medicine for thousands of years in many healing traditions. Its use in African American medicine can be traced back directly to Africa and its origins as a medicine in Native American healing has been used for centuries.

Clay is a powerful detoxifier that absorbs certain heavy metals and toxins, which are then eliminated along with the clay during a bowel movement. As a result, ingesting clay promotes healthier digestion of food and drink and bowel regulation. Chalk or clay was also eaten to treat diarrhea, and the pharmaceutical kaopectate derives its name from the kaolinite found in clay.

Clay/chalk was also used externally as a pack or poultice to reduce inflammation and pain due to arthritis, rheumatism, muscle strains, sprains, to treat itches, rashes, skin irritations, burns, acne, chicken pox, to heal cuts, and to draw out infection. In addition, pregnant women often have the urge to eat red and white clay, which provides the body with needed minerals such as calcium, iron, sodium, phosphorus, copper, magnesium and zinc.

As African Americans moved from the South to the urban North for a better life, many women replaced eating clay with eating 'Argo' starch. Eating starch did not have the same benefits as eating clay, and ingesting large amounts blocked the body's absorption of iron leading to anemia and other problems.

Preparation and application

Eating/Ingestion

A safe location for eating clay or chalk was known by people in the community. Some people would bake clay paddies the size of small cookies and others would eat directly from the source.[141]

Today, most people buy ingestible clay (which is a liquid paste) from their natural medicine store in the form of bentonite, which is also used in many colon cleanser treatments. Directions range from taking 1 tablespoon daily on an empty stomach with a full glass of water for no more than 3 days to taking 1 tablespoon 3 times per day, also for no more than 3 days.

Externally as a pack or poultice

The moist clay was applied directly to the affected area and allowed to dry or wrapped with cheesecloth or cotton cloth.[142]

Bath

1/2 to 1 cup of clay was added to a bath or soak to treat muscle strains, pains and inflammation. Epsom salt may have also been added.

Toothpaste

White clay was used as toothpaste to keep teeth clean and help treat gum disease and inflammation.

Cod Liver Oil

The Superfood!

"Every week, when we were young, my parents would line us up and we would have cod liver oil and castor oil together, once a week. It cleaned us out and we did not get sick when we were little. This went on until some time in junior high school." Imani Ajaniku

"We took cod liver oil for maintenance and lubrication of the system but it was also brain food." Bonita Sizemore

Medicinal properties

anti-inflammatory, immune booster, protects joints

---

[141] CAUTION: Avoid eating clay or chalk found in nature because of the widespread pollution from use of pesticides, herbicides, fertilizers, and chemicals from factories and plants that find their way into groundwater, rivers, streams and the soil.

[142] CAUTION: If you are using a clay poultice today, purchase the appropriate white or red clay in a powder form from a trusted source and use as directed.

Cod Liver Oil (continued)

Health benefits

Many folks remember their parents lining them up as kids to take a spoonful of cod liver oil before heading out for school or play. Few knew exactly why and what the cod liver oil did for their health. They only knew it tasted awful.

Taking regular doses of cod liver oil was and still is today a health maintenance routine that strengthens your body's immunity and may help prevent you from getting colds, flu, and chronic illnesses like heart disease, diabetes, arthritis, mental illness, certain types of cancers, and Alzheimer's.

Cod liver oil contains omega-3 fatty acids, essential for human health but the body cannot produce. You have to get omega-3's through foods like salmon, cod, tuna, halibut, algae, herring, sardines, and tuna. Unlike other fish oils and flax oil, cod liver oil also contains Vitamin D and Vitamin A. Vitamin D is necessary to maintain strong teeth and bones, keep your immune system functioning properly, stabilize your blood sugar levels, and prevent certain types of cancers. Vitamin D deficiency may be linked to the childhood epidemics of autism, asthma, diabetes, and Alzheimer's. Vitamin A is necessary to maintain vision, healthy skin and the lining of your intestinal tract. Other foods that have high levels of omega-3s are: walnuts, tofu, flaxseeds, cloves, soybeans, kale, cauliflower, collards, and winter squash.

For more information about how cod liver oil was used to treat some of the specific ailments listed above, refer to Chapter 6.

Preparation and application - Dosage for prevention and health maintenance

A routine dose of cod liver oil in African American healing traditions ranged from 1 tablespoon 1 time per week to 1 teaspoon daily. Today's daily supplement recommendation is 600 to 1,000 mg daily, which is roughly equivalent to the traditional African American dosage.

Notes and Precautions

High doses of omega-3 fatty acids may increase the risk of bleeding. Omega-3 fatty acids should be used cautiously by people who bruise easily, have a bleeding disorder, or take blood thinning medications such as aspirin.

Epsom Salt – Magnesium Sulfate

Magnesium sulfate, better known as Epsom salt, is another multi-purpose medicine that most Southern folks would have in their home. Epsom salt soaks and tonics were used to relieve aches and pains, reduce blood pressure, prevent strokes, reduce artery hardening, treat constipation, relax the nerves, reduce swelling, kill fungus and bacteria (such as athlete's foot), promote wound healing, prevent infection, increase magnesium levels, and pull toxins from the body.

Epsom salt is not a salt. It's a mineral compound of magnesium and sulfate that got its name from a bitter spring at Epsom that is located in Surrey, England. Magnesium is one of the most important of the essential minerals our body needs to function properly and is responsible for over 350 chemical processes. A bath with 2 cups of Epsom salt puts magnesium back in our bodies.

Medicinal properties

anti-inflammatory, antiseptic, nerve tonic, sedative

Preparation and application

* 2 cups of Epsom salt used in a bath and for a foot soak, 1/2 cup to one pan of water. Soaks usually lasted for 15 to 20 minutes.
* As a temporary laxative, 2 to 4 teaspoons of Epsom salt were mixed in one cup of water and drunk. Elimination usually occurred within 30 minutes to an hour. If not, another dose was taken in 4 to 6 hours.

*   As an anti-stroke or heart disease tonic, 1 teaspoon of Epsom salt was mixed in 1 cup of water and drunk three times per week.

Lemon

Lemon has been used for centuries for it's medicinal properties to help maintain good health and prevent illness, infection, and chronic disease. In African American healing traditions, lemon medicine was used to flush out toxins and bacteria from the body, as an internal and topical antiseptic, astringent, fever reducer, diuretic, anti-inflammatory agent, and to help promote weight loss. Taking lemon medicine was as simple as drinking lemon tea, making lemonade, or adding it to foods.

Lemons are nutrient-rich and acidic but they are alkaline-forming when they come in contact with body fluids and help the body maintain a healthy pH level. Adding 1/4 to 1/2 of a lemon to your daily diet may be an effective solution to maintaining good health.

Pot Licker or Liquor
from collards and other greens

African Americans have been drinking nutrient dense pot licker for centuries. In fact, it is one of the reasons why we endured and persevered through colonization and slavery. Pot licker or liquor is the broth that's left after cooking a big pot of greens. The collard plant itself is very resilient and hardy, consequently, the greens can be tough. During slavery, African Americans cooked the greens down and seasoned them with fat back or ham hocks. Most of the nutrition in the greens was cooked out and is then contained in the broth, the liquor. The pot licker left from a pot of cooked collards contains the following: Vitamins A, C, D, E, K, B-6, folate, niacin, riboflavin, thiamin; and the following minerals: potassium, magnesium, iron, calcium, phosphorus, sodium and zinc.

Sage Bush

Burn dried sage (smudge) to purify the air and get rid of harmful bacteria and energies in your home and environment. A tea made from sage bush can be drunk year round to boost immunity and for mental stamina.

Seasonal Teas And Tonics

Tonics boosted immunity and were antiviral, antifungal, and antibacterial. Oftentimes teas were made by harvesting the herb or root and letting them dry in a safe place. The dried herb or root was placed in a mason jar, filling up about 1/4 of the jar and then filling up the jar with luke warm water. The medicine was placed in a cool, dry place or in the refrigerator and sipped on a couple times a day for several days or throughout the entire season. Teas were also prepared in the standard manner of 1 to 2 teaspoons of dried herb or 3 to 4 teaspoons of the fresh herb to 1 cup of hot water. Cover and steep for 10 to 15 minutes for herb material that is not hard, 20 minutes for berries or bark, 25 to 30 minutes for roots.

Fall-Winter

Single herbs such as catnip, mullein, peppergrass, rabbit tobacco, sarsaparilla, and yellow root were gathered and prepared as a tea. Two or more of these herbs may have been combined. Other healing herbs, such as pine needles or peppermint, may have been mixed in. Three or more cups were drunk daily during this season.

Acifidity, Astifidity, Astifis, Asifidity, Asafoetida

"Another thing we had was asfidity. Mama buy that in the store. You can buy it today but it says on the thang that it's not good for internal, but I actually eat it. Mama just put that in a little rag and put it on a string and throw it around our neck. We had to wear that to keep from catchin' colds and germs. We wore that to school even though it stunk." Levatus Gillory

Acifidity was a bag of the herb asafoetida that children wore around their necks to ward off illness and disease. The herbs were sometimes made into a healing tea by putting in hot water, covering and steeping for the standard time of 10 to 15 minutes, and drinking.

Fire Cider Tonic

Mix equal parts of chopped garlic cloves, ginger root, onion, dashes of cayenne pepper, and horseradish for congestion. Put ingredients in a mason jar and fill with organic raw apple cider vinegar (ACV) containing "the mother," the tiny, web-like ball of living enzymes and nutrients in raw, unpasteurized, unfiltered ACV that makes this liquid an active healing agent. Shake vigorously. Place jar in a paper bag and put in a cool dark cabinet for 2 to 3 weeks. Shake once or twice daily. After two weeks, strain into a clean jar and store in a cool cabinet or refrigerator. Optional additions: lemon and honey.

Using as a preventative

Take 1 to 2 tablespoons 2 times a day mixed in warm water or juice as a preventative for one week.

At onset of cold or flu

Take the preventive dosage 3 times a day for 3 to 5 days.

Elderberry root mixed with Life-Everlasting Tea

Mix 1 to 2 teaspoons of equal parts of dried elderberry root and Life-Everlasting tea in 1 cup of hot water. Cover and steep for 10 to 15 minutes. Drink 3 or more cups daily.

Upper Respiratory Tonic

Mix equal parts of rabbit tobacco, pinetop, mullein, and horehound tea together and slow boil in covered pot for 30 minutes. Let cool down in pot and drink. Pour elixir in a jar and sip on throughout the winter. Can mix with honey and make a cough syrup.

Sarsaparilla and Catnip Tea

"Growin' up we would take sarsaparilla tea, catnip tea. It grew wild out there in the woods. That sarsaparilla, it was a vine. We would pick it and hang it up and then dry it for the winter time. And when we get a cold or we wanted somethin', some kind of tea, we go out there in the barn and get the tea and drink it. It keep you goin' and get the colds outta ya or stopped it from comin'. But we really didn't get no colds." Ms. Etta Minor-Williams

Mix 1 to 2 teaspoons of equal parts of sarsaparilla and catnip tea in 1 cup of hot water. Cover and steep for 10 to 15 minutes. Drink 1 to 3 times daily until cold is gone.

Mr. Red's Yellow Root Winter Tonic
(to cleanse blood and strengthen immune system)

* Clean the root and you can let it dry or use it immediately.
* Chop the stems and root and put 1/4 to 1/2 cup in a mason jar.
* Pour cold water over the yellow root to cover it one inch.
* Pour lukewarm water to the top and let sit until the water turns yellow. Sip on it twice daily.
* Refrigerate or leave in a cool dry place.

Spring

Sassafras Tea

"Sassafras, drink it in the spring. We use the red, not the white, the white will run you blind. We would dig it up in the end of October or November, when the leaves started falling and we would make a tonic for winter." Mrs. Patterson

Recipe

Dig up the root, wash and let dry for 3 to 5 days. Cut the root into small narrow pieces, approximately 2" long and 1/4" wide. Place approximately 1/4 to 1/2 cup in a pot with 1 quart of water. Bring to boil and let simmer for 15 to 20 minutes. Strain the tea, removing all roots, and pour into a glass container with an air-tight lid. Sweeten with honey and drink 1 cup a day as a tonic for 1 week.[143]

---

[143] An important warning note about sassafras and safrole: Sassafras contains safrole, which is known to have harmful effects if ingested over a period of time in large and concentrated quantities. See warning and instructions in the Sassafras section on pages 319-320 before using.

Chapter 6 – The Ailments And Their Remedies

Treatment Of Ailments

Notes to help the reader use this resource

1. Refer to the "Standard Medicine Preparations" section below to review and understand how the medicines may have been prepared and applied as a tea, poultice, tincture, pack, syrup, powder, wash, bath, or salve.
2. As you read through this chapter, "The Ailments And Their Remedies," you may wonder how certain medicines were prepared. Chapter 8, "The Medicines," offers insight into each medicine's healing properties and how that particular natural medicine or medicines may have been prepared to use as a treatment or mixed with other natural medicines.
3. Remedies, recipes, and their directions are written in both present and past tense. Their inclusion is not a validation for their effectiveness or an encouragement for the reader to follow.

IMPORTANT: Before taking any of these medications, you should consult the "Precautionary Note On Self-Treating, Recommended Dosages, and Regimens" at the beginning of Section II.

Standard Medicine Preparations

Most natural medicines (from plant, mineral and animals) were made into a tea, poultice, salve, powder or soak. Below are standard recipes that can be applied when using traditional medicine for healing.

Internal Preparations

Teas – Hot Infusion

Pour boiled water over an herb or mixture of herbs and let this steep while covered. It is best to use leaves, flowers, and green stems for infusions. For harder herbal matter like seeds, barks, or roots, it is best to use a decoction method of preparation (see *Tea — Decoction* in this section below). However, if you are using harder material in an infusion it is best to powder, grind, or bruise the material so that the medicinal properties are more accessible in the infusion. Keeping the tea infusion covered while steeping will keep medicinal volatile oils from evaporating, so that you benefit more from your tea. General medicinal dosage requires drinking 1 to 3 cups of tea each day. If storing larger quantities of brewed tea, keep covered and cool, and drink within 3 days. Some herbs require a different ratio of herb to water, and the directions below are just a general guideline.

Directions:
1. 1 to 2 tsp of dried herb for every 1 cup water
2. 3 to 4 teaspoons of fresh herb to 1 cup water
3. For larger quantities: 1 oz dried herb for 1 pt of water
4. Pour boiling or hot water over herbs
5. Cover and steep 10 to 15 minutes
6. Strain and serve

Teas – Cold Infusion

Some herbs' medicinal qualities are deactivated by heat from boiled water. In that case, it's best to make an alcohol extraction like a tincture, but you can also do a cold water extraction or infusion.

Follow the directions and ratios for a Hot Infusion above, but use cold water. Cover your tea and let sit for 6 to 12 hours before drinking. Can be left to steep in the sunlight to create sun tea, or in the moonlight to create moon tea.

Standard Medicine Preparations—Internal Preparations (continued)

Teas – Decoction

When making tea with any herbal material that is hard and woody, the herbs should be prepared as a decoction. Seeds, nuts, bark, roots, some berries, and woody stems need to be simmered, or decocted, in order to extract the medicinal qualities. If you are brewing a mixture of herbs and some are more delicate (like leaves or flowers) then add these to the tea water to steep only after the heat has been turned off.

Directions:
1.   Use the same ratios of herb to water as in an infusion.
2.   Cut or break herbs into small pieces.
3.   Place in non-aluminum saucepan and pour cold water over.
4.   Simmer for 20 to 30 minutes.
5.   Remove from heat.
6.   For any herbal material that includes roots, cover and steep for 25 to 30 minutes. If hard and woody material contains no roots, cover and steep for 20 minutes.
7.   Strain herbs and serve.

Powders

To make a powder of any herb or root, use plant material that is completely dry. Blend or grind in a coffee grinder, blender, or food processor until fine.

Capsules: If you would like to take the powder in capsule form, purchase empty capsules and fill with the powder.

Syrups

*   Prepare an infusion or decoction of the desired herbs and strain well. (You may desire to increase amount of herb used, and steep infusions longer or simmer decoctions longer in order to increase potency of your syrup.)
*   Pour an amount of honey or sugar equal to the volume of the infusion or decoction. (For 2 cups infusion, add 2 cups sugar.)
*   Warm on low heat and stir until sugar or honey is dissolved and the mixture becomes thick and syrupy.
*   Remove from heat, and let cool.
*   Store in sterilized containers with sealed lids in a cool place.
*   Watch for any spoiling or fermentation, and be aware that fermented syrups can cause jars to explode.

Tinctures

Herbal tinctures are very concentrated medicine with high potency. Alcohol or glycerine based tinctures are the two types made most often. Everclear is a popular alcohol used for tinctures. Glycerine tinctures are naturally sweet and better for children and anyone who wants alcohol-free medicine.

Alcohol: Fill a clean mason jar 1/3 to 1/2 full with the dried herb. Pour pure grain alcohol (80 proof or more) over the herbs, filling the jar to 1/4 inch before the top and close the jar tightly. Store in a cool, dry place for 3 to 8 weeks, shaking the jar daily. Optional: place jar in a paper bag. Strain the liquid through cheesecloth and store in a glass jar or colored or clear dropper bottle. Label and store in a cool dry cabinet.

Glycerine: Fill a clean mason jar 1/3 to 1/2 full with dried herb. Moisten or saturate herb with hot water, making sure minimal water accumulates in the jar. Fill the rest of the jar with vegetable glycerine and close the jar tightly. Put the jar in a crockpot, putting a towel underneath the jar first so it does not break. Fill the crockpot with water to right below the top of the jar so water cannot seep into the jar. Cover the crockpot with a towel and cook on the lowest setting for 3 days. Add water as necessary. After 3 days, strain the liquid into a clean glass jar or dropper. Label and store in a cool dry cabinet.

Standard dosage for tincture is 1/2 to 1 teaspoon 3 times daily, or 1 dropper full 3 times daily.

General instructions for steeping

* If drinking a tea for pleasure only, such as green or black or mint tea, cover and steep tea bag in hot water for 3 minutes, squeeze the excess out of the tea bag into the cup of tea, and drink. The teabag can be used as often as it retains its potency and flavor.
* If drinking for medicinal purposes, for most herbs, put in hot water, cover and steep for 10 to 15 minutes. For slightly harder matter such as berries, seeds,[144] or bark, cover and steep in hot water for a slightly longer time, 20 minutes. For roots, cover and steep in hot water for 25 to 30 minutes.
* Watch for any spoiling or fermentation, and be aware that fermented syrups can cause jars to explode.

External Preparations

Baths

Add 2 T to 2 cups of herb(s) to a bath by tying up in a muslin, double-layered cheesecloth, or thin cloth. Relax and breathe deeply.

Compresses

Soak a clean cloth or washcloth in a hot infusion or decoction. Wring out the cloth and place on affected area.

Creams or lotions

Creams are made by blending or emulsifying an oil or fat with water. There are many ways to prepare creams or lotions. Below is a general recipe.

Directions:
* Prepare an infusion or decoction of herbs. If desired, distilled water can be substituted for the herbs.
* Place 1 cup oil in saucepan on low heat, or in double boiler. (Use any high quality oils like olive, almond, coconut, or grapeseed. You can also make and use an oil infused with herbs to increase the medicinal value of your cream.)
* Add 1 ounce beeswax. Stir until beeswax is melted into oil.
* Pour mixture into blender and let cool for 2 to 5 minutes.
* Start blender on low speed and add 6 tablespoons of your infusion or decoction or distilled water.
* Optional: Add essential oils for fragrance, added medicinal value, and to help preserve.
* Pour mixture into jars and let cool.
* Apply topically to affected skin areas.

Gargles, mouthwash, or wash

Prepare the herb as an infusion or decoction. Pour into sterilized jar and store in cool place or in refrigerator.

Poultices

A poultice is a mixture of solid plant material applied directly to the skin to relieve nerve or muscle pain, sprains, and to draw pus out of the skin. Depending on the type of herbs used, you can either crush and mash the plant material into a pulp, steep herbs in a small amount of hot water (making sure to cover while steeping), or simmer them for 2 minutes. To apply, place the herb material directly on affected area and tape a bandage over to hold it in place. Alternatively, you can place the herbs in a piece of cloth, or even a sock, to hold them in place over the affected area. Another very simple method is to soak a tea bag of the desired herbs and hold the tea bag over the affected area.

---

[144] Seeds are usually crushed slightly before steeping to release the medicine within them. However, instructions for preparing seeds may vary within the various medicines and remedies.

Standard Medicine Preparations—External Preparations (continued)

Salves or ointments

1. Collect 1 to 2 ounces of dried herb(s), 1 cup & 1 to 2 tbs of fixed oil (olive oil, sesame oil, almond oil, coconut oil), and approximately 1 ounce shaved beeswax. (If making a larger quantity, keep the same ratios: 1 to 2 oz herb, 1 cup oil, 1 oz beeswax.) (***Warning!*** This recipe calls for baking the beeswax in a bowl or pot. This will cause a residue of beeswax to be left in the cooking vessel, which is almost impossible to clean entirely off. Keep this in mind when choosing the bowl or pot to cook this recipe in.)
2. Mix oil and herbs in an oven-safe container
3. Place container in oven at lowest temperature (between 100 to 140°)
4. Leave oven door ajar to keep temperature down
5. "Bake" for 3 to 5 hours, checking temperature and stirring periodically
6. Line a strainer with muslin, cheesecloth or a thin, old cotton T-shirt. Place strainer over a heat-safe bowl or pot.
7. Remove mixture from oven and pour into lined strainer to separate herbs from infused oil. Let this sit until well-drained and press the remaining oil out if you want to.
8. Measure the amount of oil in the bowl or guess the approximate volume. Should be around 1 cup.
9. Place bowl or pot either over flame on the stove or over a double boiler on low heat. Add shaved beeswax and mix until fully melted.
10. Place metal spoon in mixture and then place spoon in freezer. This sample will cool quickly so that you can see the consistency of your salve. When cool, test the salve. If it is too soft, add more wax to your mixture on the stove. If too hard, add a bit more oil to the mixture.
11. When you've reached the desired consistency, pour the liquid salve into appropriate containers and let it cool and harden.

Treatments For Specific Conditions

Allergies

Mullein tea

Use 1 teaspoon of dried leaves or 2 teaspoons of fresh leaves in 1 cup of hot water, cover and steep for 10 to 15 minutes. Drink at least 3 times daily.

Stinging nettles

1 teaspoon of dried leaves or 2 teaspoons of fresh leaves in 1 cup of hot water, cover and steep for 10 to 15 minutes. Drink 1-3 cups daily.

For heightened treatment: Make a tonic adding onion, ginger, cayenne, horseradish, and beets to the above tea mixture and/or add the listed ingredients (except the stinging nettles) to your daily diet.

Cod liver oil

Regular doses of cod liver oil added Omega 3's to the diet which increased immunity to conditions like allergies.

Anemia

Beets

Eating beets and their tops and drinking beet broth boosted and cleansed the blood. Beets were boiled or baked. Boiled beet broth, which contained many nutrients, was drunk.

Molasses, liver, eggs, legumes

Adding molasses to the diet and eating liver, eggs, and beans (legumes) were a few ways to increase the red blood cell count and treat anemia.

Arthritis and Rheumatism

(see also "Swelling" this chapter)

Apple cider vinegar

Apple cider vinegar (ACV) was taken externally and internally. ACV with honey was thought to dissolve crystal deposits left by uric acid that collect in joints and in muscles, causing pain and inflammation. Drinking a lot of water following taking the ACV dose helped to flush the dissolved crystals from the body. The standard dose for ACV was 2 tablespoons of ACV in 1/4 to 1/2 cup of warm water or juice, 1 to 2 times daily. 1 tablespoon of honey was sometimes added to sweeten. Both the ACV and honey have anti-inflammatory properties.

ACV was rubbed on the affected area so the skin can absorb its healing properties. A cloth soaked in warm ACV and wrapped around affected area also helped.

Apple cider vinegar and nine sewing needles recipe for arthritis pain

Nine sewing needs were put into a quart of apple cider vinegar (ACV). The vinegar "ate up," or dissolved, the needles. After all the needles were dissolved in the vinegar solution, the solution was rubbed on the arthritic area.

Alternative: The solution was warmed. A cloth was soaked in the solution and wrapped around the affected area. A dry woolen cloth was then put on top of and around the solution-soaked wrap so the heat and moisture would stay in.

Camphor

Camphor salve, cream, or oil was rubbed on affected area. If solution was too strong it was "cut" with coconut or olive oil. Sometimes a warm towel or heating pad was placed on the camphor-treated area for 20 to 30 minutes.

Castor oil

Rubbed into the skin and/or used as a pack (poultice), castor oil penetrates deeper than any other plant oils and reduces inflammation and pain.

A warm castor oil pack was made by soaking a cloth in castor oil, warming and placing over affected area. A hot water bottle may have been put on top of the castor oil-soaked cloth. The castor oil may have been warmed slowly on a stove and then rubbed on your hands and applied. A warm cloth was placed over the area to help the castor oil penetrate the inflamed tissue and joints. For feet and hands castor oil was rubbed on affected area and covered with socks or gloves. The upper body was covered with thermal underwear. This was done mostly at night.

Cod liver oil

Taken internally, it was said to reduce chronic inflammation. One teaspoon to one tablespoon was taken daily at least once, and up to 5 times, weekly.

Clay/chalk

Pack was applied externally and taken internally.
  * External: moistened clay pack or poultice was applied to affected area and left on for at least 1 hour one to two times per day. The area was wrapped with a wool or cotton cloth to make sure it stayed in place.
  * Internal: oven-baked clay paddies were eaten monthly or when the urge hit to detox the body and reduce inflammation. Plenty of water was drunk throughout the day after ingesting the clay.

Treatments For Specific Conditions - Arthritis and Rheumatism (continued)

Ginger

Ginger is a powerful antioxidant that reduces inflammation in affected areas. While it is often in use among African Americans today, it was not a staple in early African American healing tradition.

Add 1 teaspoon of fresh ginger daily to your food, tea, or juice or take a ginger pill as a supplement.

Mullein leaf bath, poultice or tea

Bath: Cut 4 to 6 dried leaves per 5 cups of water. Boil in a pot and soak your feet or whole body in a bath for at least 20 minutes.

Poultice: Mix 4 parts dried and finely chopped mullein leaf to 1 part water to 1 part apple cider vinegar (4:1:1). Heat up and put in a cotton cloth to make a poultice and place on affected area.

Tea: 1 to 3 cups of mullein leaf tea per day was drunk to reduce inflammation and pain internally.

Oak bark soak and poultice for joint pain and swelling

Oak bark was rubbed on joints and muscles. The bark was shaved off with an ax, peeled off the tree, and rubbed on swollen and aching parts.

Bath or soak: 5 to 10 pieces of oak bark were placed in a bath or soaking pan and covered with hot water. The affected area was soaked for 30 to 60 minutes until water became cool.

Pokeberry or pokeberry wine for arthritis

Poke is a very powerful healing agent. People were very careful when using any part of the poke plant for healing; if used incorrectly, it is *toxic*.

Many people drank pokeberry wine or ate the berries to relieve pain and inflammation associated with arthritis, rheumatism, and achy joints. Some claimed that poke medicine had even reversed their disease. One person reported that eating 3 berries a day reversed their arthritic condition while another said eating 5 a day relieved the pain. I was told in order to determine the dosage of pokeberry that will work for each person's body, start by swallowing 1 pokeberry daily per week and increase by 1 pokeberry each day (but usually no more than 3) until you notice loose stools, or stomach or bowel discomfort. When that occurs, take one less than the dosage that resulted in the loose stools or discomfort, and that is the dosage for your body. Pokeberries would be taken consistently for several weeks (4 to 6) and then folks would "give their body a break" by stopping for 1 or 2 weeks, resuming afterwards if necessary.

Note: People did not chew the seeds of the pokeberry (which are toxic to mammals), but swallowed the pokeberry whole, allowing the seeds to come out in their poop. Birds safely eat pokeberries this way.

Pokeberry and root tinctures were made by placing the root or berries in a mason jar, covering with grain alcohol, closing lid tightly and placing in a brown paper bag, allowing to soak for 30 days. Shake the jar at least once daily. After 30 days, strain liquid through cheesecloth or sieve into a clean glass jar, making sure no seeds get into the liquid that passes into the jar. One dropperful of this tincture was taken daily to treat arthritis and rheumatism. After 3 weeks, stop for 1 week and then start again.

Another recipe called for soaking the berries in wine for 30 to 60 days, straining and taking one tablespoon every evening.

Potatoes (raw)

Raw red potatoes were sliced, put in a glass bowl or jar, and covered with water. The container was covered with a towel or a top. This mixture sat overnight then strained and 1 cup of the liquid was drunk.

Red clay and vinegar cast

Red clay was moistened with vinegar and a little water was mixed and applied to affected area. This was wrapped with a linen, wool or cotton cloth to hold in place. It was applied twice daily and left on for 30 to 60 minutes during each application.

Sardine oil

Sardine oil was rubbed on affected area and covered with a cloth each night.

Turmeric

Turmeric is both a spice and an herb that has been used in Aryuvedic (India) and Chinese medicine for over 2,000 years and is purported to ease pain, inflammation, and stiffness associated with arthritis and rheumatism. While it is often in use among African Americans and people of all other cultures today, it was not a staple in early African American healing tradition.

Add turmeric spice to foods you cook such as rice, vegetables, and stews. Alternatively, make a tea from the turmeric root by crushing it first to release the medicine, then putting it in 1 cup of hot water, covering and steeping for 10 to 15 minutes, adding ginger if more potency is desired. Another method for taking turmeric is to purchase it in capsule form (powdered turmeric), taking 250 to 500 mg up to 3 times per day.

Turpentine oil

Equal parts of turpentine, olive oil or lard were mixed and rubbed on affected area twice daily. Pure gum spirits turpentine made from pine resin (with no added ingredients) was and still is used for various medicinal purposes.

Athlete's Foot

(see also "Fungus" or "Foot Health" this chapter)

Apple cider vinegar and baking soda

Vinegar makes a hostile environment for fungus and restores healthy acidity to the skin.

Direct application: Clean feet and dry thoroughly. Apply a generous amount of apple cider vinegar (ACV) with a cotton swab to affected area. Let dry and powder feet with baking soda, which absorbs moisture and helps to maintain a healthy pH[145]. Use 2 to 3 times daily.

Soak: Pour 3 cups of ACV into a tub large enough to hold your feet or foot. Add 4 to 6 cups of warm water and sprinkle in 3 to 4 shakes of baking soda. Let feet or foot soak for 10 to 20 minutes until water becomes cool. Dry feet or foot and scrub off dry, affected skin. Powder feet or foot with baking soda to absorb moisture. Use at least 2 times daily.

Black tar/coal tar soap

Black tar soap was used for its antibacterial, anti-inflammatory, and antiparasitic properties. Gently wash affected area with the soap and rinse. Wash affected area 1 to 2 times daily. Apply baking soda powder to absorb moisture. Do not use black tar soap on blistered, open, or raw skin.

Walnut - black or green walnut hull poultice or wash

Take the meat from the hull of the walnut and use as medicine. The meat (inside of hull) was rubbed over affected area, made into a poultice, or put in warm water and feet soaked.

Yellow root soak or salve

Soak your feet twice daily in a yellow root wash, apply a salve or make a poultice to treat affected area.

---

[145] pH is the level of acidity or basicity/alkalinity in your body or any aqueous solution. The pH scale ranges from 0 to 14. The best acid-alkaline balance for the body is a pH of 7.4. Anything below 7 is acidic, 7 is neutral, and above 7 is more alkaline or "basic." An acidic environment in your body makes you more prone to chronic disease, cancers, and other modern diseases. Stress is one of the conditions that creates an acidic environment in your body. An overly alkaline (or "base") environment in the body can create an imbalance and make you more be prone to illness. Over-acidity is particularly harmful to an individual. Oxygen levels in the body are low in such an environment, which can create inflammation, fatigue, organ breakdown, and other problems.

Treatments For Specific Conditions (continued)

Babies' Conditions

Colds

Castor oil for colds and babies

Rub castor oil on the top of their heads in the mole spot to draw out fevers and cold.

Cod liver oil given to newborns to ward off colds

"We took cod liver oil for maintenance and lubrication of the system but it was also brain food." Bonita Sizemore

Dosage was approximately 1/4 less than the adult dosage and was given in a syringe or mixed in with solid food or with the milk or other liquid in the baby's bottle.

Colic

Acifidity, astifidity, astifis, astificity, asafoetida

"If somebody drink liquor, put some asfidity in the bottle, you know a little bottle, then when the baby get the colic, you take this asfidity and liquor and put about two drops in it with some milk and give it to em. I put about a whole bag of asfidity in a pint-size liquor bottle and just keep it. I give it to the children to put 'em to sleep. They go straight to sleep." Levatus Gillory

Castor oil

Gently massage hand-warmed castor oil on baby's stomach.

Catnip leaves and breast milk

Mix warm breast milk with catnip leaves, put in a bottle, and give to baby.

Horehound tea and breast milk

Squeeze some breast milk in a teaspoon of tea and give to baby.

Tobacco smoke

Blow non-mentholated tobacco smoke in the mole of the baby's head, then blow in a teaspoon 3 times and put teaspoon in baby's mouth.

Hives and Rashes

Aloe

Rub the meat or gel from the aloe leaf directly onto affected area, 2 to 3 times daily.

Flour and grease

"When the babies be rashed, you brown flour and rub it on with some kind of salve or grease (fatback or tallow) and that clears it up." Levatus Gillory

Other grease-like substitutions may have been coconut oil, olive oil, aloe gel or shea butter.

Moisturizer/skin softener

Aloe vera gel: rub the meat of an aloe leaf on dry areas.

Watermelon rind (see also "Skin conditions" this chapter): rub the meat side of the watermelon rind on your dry skin areas.

Oatmeal bath or paste

Bath: using a coffee grinder or mortar and pestel, grind up one cup of dry oats. Mix in 2 cups of warm water. Pour this solution into the baby's bath and let baby soak for at least 10 minutes, gently pouring solution over parts of body not covered in tub.

Paste: grind dry oats and mix with aloe gel and rub on affected area. Let stay on for 30 minutes and wash off with warm water.

Navel Protrusion

Get a silver dollar or half dollar and tape on herniated navel, pushing the navel in so it is flush with the belly. Use medical tape so it does not hurt baby's skin when it is removed. Remove when bathing and change tape when dirty. Leave on until navel goes in.

Teething

Birdbill tea

"You got a baby that's teething, you give it birdbill. It's a weed made just like a birdbill. Just get you some of that there, bring it in the house and wash it and put it in a jar with some water and we put it in the bottle. We brews it up and when you put it in the jar, you can go ahead and give him some of it. You can keep it for a long time, just keep adding fresh water to it. It will kill that diarrhea too." Ms. Oscelena Harris

Hornet or wasp's nest

Give this to baby to chew on. The hornet and wasp make these nests out of pulped wood and bark which they gnaw, chew up, and turn into a pulp by mixing it with their own saliva. The texture of the nest is papery and an excellent object for babies to gnaw on to relieve teething pains.

Titiweed (other names: blood root, tetterwort, coon root)

This weed was given to babies to chew on to strengthen their gums and as an anesthetic.

Bee Stings

(see also "Insect Bites And Stings" this chapter)

If you got stung by a bee, the stinger was removed and any one of the following treatments below was applied to affected area. Note: These remedies were not effective with allergic reactions.

Garlic juice

Apply the juice from a crushed garlic on affected area or apply a piece of the crushed garlic on affected area and cover with an adhesive bandage.

Lavendar oil

While lavender is often in use among African Americans today, it was not a staple in early African American healing tradition.

Apply two drops of lavender oil on affected area 2 times daily. If you harvest lavender from nature, rub the leaves on the affected area. Lavender will reduce the itching, pain, and inflammation.

Tobacco or snuff

Apply chewed tobacco that has been moistened by saliva on the affected area, or apply moistened snuff to the affected area. Cover with an adhesive bandage and leave on for at least an hour.

White or red clay

Apply a paste of clay to affected area and cover with an adhesive bandage. If you harvest from a natural location, make sure that the site is not contaminated.

Blood Toxins

(tired, dirty, sluggish blood)

Blood cleansers have a powerful impact on overall health. They act to detoxify and purify the blood by removing toxins, fungus, bacteria and viruses from the bloodstream. Blood cleansers also strengthen the liver and clean the kidneys so these two organs can efficiently remove waste from the body. In

Treatments For Specific Conditions - Blood Toxins (continued)

traditional African American healing, herbs were used to "cleanse the blood" (remove toxins from the blood) routinely, as a preventative, or whenever one felt sluggish, low energy, the onset of a cold, or a "little queer" as one healer expressed. Below is a list of blood cleanser remedies and routines.

Queen's Delight tea

Make a tea by steeping 1 teaspoon of the dried Queen's Delight root in hot water for 10 to 15 minutes, covering the water while steeping, or soak the roots overnight in cold water and drink in the morning. Drink 1 to 3 cups daily for 1 week then stop. Resume after 1 month.

Red Shank tea

Make a tea from the Red Shank root using 1 teaspoon of fresh root to 2 cups of water. Drink 1 cup daily.

Sassafras tea (red)

Steep 1 teaspoon of the dried root in 1 cup of hot water for 10 to 15 minutes, covering while steeping. Drink 1 cup daily for 7 days.[146]

Beets and morning dew

"My mama used to take fresh beets and spices and put it in the pan and let it out over night and get the dew on it, and they would use that for treatment. Beets and morning mist." Eveline Prayo-Bernard

Today it is not wise to let beets sit out overnight to collect the dew because of environmental pollution. However, eating beets by boiling them and drinking the broth, eating beet greens, and/or baking the beets and greens is an effective way to get the nutritious benefits. Soaking the beets in apple cider vinegar gives them extra medicine.

Castor oil

Taken internally or applied as a pack on abdomen to help flush out toxins in liver, kidneys, and colon and to ease lymphatic congestion.

Clay, bentonite

Eating the white clay (kaolin clay) which is also called chalk removes toxins, heavy metals, and chemicals from the body, cleans the colon, supports liver and boosts immunity. It's important to determine the best dosage for your health needs. Dosages can range from taking 1 teaspoon daily for 3 days to 1 tablespoon a month. For an initial dosage, take 1 teaspoon to 1 tablespoon 1 to 3 times a week for 1 week. After each dosage, drink 1 big glass of water and plenty of water throughout the day, otherwise the clay may create constipation.

Garlic

Eat three cloves daily by blending them in a drink or adding them to food. If you add garlic to food as a cleansing agent, add them to the last 5 minutes of cooking or after the food is cooked. This can be chopped, sliced or a whole crushed garlic clove. Crushing the whole clove releases the medicine and flavor. Alternatively, you can sprinkle raw chopped garlic on your meal after it is cooked or saute raw chopped garlic in olive oil for 3 to no more than 10 minutes and add as a garnish to your meal. As another alternative, you can cook the whole garlic clove or bulb by baking in a 300 degree oven until it is soft, or wrapping in foil and placing on a grill until it is soft. However you decide to prepare garlic separately from your meal, it can be eaten on the side like a relish or chow-chow or however to fit one's taste.

(*Note*: Cooking garlic on high heat for longer than 10 minutes reduces its medicinal benefits.)

---

[146] An important warning note about sassafras and safrole: Sassafras contains safrole, which is known to have harmful effects if ingested over a period of time in large and concentrated quantities. See warning and instructions in the Sassafras section on pages 319-320 before using.

Lemon

Drink a lemon juice tonic daily using 1/2 to 1 whole lemon to flush out toxins and harmful bacteria.

Mulberry fruit

Raw: eat fresh mulberries when they are ripened to a dark purple color.

Juice: make a juice by blending the fresh ripened mulberries into a gel-like consistency, strain the mixture in a mesh cloth or sieve, and drink the liquid.

Syrup/tonic: slow cook 1 cup of fresh mulberries until all the liquid is extracted, stirring and mashing the fruit often. Let sit overnight, then reheat. Strain the mixture into a mesh cloth or sieve until all the liquid is out. Take 1 to 2 teaspoons daily for a blood tonic or to treat colds.

Onion syrup

"My mother did onion syrup. Slicin' up them onions and sprinklin' some sugar and she'd always cover it and sit it on the mantlepiece. We took onion syrup for a whole bunch of things, especially for a general cleanser if she's worried about colds and that kind of stuff. She'd slice the onions real thin and lay some onions in a bowl, sprinkle sugar, lay some more onions, sprinkle some more sugar. She would cover it with a tea towel and she'd always set it up on the mantlepiece. I guess it had to be in a warm place. She'd leave it there a certain period of time, checking on it until there was this white syrup from the onion juice and the sugar. It was for colds, cleansing and general maintenance." Luisah Teish

Onion is such a powerful healing agent. Today, sugar can be replaced with honey, which also has antibacterial and anti-inflammatory properties.

Steam bath for congestion and toxic cleansing

"My mother would fill a tub with steaming hot water and you sit in the chair or soak in the tub, cover your whole head with a towel and inhale all of that steam and everything and whatever was wrong with you would come out." Eveline Elizabeth Prayo-Bernard

Yellow root (goldenseal)

Harvest the root, clean it off, break it into small pieces, put about 1/4 cup of root pieces in a mason jar no more than quart size, fill the jar with water, let sit for a day, then begin drinking. Take sips or small cup full, 3 times a day. Keep remaining yellow root refrigerated. Do not use continually for more than 7 days, then stop for 7 days and resume until medicine is finished. Most people did not take yellow root either long-term or on a regular basis year-round. The root was most used seasonally or to treat an illness.

Boils and Cysts

Castor oil pack

Rub a generous amount of warm castor oil on affected area and wrap with a cloth. Change twice daily. Keep in place until boil or cyst disappears.

Comfrey and aloe

Make a paste or poultice from the leaves, stems and/or root of comfrey and mix with aloe gel. Apply to affected area.

Egg shell

"When you get a boil, put the skin of the egg shell on top of it to make it go down. If the boil ain't open, get you some fatback and put it on there and it'll jus' open it on up and draw that infection on out." Ruth Patterson

Garlic

Make a thick garlic paste by crushing 3 garlic cloves and mixing with tallow, olive oil, or aloe gel. Apply to affected area and wrap with a bandage. Remove when mixture is dry, wash area with warm water, and replace garlic paste again until boil is gone.

Treatments For Specific Conditions - Boils and Cysts (continued)

Yellow root

Make a salve or poultice from the dried root and apply fresh, 1 to 2 times daily.

Poke root

Apply a salve or poultice made from the poke root 1 to 2 times daily.

Bronchitis

(see also "Coughs" this chapter)

The following herbs will help treat bronchitis. See "Coughs" to read how the medicines were made and applied or refer to "Standard Medicine Preparations" at the beginning of this section.
Mullein (either taken as a tea or smoked in a pipe)
Rabbit tobacco (either taken as a tea or smoked in a pipe)
Onion cough syrup
Pine and horehound tea
Garlic and pine rosin syrup
Eucalpytus tea
Bay leaf tea
Mustard plaster cast

Burns

(see also "Skin Conditions" this chapter)

All burns were cleaned before applying any medicine. If available, medical attention was sought for severe burns.

Aloe vera

Find an aloe vera plant, break a leaf, and rub the gel inside the leaf on the burn several times a day until healed.

Clay

Apply a red or white clay poultice to affected area. Change every two hours and keep moist.

Cold water and butter

Rinse affected area with cold water to stop the pain and pull the heat out, dry affected area, and then rub butter on burn.

Egg whites

Spray cold water on the affected area until the heat is reduced and burning stops. Then, rub or dip egg whites on the affected area. Let the whites dry and form a protective layer. Then add more egg whites until dry. Do this for one hour or longer until pain is gone. Egg white is a natural collagen full of vitamins and helps regenerate burned skin.

Potato

Slice a raw potato so that one side is potato skin and the other is raw potato. Place the potato side on the burn and wrap to keep in place. Leave on until the potato is no longer moist or turns brown. Replace with fresh potato until pain is gone and area heals.
Alternatively, grate a raw potato to create a type of mush. Do not drain the liquid or moisture. Place the raw potato mush over burn area and wrap in place. Leave on until mush dries out and/or turns brown, then replace.

Sweet gum tree home remedy for severe burns

The sweet gum tree remedy for burns below was given to me as a beautifully written three page narrative by a Georgia minister I knew only by the name of Reverend Cook.

"In late 1917 or early 1918 when I was about 4 1/2 years old, I remember my sister Cora being burned very severely on her hand. A lot of different people recommended a lot of different medicines for her burn but the burn didn't heal and it didn't go away. In all of this my mother remembered a home remedy her own mother used to heal severe burn wounds. My grandmother used the balls (cones) from the sweet gum tree.

"Immediately the burn quits aching and the healing process begins. In a few days you can see the burn wound is getting better and a noticeable healing is taking place.

"This remedy was used on me after my own mother passed on. It was the spring of 1920. My sister-in-law had fried some bacon in the frying pan on the stove and told me, a 7-year old child, to remove the grease from the stove. While removing the hot frying pan containing the hot bacon grease, I accidentally spilled the grease on my foot. I was in such shock and pain that I ran outside and around and around the house until I collapsed.

"In a short time (a few days), the burn turned into a blister. The blister turned into a severe sore that was so deep it appeared the wound was exposing the bone in my foot.

"It was then that I remembered my mother making my grandmother's burn remedy. We lived in the country and the nearest neighbor with a milking cow lived about 5 miles away. My brother walked that 5 miles to get the cows milk with the cream on top. He followed the instructions as I remembered them. He burned the balls (cones from the sweet gum tree) until they turned to ashes and mixed the ashes with the sweet cream to make a poultice/salve. He applied this poultice to my burn wound and immediately the aching ceased. In just a few short days you could see the wound heal up. In about 2 weeks after using this remedy, I was able to walk again.

"I had to use this remedy for a burn on someone else in 1954. It still worked!"
Reverend Cook (Georgia)

Here is Reverend Cook's recipe for the remedy:
* Collect the balls (cones) from the sweet gum tree and put them in a pan or skillet over heat and cook them until they turn to ashes.
* Take fresh cream collected from the top of fresh milk. (In the old days the milk from just milked cows was used. You would take the milk from the cow and let it sit until the cream rose to the top and this was the cream that was used.)
* Make a poultice (salve) by mixing the ashes and the cream together.
* Apply to the burns several times daily.

Calluses On Feet

(see "Foot Health" this chapter)

Chicken Pox

"For chicken pox, go in the chicken coop, face forward and leave walking backward. Do this before 5 a.m. sunrise." Ms. Jacobs[147]

Corn shuck tea

Take dried corn shuck. Put leaves and silk in a pot, cover with water. Bring to a boil and let sit for 15 minutes. Strain and drink 3 times a day. Pour remainder in a jar and keep refrigerated.

---

[147] See Ms. Jacobs' full interview in the "Strong Medicine, Beyond The African American" section.

Treatments For Specific Conditions - Chicken Pox (continued)

Aloe vera gel and white clay

Apply aloe vera gel or white clay to affected area 2 to 3 times a day to treat itching and pox sores. Make sure area is cleaned before application.

Circulation

Cayenne

Cayenne or hot peppers were consumed daily with meals to increase circulation. 1/4 to 1/2 of a teaspoon of cayenne was added to meals during cooking. Cayenne was also used to improve circulation.

* Make a tea by using 1/4 teaspoon of cayenne spice in a cup of warm water. Sweeten with honey. Optional: make your favorite herb tea, such as mint or chamomile, and add the cayenne while steeping.
* Apply a cayenne poultice to an area needing improved circulation. Leave on for 30 to 60 minutes and apply twice daily.

Timtyme Weed or Thyme

Used to increase blood circulation and acted as a stimulant. Crush up the entire weed with the flower and make a tea by steeping 1 teaspoon of the herb in hot water for 10 to 15 minutes, covering while steeping, and drink when the steeping is completed.

Cold Sore

(see "Fever Blister" this chapter)

Colds and Flu

The single herbal medicines listed below were often mixed with other herbs to help treat symptoms of cold and flu—mostly cough, fever, and congestion. For example, mixing mullein, a mint, or pine needles helped treat congestion. The standard preparation for making a tea was by steeping 1 to 2 teaspoons of the dried herb in hot water, covering while steeping, or by placing about 1/4 cup of the dried herb in a mason jar and filling with luke warm water, letting sit overnight and sipping on several times a day. Drinking 3 cups per day of hot tea or "sipping on" the tea made in the mason jar several times a day was common practice.

Boneset tea

Boneset tea was drunk to treat symptoms associated with the common cold and flu, including fever and congestion, and to boost immunity in order to shorten the length of the ailment.

Buttongrass tea

Buttongrass tea was drunk to treat fevers, respiratory ailments, and aches and pains associated with colds and flu.

Buzzard weed tea

Buzzard weed tea was drunk to treat general pain and discomfort associated with colds and flu.

Cow chip tea

Mostly prepared to treat cough, congestion and pneumonia.

Scoop up a cow paddie and place in a pot. Fill the pot with water and bring to boil, then simmer for 30 minutes. Strain several times in a cheesecloth until there are no sediments. Drink one cup daily until symptoms subside.

(Note: This remedy is not recommended for use today. During the time this remedy was a common

practice, the environment was not as polluted as it is today and most cows were free range and fed a healthy grain.)

Goldenrod

"Them goldenrod is good for colds. It's gotta leaf bought yeah long, look like a sage leaf, only it's shiny and it has a heap of leaves grows up on it, and the stem go straight up, jus 'bout dat high. Dat's bitter." Ruth Patterson

Hog hoof tea

Cut off the hoof from the carcass. Wash it and dry it. Boil the hoof in a big pot of water for at least 1 hour, then drink 1 cup of the steaming hoof water tea to cure a cold. Pour the remainder in a mason jar, refrigerate, and sip on daily.

Rabbit tobacco tea

Rabbit tobacco tea was drunk to treat congestion and coughs and to combat bacteria and infections due to colds and flu.

Sassafras tea (red)

"Pick the red sassafract leaves, not the white. The red leaves have red streaks in it, kinda brown lookin leaf, a dark leaf and the white sassafract, it gotta shiny leaf on it. You can get them red leaves and boil em and the water be kinda brown lookin. But the white leaf, it ain't no good. It's pretty much used for the scent, the smell, that's all. You don't use white for cookin, you use red sassafract. It's good too if you make tea outta that for colds. It grows out in the old field and peoples ain't tend it in a long time. Go out into that field and break a lil stem offa it and smell it; if it's sassafract, you cain't tell it's red sassafract til you dig down in dere and pull up a sprig and its white, but if you pop that end loose and it's red, that be the red sassafract, and if you pop it loose and it's white, that's the white sassafract.

The white will run you blind, stay away from that. You wanna take the red. You can drank the red for coffee or you can take it and make medicine outta it for different thangs. It surely is good for colds." Ruth Patterson

Miss Hazel's Sassafras root tea recipe for colds – use only the red roots:
  * Dig up the roots, clean and let dry.
  * Cut dried roots into four to six-inch lengths and split several times lengthwise.
  * Place the chunks of roots (with bark) in a pot and cover with cold tap water.
  * Bring to a slow boil and let simmer for 15 minutes.
  * Strain with cheesecloth and sweeten with honey. Drink 2 or more cups daily.
  * Can add lemon. Roots not used can be tied in bundles and used as an air freshener or medicine for a later date.[148]

Yellow root tea

Drink up to 3 cups daily. After one week, stop for one week and then resume if necessary.

Herb tea combinations

Boneset, calamus and yellow root

"You can find all of these up in this place (the woods). Boneset and calamus is a weed and yellow root is a root. It got a top. That's the only way I can find it by the top of it. It grows up and you can get the root. They say the root is better than the top. But the top is just as green as the root is yellow. And, you can break it and see the root, that's how I finds it. When I get a streak in the woods, I break it to see

---

[148] An important warning note about sassafras and safrole: Sassafras contains safrole, which is known to have harmful effects if ingested over a period of time in large and concentrated quantities. See warning and instructions in the Sassafras section on pages 319-320 before using.

Treatments For Specific Conditions - Colds and Flu (continued)

if it's yellow. That's it. I use all of it. I don't throw the tops away, the tops just as good as the root. I chop up all of it and boil it down. And, I don't make it all at one time. I make some of it and then I tie it up and save it and let it dry and if I need it again, or somebody else need some of it, I get it and give them some." Mrs. Sally McCloud

Get equal parts, put in a pot, fill pot with water, bring to boil, cover, and slow simmer for 30 minutes. Strain and drink 1 to 3 cups a day. Put remainder in a glass jar and refrigerate.

Pergiegrass (peppergrass or pennygrass), rabbit tobacco, and horehound tea

Mix equal parts pergiegrass (peppergrass or pennygrass), rabbit tobacco, and horehound, cover and steep in a pot covered in water for 30 minutes. Drink 1 to 3 times a day.

Rabbit tobacco, pine tar, pine tops and lemon

* Rabbit tobacco (use the brown silvery leaves which are most potent)
* Pine tar (sap from pine tree)
* Pine tops
* One lemon cut in half, drain juice in pot, and drop lemon in.

Use equal parts and slow brew in a covered pot for 15 to 20 minutes. Let sit and drink as tea or sip on at room temperature. Store in a glass jar and put in refrigerator. Drink 1 to 3 cups a day or just sip from jar.

Tonics to sweat out colds

Garlic, pine rosin or needles, and lemon

In a pot add 3 to 4 cloves of crushed or chopped garlic, 2 tablespoons of pine rosin or pine needles, and 2 cups of water. Bring to a boil, cover and remove from fire. Add honey to sweeten, 1/2 lemon (squeeze juice in first), cover and let steep for 20 to 30 minutes. Optional: Add 1/4 teaspoon of cayenne and fresh ginger. Strain and drink 2 to 3 times a day.

Hot totty

Ingredients: whiskey or brandy, peppermint, lemon, honey, cayenne.
Make a strong peppermint tea (cover and let steep for 15 minutes) and add honey, lemon and 1/4 teaspoon of cayenne. Add 2 to 4 tablespoons of whiskey or brandy to mixture. Drink right before bedtime. Sleep in warm clothes and cover up with blankets to make sure you get a good sweat.

Raw apple cider vinegar with the "mother", ginger, garlic, onion, peppers

Winter tonic to boost immunity

(Antiviral, antifungal, antibacterial)
Use equal parts of chopped garlic cloves, ginger root, onion, cayenne pepper, and apple cider vinegar (ACV) containing "the mother." "The mother" is the tiny, web-like ball of living enzymes and nutrients in raw, unpasteurized, unfiltered ACV that makes this liquid an active healing agent.
Mix equal parts:
* 1 part chopped garlic cloves
* 1 part fresh chopped white onion (or hottest onions)
* 1 part fresh grated ginger root
* 1 part fresh chopped cayenne peppers or 1 to 2 teaspoons cayenne powder
* Optional: horseradish for congestion, the juice of 1 lemon, honey to sweeten

Put ingredients in a mason jar and fill with the organic raw ACV. Shake vigorously. Place jar in a paper bag and put in a cool dark cabinet for 2 weeks. Shake once daily. After two weeks, strain into a clean jar and store in a cool cabinet or refrigerator.

Preventative

Take 1 to 2 tablespoons 2 times a day as a preventative for 1 week.

At onset of cold or flu

At the onset of illness, take the preventive dosage 3 to 5 times a day for 3 to 5 days.

Illness

If you have cold, flu, congestion or an infection, take 1 to 2 tablespoons 6 times a day, making sure you flush your body with water.

Castor oil dose

Often a dose of castor oil at the onset of a cold or flu successfully purged out or reduced its duration and boosted the immune system. Castor oil's medicinal properties may have also helped prevent the growth of numerous types of viruses, bacteria, yeasts and molds. Take one tablespoon followed by a shot of lemon or orange juice to offset the awful taste.

Snakeweed tea

Put 1 teaspoon of dried snakeweed or 2 teaspoons of fresh snakeweed in 1 cup of hot water, cover and steep for 10 to 15 minutes. (For a stronger snakeweed tea, add 2 to 4 tablespoons of whiskey.) Sweeten with honey. As an option, add lemon and/or 1/4 teaspoon of cayenne. Drink 2 to 3 cups daily throughout duration of the cold. Sleep in warm clothes and cover up with blankets to make sure you get a good sweat.

Store-bought cures

(Common cures for colds, flu, and prevention bought at drug stores throughout the South and advertised as early as the beginning of the 19th century)

666 – 3 Sixes for colds

"We took onion syrup for a whole bunch of things, especially for a general cleanser if [Mama was] worried about colds and that kind of stuff. ... I wasn't crazy about the taste of onion syrup. But when [Mama] found a substitute for it I wish we had gone back to the onion syrup, because she substituted it with a compound you bought in the store called Three Sixes. 666. It was awful. I wanted the onion syrup because it had a sweet kick to it." Luisah Teish

Black Draught tea

Black Draught tea was commonly used as a folk medicine for many ailments. Like 666, it has been sold commercially since the late 19th century. It was a cathartic or purging medicine, like castor oil, and was composed of a blend of magnesia and senna.

Congestion

(sinus, nasal, chest and head colds)

Bay leaf tea, inhalant, and steam bath

Tea

Add 1 to 2 dried bay leaves per one cup of hot water. Sweeten with honey if desired. Cover and steep 10 to 15 minutes. Drink 3 times per day to relieve congestion.

Inhalant

"My mother would boil things to put up under the bed. It would smell like lavender but it was a little different. You could really smell the oil in it. She'd put it in the room like people use Vicks Vapor to help. It would be her version of aromatherapy to keep the air with something medicinal in it so you could breath, open up your sinuses. We didn't live in an area where there was bay leaves on the trees so she just took whatever she had." Anita Poree

Add 5 to 10 dried bay leaves and 2 teaspoons of sage to a pot of boiling water. Remove from heat and cover. Put a towel over your head, remove pot cover, and lean over pot and inhale the steam. Make sure you create a tent-like effect with the towel so you can direct the steam toward your nostrils. Inhale for 15 to 20 mintues.

Steam bath

Add a bunch (10+) leaves to a hot bath. Close bathroom door. When water is cool enough to soak, get in and soak for at least 10 minutes. You are essentially creating a sauna-type environment.

Buzzard weed, rabbit tobacco, and pine tar

"Buzzard weed is a good medicine. Take rabbits tobacco and pine tar with buzzard weed, put it all together in a pot, pour water on it and boil it down and drink it. That's good for colds, congestion, pneumonia and influenza." Mr. Pete Smith

Camphor salve

To make a camphor salve, you will need:
> 1/2 cup of beeswax
> 1 to 2 tablespoons of cutting oil like olive or coconut
> 1/2 to 1 tablespoon of camphor crystals/granules or 5 to 10 drops of essential oil[149]

Slowly heat the beeswax and cutting oil in a pot. If using crystals, add them in once the beeswax and cutting oil mixture is melted, stirring slowly until the granules are dissolved. If using essential oil, add and stir thoroughly once the beeswax and cutting oil mixture is melted. Pour entire contents into a glass container and let harden. Add more beeswax if the mixture is too oily, or more oil for a softer consistency.

Rub the salve on chest and back for congestion 2 to 3 times daily. Place a warm cloth over area after the salve has been massaged into skin to heighten the effectiveness.

You can also use as an inhalant in conjunction with the camphor salve to relieve sinus congestion.

Castor oil pack

Castor oil packs were placed on the chest to treat congestion and upper respiratory infections, applied twice daily especially right before bedtime.
* Rub a generous amount of castor oil on your chest and back.
* Cut a piece of flannel or woolen cloth large enough to cover your chest and saturate the cloth with castor oil.
* Place the cloth on top of your chest and/or back.
* Wrap a towel around to keep cloth in place.
* Place a heating pad on top of the towel and relax for one hour.
* Optional: Place a piece of plastic garbage bag between heating pad and towel.

After treatment, put cloth in a plastic bag or container and place in the refrigerator. Warm it up before its next use and refresh with one to two tablespoons of fresh castor oil.

Cedar wood tea

Chop pieces of cedar, rinse and put in a pot and cover with water. Slow simmer for 30 minutes and drink as a tea. Let cool, strain, place in a glass jar, and refrigerate. Sip on freely.

Cow chip tea (also for pneumonia)

"Mama used to fix a tea with cow manure after she dried it out. We drank it. This helped to clear our chest so we wouldn't get no colds." Levatus Gillory

---

[149] As an alternative to the ingredients on this line, you can substitute 1/2 tablespoon of camphor and 1/2 tablespoon of menthol or another soothing/healing agent such as camphor

Spread out cow dung/manure and let it dry out. Make a tea from one teaspoon of cow chip to one cup of boiling water. Cover, let steep for 30 minutes, then strain. Add peppermint tea or candy, sweeten and drink.

(*Note: This remedy is not recommended for use today. During the time this remedy was a common practice, the environment was not as polluted as it is today and most cows were free range and fed a healthier grain.*)

Eucalyptus tea, inhalant, and steam bath

Tea

Use 1 teaspoon of dried eucalyptus leaves per 1 cup of hot water. Cover and steep for 10 to 15 mintues. Drink 3 times daily to relieve congestion and to prevent colds and flu.

Inhalant

Add 3 to 5 eucalpytus leaves to a pot of boiling water. Remove from heat and cover. Put a towel over your head, remove pot cover, and lean over pot and inhale the steam. Make sure you create a tent-like effect with the towel so you can direct the steam toward your nostrils.

Steam bath

Add a bunch (10+) leaves to a hot bath. Close bathroom door. When water is cool enough to soak, get in and soak for at least 10 minutes. You are essentially creating a sauna-type environment

Liniment

Use healing herbs and oils to make a liniment and rub on chest and back to relieve congestion. See "Liniment" in the "Medicine" section, Chapter 8.

Mullein/Mullet

Tea

Put 1 to 2 teaspoons of dried mullein leaves or 2 teaspoons of fresh mullein leaves in a strainer and let steep in 1 cup of covered hot water for 10 to 15 minutes. Remove the cover and strainer and drink the tea. Alternately, put the dried or fresh mullein leaves in 1 cup and pour hot water over them, cover and let steep for 10 to 15 minutes, then pour the liquid through a strainer and drink.

For a more potent cup, steep 2 to 3 teaspoons of dried mullein in 1 cup of hot water for 20 minutes.

Optional: Sweeten with honey, add cayenne, lemon and blend with peppermint, eucalyptus or bay leaves. Drink 2 to 3 times daily.

Mullein leaf smoke (for pulmonary and chest congestion)

Pack a pipe or make a cigarette out of dried cut-up mullein leaves. Smoke and inhale 3 times to relieve pulmonary and chest congestion. Do twice daily.

Mustard plaster

"Every once in a while we would get a cold and Mom would do mustard rolls. She'd actually get the mustard seed and she would pound it. And then mix it with some oil, I think talla or pig fat. She'd rub that on our chest and on our back and cover it with a piece of cloth for warmth." Imani Ajaniku

Mix powdered mustard seeds with water and spread over a sheet or cloth, then place the cloth on the chest. The skin warms up, the lungs open, and congestion seems to clear up. The same treatment can be used on achy joints caused by overuse or arthritis. Don't apply a mustard plaster directly to the skin—the oils may cause blisters on the skin. Remove the plaster when you start to feel uncomfortable, and wash the area thoroughly with cool water. Apply twice daily.

Pine cone or pine bark, pine tar (sap), and whiskey

Take a pine cone or bark with sap on it, cover with water in a pot and low simmer for 30 minutes. Let sit in pot until water cools. Use 2 tablespoons whiskey or brandy to 1 cup of pine tea. Add honey to taste and one lemon. For stronger medicine, let sit for 24 hours, then use. Keep in an airtight jar, cover

Treatments For Specific Conditions - Congestion (continued)

with a paper bag and store in a cool and dry cabinet. Refrigerate after 7 days. Take 1 tablespoon 3 to 4 times a day.

Pine tree limb, mullein, and horehound tea

"Gather limbs from the pine tree that has pine rosin. Put the pine limbs, mullein and horehound in a pot, cover with water and cook down. Drink three times daily and right before bed to sweat out the fever." Author unknown

Rabbit tobacco

Smoke

Fill a pipe with the dried leaves from rabbit tobacco plant, or make a cigarette. Inhale the smoke deeply two times. Hold the smoke in for 10 seconds and blow the smoke out. Do this 3 times in a row. It will bring up the phlegm, open sinuses, and clear lungs. Do this treatment 3 times a day for no more than 7 days or for the duration of the congestion and cold, whichever comes first. If condition worsens during use of this treatment, discontinue and seek advice from your health care professional.

Tea

Drink rabbit tobacco tea 3 times a day for the duration of the congestion and cold.

St. John Poultice for chest congestion

"[Mama] also used something called St. John to clean your chest area out. It was made with pure oil and had a little sweet top to it and was brown. She mix that up, rub on your chest and put a warm wool cloth over it." Anita Poree

Steam bath for congestion cleansing

"Mama would fill a tub with steaming hot water and put whole bay leaves in it. She'd make you sit in a chair right next to the tub and cover your whole head with a towel. You'd inhale all of that steam and everything and whatever was wrong with you would come out." Eveline Prayo-Bernard

Alternative: Adding herbs such as eucalyptus, sage, and Epsom salt in the steam bath described above makes the bath more effective.

Tallow for chest congestion

"They took (talla) and fried it, let it get cold, cut it in blocks. Grandma made a sack and tied it around our neck and that was supposed to pull the mucous and congestion out." Author unknown

Tallow (sometimes spelled tallah or talla) is used to relieve chest congestion. Tallow is the fat from cooked beef or pork. After you cook the meat, put the pan with the fat in the refrigerator or leave out overnight if it is cool. The next day the fat will settle at the top. Scrape it off and put in a separate bowl. Slowly heat up the tallow in a small pot until it is warm. You can add pine tar or Vicks salve. Spread the tallow salve on chest and cover with a woolen cloth. It will draw out the cold and loosen up the congestion.

Turpentine salve

Mix 1 tablespoon of turpentine into 2 tablespoons of olive oil, lard, coconut oil, or shea butter. Spread on chest and place a warm woolen cloth over area.

Vicks salve and strong snuff for chest congestion

Make a paste from the Vicks salve and snuff. Rub on chest and put a heavy flannel or wool cloth on the area. Best to do right before bed.

Vicks salve and olive oil poultice for chest congestion

Mix 1 teaspoon olive oil with 1 tablespoon of Vicks salve and rub on chest and back to relieve (break-up) congestion and pull out the cold.

Constipation

"Here again, people isolated out in the country had to stay on top of this and make sure the kids are not constipated, making sure the colon is clean. They knew on a more practical level that if you got backed up, it would cause pain and pain was an indicator that something was going on and pay attention to where it is. They didn't have all this scientific data that says good health is connected to a clean colon. They knew on a preventive level as opposed to reading it out of a book. That's where spring tonics came from... My grandmother said there was one thing that I needed to remember, "If you always wanted to be healthy, don't be full of shit." Anita Poree

Aloe vera

Gel

Take 2 tablespoons of aloe vera gel twice daily on an empty stomach. Scoop the gel from a leaf and mix with juice.

Juice

Drink two cups of juice daily on an empty stomach or in between meals.

Cascara Sagrada

Bring to boil 1 teaspoon of dried bark in 3 cups of water. Simmer for 30 minutes. Let cool to room temperature, then drink 1 to 2 cups per day, close to bedtime. Bowels should move within 6 to 8 hours. Cascara sagrada can also be used in capsule or tincture form. Not for long term use (longer than 3 to 5 days) or if you are pregnant or have ulcers or gastrointestinal problems.

Castor oil

Internal

Take 1 tablespoon (chased with lemon or orange) in the morning or evening. It also eliminates tapeworms and other intestinal worms.

External pack/poultice

Put on chest and abdomen before bedtime. Saturate a piece of wool, flannel, or cotton cloth in castor oil. Make sure the cloth is cut to the size you need to cover. You may want to warm the oil first by putting bottle in a bowl and pouring boiled water in bowl, letting the bottle sit for 5 to 10 minutes. Place the pack over the affected body part. Cover with plastic. Place a hot water bottle or heating pad over the plastic and cover that with a towel to insulate the heat. Leave it on for 30 to 60 minutes, resting and being still while the pack is in place. Remove the pack and cleanse the area with water and baking soda. Store the pack/cloth in a covered container and keep in refrigerator until next use.

Elderberry root and Life-Everlasting tea

Drink 2 to 3 times daily.

Maypop tea (Passion Flower)

Put 1 teaspoon of the dried herb in 1 cup of hot water, cover and steep for 10 to 15 minutes. Drink 2 to 3 cups daily.

Senna tea

Put 1 teaspoon of dried senna in 1 cup of hot water, cover and steep for 10 to 15 minutes. Drink right before bedtime.

Treatments For Specific Conditions - Constipation (continued)

Yellow root, buzzard weed, and pudgegrass teas

Blend 1/2 teaspoon of each dried herb in 1 cup of hot water, cover and steep for 10 to 15 minutes. Drink 2 to 3 times daily until relieved.

Coffee grounds

Mix 1 teaspoon used coffee grounds with 1 to 3 teaspoons black strap molasses. Eat 1 tablespoon of mixture.

Epsom salt

Mix 1 teaspoon of Epsom salt in 1/2 cup of water and drink.

Epsom salt and Black Draught tea for constipation

Mix 1 teaspoon of Epsom salt and 1 teaspoon of Black Draught in 1 cup of warm water and drink at bedtime.

Okra

"The only time I use okra is as medicine" Luisah Teish

Eating okra or drinking okra water is a great choice for treating bowel irregularity. Okra is a natural cleanser. It is rich with mucilage, a thick, gooey substance that gives okra its slimey texture. Mucilage lubricates the intestines as it passes through, soothing inflamed areas and absorbing toxins and excess water while flushing out the colon.

To make okra water: soak 2 pods overnight in a glass of water and drink first thing in the morning.

Turpentine

"They'd sit you over hot water and you'd have to sit there for a while and you had to get up and walk around and sit down and get up and walk around and they gave you a drop of turpentine for the stomach." Anita Poree

Corns On Toe

(see also "Foot Health" this chapter)

Salt pork or bacon

"To get rid of corns, cut off ... any kind a piece of salt pork or bacon before it get dried hard [and] put a piece [on the corn]." Etta Minor-Williams

Hold the moist salt pork or bacon in place with guaze or a large adhesive bandage. Cover foot with sock. Remove daily, wash area and then replace as needed.

Tallow/talla

Apply a generous amount on calloused skin and cover with cotton socks. Apply at nighttime to let the tallow soften skin overnight. Once it has softened scrub callus with a pumice stone or foot shaver to remove dead skin. Tallow can be mixed with another oil like olive oil or shea butter.

Coughs

(see also "Whooping Cough" this chapter)

Syrups and lozenges

Garlic and pine rosin

Chop 1 garlic bulb. Get 1/2 to 1 cup of sap/rosin from the pine tree. Add the chopped garlic, rosin and 1/4 to 1/2 cup maple syrup or cane sugar to a sauce pan. Cook and stir mixture no longer than 10 minutes until there are no more clumps of pine rosin. For drops, pour mixture into a flat pan or cookie sheet, let cool and harden, and break off pieces to suck on as needed. For syrup, pour mixture into a thick glass jar and take 1 teaspoon as needed for cough, approximately 3 times a day.

Horehound

Place 1 cup of dried herb or 3 cups of fresh herb in a large glass bowl. Pour 1 and 1/2 cups of boiling water over herb, cover and let steep for 10 to 15 minutes. Place liquid in a saucepan and turn fire on low. Add 1/2 to 3/4 cup of honey, stirring slowly until honey dissolves. Simmer slow for 10 minutes. Let cool, place in an airtight jar, and refrigerate. Take 2 teaspoons 3 to 4 times a day.

Horehound drops

Follow directions for horehound syrup except add 1 to 2 cups of cane sugar instead of honey. Pour mixture into a flat pan lined with wax paper and allow to harden. Cut into small pieces before it hardens completely. Optional: Add peppermint or pine rosin. Take as needed.

Onion

Chop 1/2 to 1 whole onion and "rub" in a saucepan with 1 tablespoon cane sugar. Cook down to a syrup and take for cough. Bottle and use as necessary. Refrigerate when not using.

Pine cone or pine bark, pine tar (sap) and whiskey

Take a pine cone or bark with sap on it, cover with water in a pot, and low simmer for 30 minutes. Let sit in pot until water cools. Use 2 tablespoons whiskey or brandy to 1 cup of pine tea, add honey to taste and 1 lemon. This time-honored recipe acts as an expectorant and expels mucous. For strong medicine, let sit for 24 hours then use. Take 1 tablespoon 3 to 4 times a day. Keep in an air-tight jar, cover with a paper bag and store in a cool and dry cabinet or refrigerate.

Herb teas

To make any of the teas below, follow the standard recipe for making herb teas in the Internal Preparations section at the beginning of this chapter. For stronger brew, add 1 teaspoon more of herb to each cup of water, cover and steep for 20 to 30 minutes. Optional: add peppermint, lemon and/or honey. Drink 3 times daily. Use double the amount of herb if fresh and not dried.
  Bay leaf
  Eucalyptus
  Horehound
  Mullein
  Rabbit tobacco

Herb tea blends

Bay leaf and sage

Use 1 teaspoon each of bay leaf and sage per 1 cup of hot water, cover and steep for 20 minutes. Sweeten with honey and drink.

Pine, mullein, and horehound

Boil 4 to 6 cups of water. Add a handful of pine needles, 2 tablespoons of mullein, and 2 tablespoons of horehound. Cover and let steep for 30 to 60 minutes, then strain. Drink 3 times daily.

Smoke/Inhalants

Mullein

Place dried and packed mullein in a pipe or roll in a cigarette. Inhale deeply 2 to 3 times.

Rabbit tobacco

Place dried and packed rabbit tobacco in a pipe or roll in a cigarette. Inhale deeply 2 to 3 times.

Chest salves

Mustard plaster cast

(see also "Congestion" this chapter)

Use Vicks salve or make your own healing liniment using herbs like menthol, camphor, and eucalyptus. Rub on your chest and back.

Cramps

(for menstrual cramps see "Female Health" this chapter; for muscle cramps see "Muscle Strains And Cramps" this chapter)

Cuts And Wounds

Cuts and wounds were always cleaned first with cool to warm water and a mild soap if available before applying any of the medicines below.

Aloe vera

Wash the cut or wound with cool water. Pick a leaf from an aloe plant, scoop out the gel, and apply a generous amount to affected area. For deep cuts or wounds, pack aloe into the opening. Wrap with a sterile gauze or bandage. Change 1 to 2 times daily until area is healed. Applying aloe vera to cuts and wounds was done to prevent infection and speed the healing.

Aloe vera and spider webs

(also see below for use of spider webs without aloe vera)

For deep cuts or wounds that required sutures, the wound was squeezed closed as much as possible with fingers, the wound packed inside through the small opening with clean spider webs, and then spider webs spread across the top of the wound. The wound and web were then saturated with aloe vera gel and wrapped tightly. Wrapping was changed daily and the wound cleaned with water, the cleaning done carefully so as not to displace the spider web. Fresh aloe was reapplied 2 to 3 days later but the spider web was not removed. Sometimes cobwebs (abandoned spider webs) were used if spider webs could not be found.

The following account from a Northern California woman named Anon Forrest extols the power of the use of aloe vera and spider webs to heal deep wounds:

"When my daughter was 4, she severed her little toe on a split Manzanita branch while runnin' around in her flip flops. I mean, that toe was hanging by a thread, so I decided to just take it off. My daughter thought differently. So, instead of amputating, I cleaned the stub and toe by soaking them in a strong salt water solution of tepid water. I found a brand new cobweb about 4" wide, folded it until I had a nice wad of clean cobweb, applied it to the toe and stump, lined up the parts and mitered them, then squeezed Aloe vera leaves, soaking the cobweb. Then I wrapped the toe in sterile gauze, closing the gap between the foot and the rest of the toe, and bound her little toe to the neighboring toe to prevent the re-attached toe from moving away from the foot. I took this wrap off every 3 to 4 days to make sure it was clean and to reapply the Aloe vera by squeezing the juice over the gauze of the first wrap.

"About a week later, my neighbor, who's a doctor, looked at it with her flashlight and magnifying glass, and she saw connective tissue growing between the little toe and the stump. I waited about 6 weeks to make sure the toe had completely re-connected. The toe was fine, and my daughter went on and played soccer and everything else.

"I learned about using Aloe vera gel from my mother-in-law, whose own mother reconnected a

finger bone that was completely severed in a lawn mower accident. Even the bone and nerves reconnected!"

[Quoted by Dianne Durham in the article "The Allure of Aloe Vera" written specifically for my blog, Working The Roots. Dianne describes Anon Forrest as an earthy wise woman in her late 60's who is adept at natural healing and has lived remotely on a mountain in Northern California for 41 years.]

Baking soda packs

"Mama would put baking soda on a cut. She would pack it in there and keep it from bleedin and it would boil all those germs out of there." Levatus Gillory

Bay leaf

Clean wound. Gather a few fresh bay leaves and bruise to release the oil. Rub the leaf on affected area, apply leaf to wound, and wrap with a sterile bandage. Change daily.

Camphor

Used on cuts to prevent infection and stop pain and scarring.

"My grandmama used a lot of camphor from the trees. ... She'd boil it down and make a salve, like mentholatum, really potent. She put camphor on cuts and scars and that camphor would pull out the pain and infection." Bonita Sizemore

Castor oil

Apply castor oil drops or a castor oil pack to aid in healing. Wrap wound with a sterile bandage or wool cloth after application. This was done often at bedtime and left on overnight.

Chimney soot or coal ash

Cuts and wounds were packed with chimney soot or coal ash and wrapped with a clean cloth to stop bleeding and reduce infection. When bleeding stopped cut was rinsed off and repacked with ash.

Clay or "chalk" (white/bentonite)

Moist clay was applied over affected area and wrapped with a sterile bandage. Bandage was changed 2 to 3 times a day or when clay became hard. Good to stop bleeding.

Comfrey root

The root and leaves were mashed in their natural oil until it looked like jelly. Tallow, lard, or olive oil may have been added for smoother consistency. Medicine was rubbed on affected area and the affected area was then wrapped. Wrap was changed and fresh medicine applied 1 to 2 times a day.

Epsom salt

Wounds were soaked in warm/hot water and Epsom salt for 20 minutes to promote healing and prevent, reduce, and/or stop infection. After soaking, rinse with cool water and apply one of the other medicines suggested. Do Epsom salt soaks twice daily until healed.

Eucalyptus leaf oil

Clean wound. Gather a few fresh eucalyptus leaves and bruise to release the oil. Rub the leaves on affected area, apply leaves to wound, and wrap with a sterile bandage. Change daily.

Fire

Wrap cut with a woolen material and hold over a fire to draw out the poison.

Honey and Sulfur

Mix 1 teaspoon of honey with 1 teaspoon of sulfur, apply to wound/cut, and cover with a sterile bandage. Repeat once daily until healed.

Treatments For Specific Conditions - Cuts and Wounds (continued)

Onion poultice

Cut a slice of onion large enough to cover cut or wound. Apply directly to affected area and wrap with a sterile bandage. Change once or twice daily with a fresh onion slice until healed.

Sassafras root

Make a poultice or salve and apply to cut or wound and wrap area with a sterile bandage. Used to promote healing and reduce infection.[150]

Spider webs

"For puncture wounds, because we were always barefoot and stepping on nails, I remember my grandmother would make the wound bleed, and she would paddle it until it bled, we'd get all the poison out and cover it with spider webs and smut from the stove and wrap it up on your foot and then you'd be walking around." Ms. Etta Minor-Williams

Used to stop bleeding, to aid in healing and regeneration of cells, and to prevent infection. Gather clean, abandoned webs. Squeeze the wound was closed as much as possible with fingers, pack inside through the small opening with the spider webs, then spread remaining spider webs across the top of the wound. May be helpful to gently roll webs into a bundle before packing into wound.

Sugar Pack

To stop bleeding, sugar was used to pack cut or wound. When bleeding stopped, area was rinsed thoroughly and medicine was applied.

Sulfur and honey

Mix pure unadulterated sulfur with honey, apply to cut or wound, and cover with bandage. Reapply fresh sulfur and honey and change bandage once or twice daily.

Turpentine

Apply a few drops of pure gum turpentine to a wool patch that is large enough to cover cut or wound. Place patch over affected area. Use a bandage or tape to keep in place. Change once daily.

The turpentine can also be mixed with castor oil. To do so, add 4 drops of turpentine to 1/2 teaspoon of castor oil, mix well, and apply.

Diabetes

("High Sugar or Sugar")

Banana peel tea

Put a banana peel in a pot with water just enough to cover the peel. Bring to a slow boil, turn off the heat, cover, and let sit for 30 minutes. Drink three times a day.

White Mulberry leaf tea

Put 1 teaspoon of dried white mulberry leaves or 2 to 3 teaspoons of fresh white mulberry leaves in 1 cup of hot water, cover and steep for 15 to 20 minutes. Drink 1 cup of the brewed tea prior to each meal to help reduce blood sugar levels and maintain them at a healthy level.

Yellow root tea/tonic

Put 1 teaspoon of dried yellow root in 1 cup of hot water, cover and steep for 30 minutes. Drink 2 to

---

[150] An important warning note about sassafras and safrole: Sassafras contains safrole, which is known to have harmful effects if ingested over a period of time in large and concentrated quantities. See warning and instructions in the Sassafras section on pages 319-320 before using.

3 times daily. For a larger batch, put 1/4 to 1/2 cup of dried yellow root in a 1-quart mason jar. Fill the jar with lukewarm water, close the jar. and when the water turns deep yellow, it is ready to sip. Sip 2 to 3 times a day. Keep refrigerated.

Garlic

Some Southerners believed that eating 3 or more garlic cloves daily controlled their "high sugar." Garlic would be chopped, crushed, and added to food or relish dishes like chow-chow. The active ingredient in garlic, allicin, may lower blood glucose levels and also boost the immune system. To release allicin, garlic must be chopped or crushed.

Huckleberry

(ground berries and leaves)

Leaves

Make a tea from the leaves and drink 1 to 3 times daily.

Berries

Grind the dried berries and make a tea using 1 teaspoon of powdered berries to 1 cup of hot water. Drink 3 cups daily.

Low glycemic diet

Many Southerners naturally ate a low glycemic diet rich with greens, grains, legumes. Processed foods were eaten rarely. Meat was often a luxury and added to foods for flavoring. Many hunted for their meat, eating lean wild game such as squirrel, raccoon, deer, small birds, and also fish. A low glycemic diet does not cause huge spikes in blood sugar when digested.

Mr. Red's tonic for "high sugar"

Combine equal parts of the ingredients below in a pot. Cover with cold water 2 to 3 inches above ingredients. Bring to a boil and let sit covered for 60 minutes. Cool, strain, and put in a jug or jar. Refrigerate and sip on three times a day.
  Green pine tops
  Pine straw (pine needles)
  Lion's tongue (spotted wintergreen)
  Peach tree leaves
  Yellow root

Spanish Moss

Drink 3 cups daily to treat diabetes. Gather the Spanish moss, wash it in cool water, and place enough to cover the bottom of a small pot. Cover with water and bring to a boil, remove from heat, put covering over the pot, and let steep for 10 to 15 minutes. Pour liquid in a clean glass container and store in refrigerator.

Diarrhea

Blackberry root tea

Simmer 1 tablespoon of root per cup of water for 15 minutes, then strain. Sip about 1/4 cup of blackberry root tea per hour until symptoms subside.

Clay

(white, bentonite)

Take 1 teaspoon to 1 tablespoon of white clay every 1 to 2 hours until symptoms subside. Drink 8 ounces of water after each dose.

Treatments For Specific Conditions (continued)

Ear Problems

Earache

Apple cider vinegar

Place 2 to 3 drops of diluted apple cider vinegar (ACV) in affected ear. Make the solution 1 part ACV to 1 part water. For young children, a weaker solution of 1 part ACV to 2 parts water was made. Cover affected area with cotton ball and tilt head to side for 20 minutes. Repeat one other day if necessary.

Peroxide and Water

*"My mother would get two teaspoons of water to one of peroxide and heat it up, so it's just warm. She'd tell [you] to put your head down, and dip cotton in the solution and squeeze it down the ear. You could hear the ear crackling from the peroxide bubbling up. She'd wait a few minutes, then turn [you] over and do the other side."*Anita Poree

After this treatment, the ears were plugged with a cotton ball and the person laid down for 30 to 60 minutes.

Sweet oil, garlic oil

Add 4 chopped garlic cloves to 4 teaspoons of olive or coconut oil. Place in a small saucepan and slowly warm until garlic sizzles. Turn off fire, cover, and let cool to lukewarm. Pour mixture in a small glass jar. Use an eyedropper to place 2 to 3 drops of mixture in affected ear. Plug ear up with a cotton ball and lie down for 30 minutes so oil can drain down to infection. Use right before bed. If used during daytime, do same as above and lay down for 30 minutes and leave cotton ball in ear most of day. Store mixture in refrigerator and warm the jar or bottle in a pot of hot water to warm up the mixture when using this medicine again.

Tobacco Smoke

Dried tobacco was gathered, cut, and put in a pipe or rolled as a cigarette. It was lit, inhaled, and smoke blown directly into infected ear while cupping both hands around the ear to direct smoke into ear cavity.

Earwax removal

Sweet oil/Olive oil

Put two drops of warm oil in the affected ear, cover with a cotton ball, and lie down ear side up for 30 to 60 minutes or best to do overnight. The oil eventually softens the build-up. Rinse with warm water if the clump does not come out immediately. Repeat one more time if necessary.

Hydrogen peroxide and apple cider vinegar

Make a solution of 1 part apple cider vinegar (ACV) and 1 part hydrogen peroxide. Put 2 drops into affected ear, cover with a cotton ball, and lie down ear side up for 30 to 60 minutes or overnight. The build-up should break up and be easily removed. If not, use warm water to flush it out. Repeat another day if necessary.

Edema/Water Retention/Fluid Retention

Dandelion leaf and/or root tea

Make a tea with the leaf, root, or a combination of both. Drink 3 cups a day. Dandelion acts as a diuretic and also is rich with potassium.

Stinging Nettles tea

Make a tea and drink 3 or more cups daily to remove excess water from the body.

Erectile Dysfunction

("For a strong nature")

(see also "Men's Health" this chapter)

Maintaining a "strong nature" is important to men of all cultures. Decreased libido and erectile dysfunction are becoming increasingly more common today as men age. Some of the causes of today's impotency problems may be illness or the side effects of pharmaceutical medications taken for blood pressure, high cholesterol, diabetes, obesity, lack of exercise, or one of the side effects of enlarged prostate. The natural remedies below have been used to help men maintain or redevelop a "strong nature."

Coon root tea

Put 1 teaspoon of the dried root in 1 cup of boiled water, cover and steep for 10 to 15 minutes. Drink 3 cups daily.

Horny goat weed

My father used horny goat weed until he transitioned at age 78. Prior to that, he had a healthy five-year relationship with his girlfriend who was 46 years at the time of his earthly departure. Horny goat weed has been used in Traditional Chinese Medicine for over 5,000 years as an aphrodisiac that improves male sex drive. While it is often in use among African Americans today, it was not a staple in early African American healing tradition.

Raw Oysters

Raw oysters were the traditional aphrodisiac of choice among men and women living in the southern states that border the Gulf and Mississippi River, including Louisiana, Mississippi, Alabama, and Florida. Recent scientific research has shown that raw oysters do have chemical compounds that, when eaten, release the sex hormones testosterone and estrogen.

Saw Palmetto

Successful in treating enlarged and swollen prostate and its side effects such as erectile dysfunction.

Eye Conditions

Sty in eye

Apple cider vinegar

Make an apple cider vinegar (ACV) wash, 1 tablespoon to 1/4 cup of water, and put 1 to 2 drops in eye 2 to 3 times daily. Also use a Q-tip to put ACV wash directly on sty. If it stings too much, dilute the wash solution, 1 teaspoon at a time.

Castor oil

Place 1 to 2 drops on sty or in eye 2 to 3 times daily, especially at night.

Saline wash

Make a warm saline wash, 1 teaspoon salt to 1/4 cup of water, and put 1 to 2 drops in eye 2 to 3 times daily until gone. Place remaining wash in a glass jar and store in refrigerator. Can use cold in future applications.

Eye Health

Bilberry tea

Bring to boil 1 cup of fresh dried bilberries in 2 to 3 cups of water. Slow boil for 20 minutes, let sit for 10 minutes, and drink 1 cup. Continue drinking throughout the day, refilling pot with water and reheating. Potency reduces but is still medicinal.

Female Health

The natural medicines below have traditionally been used for centuries to give women relief from menstrual and menopausal discomfort.

A NOTE OF CAUTION: *The effectiveness of any medicine—pharmaceutical or herbal—can vary greatly especially when treating women's health. This variation may depend on the use of the proper dosage catered to the unique needs of each woman, and depends entirely on whether or not that medicine is an effective healing agent for each individual body. I have found this particularly true when taking natural medicines to balance hormones to treat PMS, peri-menopause, menopause and other female related problems.*

Blue and black cohosh in particular are very potent medicines and were not taken long-term (more than 7 days) or while pregnant. These medicines were used with caution or under the guidance of a health professional. With all medicines it is always best to start with the lowest dosage, and increase to maximum dosage without adverse side effects. Adverse side effects may be headache, nausea, vomiting, or diarrhea. If one experiences adverse side effects, then dosage should be stopped. If you have any concerns, consult your health care professional.

Fertility

Drink Queen's Delight tea.

Hormone regulation and general maintenance

Chasteberry/vitex

Chasteberry/vitex is a gentle hormone regulator that works well if taken consistently over time. It is available in capsule, tincture, or fresh or dried berry. The dried berries can be found in tea bags or in bulk.

For capsule, take 200 to 400 mg twice daily for 1 month, then reduce to 1 time per day.

If taking tincture from a health food manufacturer, take suggested dosage as directed on the bottle or other package. If making own tincture from dried berries, take 30 to 40 drops (about 1 dropper full) once daily.

If tea bag is bought from the store, take as directed.

If making own tea from fresh or dried chasteberries, put 1 teaspoon of fresh or dried berries in 1 cup of hot water, cover and steep for 10 to 15 minutes. Drink twice daily for 1 month, then reduce to drinking once daily.

While it is often in use among African Americans today, chasteberry/vitex was not a staple in early African American healing tradition.

Evening Primrose Oil

While evening primrose oil is often in use among African American women today, it was not a staple in early African American healing tradition. Suggested dose: 500 to 1,000 mg daily.

Lydia E. Pinkham (Lydia Pinkham Herbal Compound)

Take as directed.

Menopause

The following remedies can be taken to ease the symptoms of menopause.

Black cohosh

Put 1 to 2 teaspoons in 1 cup of hot water, cover and steep for 15 to 20 minutes. Drink twice daily.

Alternatively, take 20 to 40 mg in capsule or tablet form twice daily, or as directed on bottle. (**A note of caution**: Black cohosh is a very potent medicine and was not taken long-term (more than 7 days) or while pregnant. This medicine was used with caution or under the guidance of a health professional.)

Chasteberry/vitex

While chasteberry/vitex is often in use among African Americans today, it was not a staple in early African American healing tradition. Take 400 to 500 mg, usually in the form of dry pill or tincture. Alternatively, put 2 teabags in 1 cup of hot water, cover and steep for 10 to 15 minutes.

Lydia E. Pinkham (Lydia Pinkham Herbal Compound)

Take as directed.

Evening primrose oil

While evening primrose oil is often in use among African American women today, it was not a staple in early African American healing tradition. Suggested dosage: 500 to 1,000 mg twice daily.

Flaxseed oil

Suggested dosage: 1 teaspoon to 1 tablespoon of flaxseed oil daily to help reduce symptoms during menopause.

Menstruation (Menses)

Cramps

Black cohosh tea

(hormone regulator, nervine/pain reducer, antispasmodic)

Drink 1 to 3 cups of tea daily to ease symptoms. Put 1 teaspoon of dried root in 1 cup of hot water, cover and steep for 10 to 15 minutes. (**A note of caution**: Black cohosh is a very potent medicine and was not taken long-term (more than 7 days) or while pregnant. This medicine was used with caution or under the guidance of a health professional.)

Catnip tea

Drink 2 to 4 cups daily. Put 1 to 2 teaspoons of catnip in 1 cup of hot water, cover and steep for 10 to 15 minutes.

Sassafras bark tea

"I used to take sassafras bark and make tea for cramps. I'd boil the bark down with little sticks a little bit longer than your finger. You put two or three of them in there and you boil that down. I remember really figuring out that if I got it soon, then I wouldn't have those cramps." Bonita Sizemore[151]

Lydia Pinkham Herbal Compound

"Now if you got some Lydia E. Pinkham and you look on the bottle you'll see Jamaica dogwood root, sassafras and these kinds of things in the formula. If we wanted to find that stuff around here, we'd have to go this drugstore on 62nd and Foothill [in Oakland, CA]. These other drugstores don't know nothing about no Lydia E. Pinkham. That compound that my mother used you could find in an old Black drugstore." Luisah Teish

Lydia E. Pinkham is a 19th century herbal tonic that was developed by Lydia Pinkham in 1875. The tonic was specifically formulated with herbs traditionally found to aid in relieving menstrual and menopausal discomfort.

The original tonic included five herbs: unicorn root, life root, black cohosh, pleurisy root, and fenugreek seed.

---

[151] An important warning note about sassafras and safrole: Sassafras contains safrole, which is known to have harmful effects if ingested over a period of time in large and concentrated quantities. See warning and instructions in the Sassafras section on pages 319-320 before using.

Treatments For Specific Conditions - Cramps (continued)

A later version of the tonic was formulated with these seven natural herbs: motherwort, gentian, Jamaican dogwood, black cohosh, pleurisy root, licorice, dandelion, and Vitamins C and E; 10% ethyl alcohol as a preservative.

Today, Lydia Pinkham Herbal Compound is marketed by Numark Laboratories and can be bought online or at selected drug stores across the country.

For more information see the Lydia E. Pinkham information in the next chapter, "Medicines," Part II, Chapter 8.

Magnesium or Epsom salt

Diets were supplemented with magnesium right before the start of the menstrual cycle to reduce cramps and edginess. This was done by an Epsom salt soak or by drinking an Epsom salt tonic of 1/2 teaspoon Epsom salt to 1 cup of water. Many women I interviewed said they didn't get cramps or have PMS. This could be due to the staple diet of many African Americans in the South being dark leafy greens and beans which are both high in magnesium. Today, many women take magnesium supplements to ease menstrual cramps or an Epsom salt bath.

Heavy bleeding (Menorrhagia)

There are many reasons why women may experience heavy bleeding during menses. Possible causes are hormonal imbalance, perimenopause, fibroid tumors, cervical or endometrial polyps, uterine or cervical cancer. The following were taken to relieve some of the symptoms.

Black cohosh tea

(hormone regulator, nervine/pain reducer, antispasmodic)

Drink 1 to 3 cups of tea daily to ease symptoms. Put 1 teaspoon of dried root in 1 cup of hot water, cover and steep for 10 to 15 minutes. (**A note of caution**: Black cohosh is a very potent medicine and was not taken long-term (more than 7 days) or while pregnant. This medicine was used with caution or under the guidance of a health professional.)

Chasteberry/vitex

While chasteberry/vitex is often in use among African Americans today, it was not a staple in early African American healing tradition. Take 400 to 500 mg, usually in the form of dry pill or tincture. Alternatively, put 2 teabags in 1 cup of hot water, cover and steep for 10 to 15 minutes.

Lydia E. Pinkham (Lydia Pinkham Herbal Compound)

Take as directed.

Other herbs many women use today that help relieve heavy menses: cinnamon bark, cramp bark, dong quai, raspberry leaf, shepherd's purse, and yarrow.

PMS (pre-menstrual syndrome)

Symptoms of PMS may include cramps, headaches, anxiety, mood swings and/or heavy menstrual flow. The following remedies can be taken to alleviate the symptoms of PMS.

Chasteberry/vitex

While chasteberry/vitex is often in use among African Americans today, it was not a staple in early African American healing tradition. Take 400 to 500 mg, usually in the form of dry pill or tincture. Alternatively, put 2 teabags in 1 cup of hot water, cover and steep for 10 to 15 minutes.

Lydia E. Pinkham (Lydia Pinkham Herbal Compound)

Take as directed.

Flaxseed oil

Suggested dosage: 1 teaspoon to 1 tablespoon of flaxseed oil daily to reduce PMS symptoms.

Eating clay for the mineral content

Three days prior to menstruation, mix 1 teaspoon to 1 tablespoon of clay in a warm cup water and drink before bedtime. This may help alleviate cramps, bloating, headaches and irritability associated with PMS.

Magnesium or Epsom salt

Diets were supplemented with magnesium right before the start of the menstrual cycle to reduce cramps and edginess. This was done by an Epsom salt soak or by drinking an Epsom salt tonic of 1/2 teaspoon Epsom salt to 1 cup of water. Many women I interviewed said they didn't get cramps or have PMS. This could be due to the staple diet of many African Americans in the South being dark leafy greens and beans which are both high in magnesium. Today, many women take magnesium supplements to ease menstrual cramps or an Epsom salt bath.

Evening primrose oil

While evening primrose oil is often in use among African Americans today, it was not a staple in early African American healing tradition. Suggested dosage: 500 to 1,000 mg 3 times daily. Because it takes natural remedies longer to effect change in the body, it may take 6 to 8 weeks before any relief is noticed, and then the dosage can be reduced to taking daily only 1 to 2 weeks prior to menstrual cycle to maintain positive effects.

Suppressed menstruation/missed periods (Amenorrhea)

The following can be taken to relieve the symptoms of suppressed menstruation/missed periods.

Black cohosh tea

(hormone regulator, nervine/pain reducer, antispasmodic)

Drink 1 to 3 cups of tea daily to ease symptoms. Put 1 teaspoon of dried root in 1 cup of hot water, cover and steep for 10 to 15 minutes. (**A note of caution**: Black cohosh is a very potent medicine and was not taken long-term (more than 7 days) or while pregnant. This medicine was used with caution or under the guidance of a health professional.)

Chasteberry/vitex

While chasteberry/vitex is often in use among African Americans today, it was not a staple in early African American healing tradition. Take 400 to 500 mg, usually in the form of dry pill or tincture. Alternatively, put 2 teabags in 1 cup of hot water, cover and steep for 10 to 15 minutes.

Lydia E. Pinkham (Lydia Pinkham Herbal Compound)

Take as directed.

Perimenopause

Perimenopause refers to the time during which a woman's body is progressing toward menopause. During perimenopause, hormone levels rise and fall unevenly, menstrual cycles are irregular, and a woman may experience menopause-like symptoms such as hot flashes, insomnia, and vaginal dryness.

Below are commonly-used and/or traditional remedies that have helped alleviate symptoms of menopause for many women.

Black cohosh tea

(hormone regulator, nervine/pain reducer, antispasmodic)

Drink 1 to 3 cups of tea daily to ease symptoms. Put 1 teaspoon of dried root in 1 cup of hot water, cover and steep for 10 to 15 minutes. (**A note of caution**: Black cohosh is a very potent medicine and

Treatments For Specific Conditions - Perimenopause (continued)

was not taken long-term (more than 7 days) or while pregnant. This medicine was used with caution or under the guidance of a health professional.)

Chasteberry/vitex

While chasteberry/vitex is often in use among African Americans today, it was not a staple in early African American healing tradition. Take 400 to 500 mg, usually in the form of dry pill or tincture. Alternatively, put 2 teabags in 1 cup of hot water, cover and steep for 10 to 15 minutes.

Evening primrose oil

While primrose oil is often in use among African Americans today, it was not a staple in early African American healing tradition. Take 250 to 500 mg twice daily.

Flaxseed oil

Take 1 to 2 tablespoons of flaxseed oil daily.

Lydia E. Pinkham (Lydia Pinkham Herbal Compound)

Take as directed.

Pregnancy support

Clay/chalk

Geophagy, the habit of eating all forms of earth such as clay, dirt, and mud, is practiced worldwide. Eating clay is usually associated with women of childbearing age. Pregnant women usually crave clay for its mineral content, which includes many essential minerals such as potassium, calcium, phosphorus, magnesium, copper, zinc, manganese, and iron, as well as many trace minerals. Most people who use medicinal clay today purchase bentonite from their natural medicine store and take as directed (usually 1 tablespoon on an empty stomach followed by a full glass of water and drinking plenty of water throughout the day afterwards).

"We used to feed women Mississippi clay dirt and I remember folks sendin for dirt from Mississippi and eat starch until they got it. I remember my Aunt Marybelle Reed, bless her heart. She was in that in-between place because she knows all this root stuff and she'd also gone to nursing school so she had a foot in both worlds. Aunt Marybelle Reed would send for Mississippi clay dirt. And she would put it on a cookie sheet and run it in a slow oven sumtin like 250 degrees and she would leave it in over night, pull it out and pound it and give pregnant women Mississippi clay dirt—for the mineral content." Luisah Teish

Induce labor (post term)

Castor oil

Take 1 tablespoon to *"help induce labor if you are past your due date."* Eveline Prayo-Bernard

Blue cohosh

Blue cohosh was sometimes used to stimulate uterine contractions to deliver babies. Black cohosh may have been used in conjunction with blue cohosh. (*A note of caution*: Blue cohosh is a very potent medicine and was not taken long-term (more than 7 days) or while pregnant. This medicine was used with caution or under the guidance of a health professional.)

Stretch marks

Women have rubbed the following salves on their stomach to successfully prevent, reduce, and eliminate stretch marks: aloe vera gel, cocoa butter, lanolin, olive oil, shea butter. Greater success if salve is used throughout pregnancy, before stomach stretches.

Fertility

(For Women's Fertility see "Female Health" this chapter)
(For Men's Fertility see "Men's Health" and "Erectile Dysfunction" this chapter)

Fever

Buttonwillow tea and cool bath or soak

Make a stronger tea than the usual method by adding 2 to 3 teaspoons of herb (instead of the usual 1 to 2 teaspoons) to 1 cup of hot water. Drink several cups until fever breaks. For soak, add 1 to 2 cups of dried herb or 2 to 4 cups of fresh herb to hot bath water. Soak when bath is cool.

Catnip tea

Drink 3 or more cups until fever breaks.

Pine tree limb, mullein, and horehound tea

"Gather limbs from the pine tree that has pine rosin. Put the pine limbs, mullein and horehound in a pot, cover with water and cook down. Drink three times daily and right before bed to sweat out the fever." Author unknown

Castor oil (also known as the oil bush plant) and castor oil leaves

"Do you all remember the castor oil tree? My mother used to rub me down with some oil and she wrapped my body in the castor oil leaves at night and the next morning those leaves would be dry like they were dried in an oven. They took all the fever out of my body. It's a tree with big wide leaves." Eveline Prayo-Bernard

Rub castor oil on chest and abdomen and cover with a woolen cloth. Alternatively, wrap the body in castor leaves and leave on until parched, remove, and replace with fresh leaves until fever breaks. The pores in the skin naturally absorb the oil from the leaves and the body will receive the medicinal benefits.

Cool water compress and wash

Place a cool compress on the head. Wash back, chest, and stomach with cool water to bring body temperature down until fever breaks.

Eucalyptus leaf poultice

Wrap eucalyptus leaves in a piece of gauze that is long enough to wrap around your forehead. Pour hot water over the gauze to release the oils in the leaf. Wrap around your head for one hour. Repeat with fresh leaves until fever is gone.

Flaxseed poultice

* Soak several wool, gauze, or cotton cloth strips in flaxseed oil. While you may need several strips for a full treatment, you will only use them one at a time. Wrap one of the strips around the forehead and leave on for one hour. If fever persists, remove the first strip and immediately replace with another. Repeat every hour until fever breaks.

* Grind 1/2 to 1 cup of flaxseeds with a mortar and pestle. Cut a layer of gauze that can wrap around your head 2 to 3 times. Place ground flaxseeds in gauze and fold a layer of gauze over the seeds. Pour hot water over the gauze and seeds to release the medicine. Wrap gauze poultice around forehead and leave on for 1 hour. Repeat every hour until fever breaks.

Treatments For Specific Conditions - Fever (continued)

Mullein leaf and chicken head poultice

"Mullein was used for fever. They would take a mullein leaf and put it on your head and it was supposed to draw the fever out of your body. My mother would wrap the chicken head in the mullein leaf and put it on your head." Author unknown

Peach tree leaf body wrap

Take a bucket full of peach tree leaves. Wet them with water and shake or strain the water off. Spread the leaves on a sheet and wrap the person up in the sheet with the leaves. When the leaves are dry and parched, remove and repeat process until fever is out.

Peach tree leaf poultice

Take one cupful of peach tree leaves. Put the leaves in a cheesecloth poultice and soak in vinegar for 10 minutes. Place the poultice on stomach. Remove and replace with fresh leaves when poultice is dry.

Pine rosin, honey, and turpentine

"There was something we called rosin. It looks like the honey out of the pine tree. Draw it out, cut it up and mix with 3 tablespoons of turpentine. Sweeten with honey and take 1 tablespoon for fever with colds." Author unknown

Quinine and castor oil mixture

Quinine has been traditionally used worldwide to treat fevers associated with malaria. It was also used in the rural South to break fevers. There are no dosages with this remedy.

Vicks salve rubbed

Vicks salve rubbed on chest and back is useful in reducing fever. Also, the salve can be mixed with castor oil to make it more effective.

Fever Blister

Aloe vera gel

Apply aloe vera gel 3 times or more daily until gone.

Ear wax

At onset, apply wax from your ear on affected area as often as possible.

Earwax and yellow root (goldenseal)

"If you get fever blisters, you take earwax and put it on the fever blister and it would go away." Levatus Gillory

Eucalyptus oil

Apply the oil with a Q-tip or cotton swab 3 to 5 times daily at onset until gone. To make eucalyptus oil, place 1/4 – 1/2 cup of eucalyptus leaves and 1 cup of olive oil in a crockpot and slow-cook for 6 hours. Cool, strain, and place oil in a dark colored glass bottle with an airtight top.

Tea tree oil

While tea tree oil is often in use among African Americans today, it was not a staple in early African American healing tradition.

Apply with a cotton swab or Q-tip twice daily until gone. Dilute with olive oil to prevent skin irritation.

Flatulence/Gas

(see also "Stomach Problems" chapter)

Drinking liquids during a meal can interfere with digestive juices your body produces and can cause gas and indigestion. Adding spices like garlic and bay leaf while cooking food helps digestion. Making Southern style chow-chow relish and eating as a side dish also naturally helps digestion (see ingredients below).

Catnip tea

Sip 1 cup of tea 30 to 60 minutes before a meal and 15 minutes after a meal.

Mint/Horsemint/Peppermint tea

Sip one cup of tea 30 to 60 minutes before and 15 minutes after a meal.

Astifidity/Asafoetida

Add a pinch of powdered astifidity to a cup of warm water and sip.

Baking soda

Completely dissolve 1/2 teaspoon of baking soda in 1/2 cup of water. Consume slowly by sipping. Drink no more than 3 times a day to relieve gas.

Castor oil

Take 1 tablespoon to alleviate symptoms and get your digestive system moving.

Chow-chow

There are numerous variations for this Southern relish side dish. The ingredients are: cabbage, onion, tomatoes, green bell peppers, red bell peppers, white vinegar, water, salt, and sugar. Variations also may add powdered mustard, horseradish, celery, hot peppers, ground ginger, and/or turmeric.

Garlic

Add garlic to food while cooking no longer than 10 minutes before meal is finished cooking. Garlic should be cooked for no longer than 10 minutes.

Ginger

While ginger is often in use among African Americans today, it was not a staple in early African American healing tradition. After a meal, eat fresh ginger slices or drink ginger tea to help alleviate flatulence/gas.

Foot Health

Aching/tired feet

Epsom salt

Soak in a hot Epsom salt bath for 30 minutes or longer. Add 1 cup of Epsom salt to small tub of water. Can also add apple cider vinegar (ACV) to bath. Then rub castor oil on feet and cover with socks.

Castor oil

Massage feet with a generous amount of warm castor oil and then cover with cotton socks. Best to do at bedtime. Optional: soak feet in Epsom salt before rubbing castor oil on feet.

Treatments For Specific Conditions - Foot Health (continued)

Athlete's foot
(see "Athlete's Foot" this chapter)

Calluses

Castor oil

Massage a generous amount of castor oil to callused area and cover foot with sock. This treatment works day or night.

Tallow/talla

Apply a generous amount on callused area and cover with cotton socks. Apply at nighttime to let the tallow soften skin overnight. Once it has softened scrub callus with a pumice stone or foot shaver to remove dead skin. Tallow can be mixed with another oil like olive oil or shea butter.

Corns
(see "Corns On Toe" this chapter)

Fungus on feet
(see "Fungus" this chapter)

Gout
(see "Gout" this chapter)

Swollen feet/edema

Mullein

Make a mullein leaf bath in a foot tub using 4 to 5 leaves and soak feet for at least 30 minutes. Repeat 1 to 2 times daily. Also drink mullein tea.

Oak Bark

Shave several pieces (4 to 5) of oak bark from a tree and place in a foot tub of hot water. Soak feet for 30 to 60 minutes. Repeat 1 to 2 times daily. Also drink oak bark tea up to 3 cups daily.

Fungus: ringworm, athlete's foot, jock itch, candidiasis

(see also "Athlete's Foot" this chapter)

Fungi are microorganisms that can exist everywhere and on everything. Fungi flourish in a warm, moist atmosphere whether in soil, air, plants, water, or on the human body, especially the skin. When present on the skin, some of these organisms can lead to infection. Common types of fungal skin infections are athlete's foot (affecting all parts of the foot but especially the sole and between the toes), ringworm, jock itch (affecting the external male genital area), and candidiasis (affecting the external vagina area). The remedies below have been used to treat topical fungal infections.

Apple cider vinegar

Soak a cotton ball or makeup pad in apple cider vinegar (ACV) and place it on the ringworm/fungus infection. Fix it with an adhesive bandage twice a day until ringworm is gone. Apply a fresh application twice a day until ringworm or other fungus infection is gone.

Black tar soap

Wash and scrub on affected area. This treatment was often used right before applying other treatments in this section.

Castor oil

Rub a layer on affected area 2 to 3 times daily. Cover with an adhesive bandage after application. Clean area with black tar soap prior to each application. Use a generous amount for night-time application and cover with a sock or bandage.

Cedar wash

Place fresh leaves, twigs, and berries in a pot of hot water that has already been boiled. Use 1 cup of cedar matter to 1 cup of water. Let soak in the hot water until cool. Strain liquid into a bowl through a cheesecloth. Pour the liquid into a jar so you can use as a wash to apply to ringworm and other skin conditions.

Coon Root

Apply coon root/bloodroot directly or make a wash or salve to treat ringworm, skin fungus, eczema, herpes, and warts and to repel insects.

Direct application: harvest and clean the root, crush to release the medicine and juice, then apply to affected area 2 times daily.

Wash: steep 2 to 3 teaspoons of root in 1 cup of hot water. Cool and then strain out the solid matter. Add and mix in 2 tablespoons of vinegar. Store in a glass jar in the refrigerator. Use 2 to 3 times daily until condition is gone.

Salve: for the treatment of warts and other skin conditions, crush the root in a grinder or in a bowl with pestle. Mix with a natural vegetable oil until it is creamy. Add 1 tablespoon apple cider vinegar to mixture. For future use, put mixture in a glass jar and store in a cool, dark, dry place or put in paper bag and store in refrigerator. After washing apply a small amount to affected area 2 to 3 times daily.

Fig Juice

Break open a fig leaf and use the milk sap from the leaf to rub on the ringworm lesion. Repeat several times a day until gone. The leaf has antifungal properties.

Green walnut hulls

Open the green outer hull of a black walnut and rub the inside of the hull on the affected area. Make a poultice by scooping out the inside of the hull, placing on affected area and wrapping with a bandage. Repeat 3 times or more daily until gone. Clean area well before each application.

Jerusalem weed

Commonly used as a wash to treat skin fungus such as ringworm or athletes foot. Make a wash by adding 3 teaspoons of leaves and flowers to hot water. Cover and steep until cool, then drain. Pour liquid into a glass jar. Use as a wash on affected area 2 to 3 times daily. Store in refrigerator when not using.

Mulberry tree

A milky juice similar to fig milk can be found in parts of the red mulberry. It can be applied to skin to treat ringworm and other fungal skin conditions.

Orange weed

Used to treat a variety of skin conditions such as body sores, ringworm, and itchy rashes like poison oak and ivy. Crush the leaves to release the medicine and rub on affected area several times a day. Make a wash by crushing or bruising enough leaves to fill a pot about 3/4ths of the way to the top. Pour in cool water, making sure the water covers the leaves about 1 inch over. Bring to a slow boil, remove from heat, and cover. Let cool and strain liquid into a clean glass container. Apply the wash/liquid on affected area several times a day.

Penny and Vinegar

Soak a penny in vinegar for 6 to 8 hours. Rub the soaked penny on affected area, then tape the penny

Treatments For Specific Conditions - Fungus - Penny and Vinegar (continued)

to the area. Do this twice daily, cleaning area each time. When the copper reacts with vinegar, it creates a fungi-killing effect.

Pokeberry

Wash area with cool water, then rub the juice of a pokeberry on affected area 1 to 2 times daily until condition is gone.

Poke root

Make a poultice or a salve from the poke root and apply to affected area twice daily after washing with cool water.

Sarsaparilla root poultice

Chop and mash the sarsaparilla root and apply mixture to affected area twice daily after cleaning. Wrap with a gauze or bandage to hold the mixture on.

Sweet gum tree sweet gum balls

Gather sweet gum balls/fruit and crush them to break them into small pieces. Put them in a saucepan or skillet and cook them on medium heat until they soften. Add a natural vegetable oil or tallow to make creamy. Mix well and let cool. Apply to affected area 2 to 4 times daily after washing with cool water. Store remainder in a glass jar in a cool dark place or in refrigerator if you use tallow.

Gas

(see "Flatulence/Gas" this chapter)

Gout

Gout is a painful health problem that is usually felt in the big toe. Gout is caused by the body's inability to break down uric acid resulting in uric acid crystals accumulating in tissues and joints causing pain and inflammation.

Apple cider vinegar

Mix 1 teaspoon to 1 tablespoon of honey in 1/8 cup of warm water with 1 to 2 tablespoons of raw apple cider vinegar (ACV) containing "the mother," the tiny, web-like ball of living enzymes and nutrients in raw, unpasteurized, unfiltered ACV that makes this liquid an active healing agent. Drink twice a day. Works best as a preventative and also at the first onset of a gout attack.

Black cherry juice

Make a juice from 1/2 to 1 cup of black cherries and drink daily to prevent and treat gout.

Castor oil poultice

Use a castor oil pack. Soak a piece of white flannel in warm castor oil, wring out excess, and place over the affected area. Cover it with plastic wrap and apply heat using a heating pad or hot water bottle. Do this 2 times a day, leaving on for 30 to 60 minutes.

Celery

Seeds

Boil 1 tablespoon of celery seeds in 2 cups of water until seeds are soft. Cool and strain. Drink 1 cup of the broth four times a day until symptoms are relieved.

Stock broth

Chop up one entire bunch of celery, put in a pot, cover with water, and bring to boil. Turn off water and let cool. Drink the broth freely and eat the celery.

Cod liver oil

Take 1 teaspoon to 1 tablespoon per day of cod liver oil.

Mullein/Mullet

Soak your feet in a mullein bath, drink the tea, and make a poultice to treat gout.

Mullein foot soak

Take 2 to 3 large leaves, cut them up, and place in hot foot bath. Soak feet for 30 minutes in the bath. Optional: add Epsom salt.

Mullein tea

Add 1 teaspoon of dried mullein leaves to 1 cup of water. Cover and steep for 10 to 15 minutes. Drink 3 times daily. This tea reduced swelling and helped dissolve and eliminate the uric acid crystals through urine.

Mullein poultice

Soak leaves in warm water about 5 minutes, until soft and saturated. Take the leaf and wrap around affected area and secure with a damp, warm cloth (cheese cloth, cotton, or wool). Leave on for 30 minutes. Sometimes castor oil was rubbed on affected area prior to the leaf application.

Hair and Scalp

Apple cider vinegar

Saturate the scalp with apple cider vinegar (ACV) to treat dandruff and an itchy, flaky scalp. Leave on for 30 minutes and then rinse. ACV helped normalize the hair's natural pH.

Castor oil

Use castor oil to moisturize hair and treat scalp conditions.

Horsemint Salve

"When we was kids, we used to add some lard or Vaseline or whatever you want to haasmint (horsemint) and let it cook down, and oooh, it smell good. We used to put it in our hair. It make your hair grow too, we had the softest hair." Valena Noble

Olive oil, Coconut oil or Lanolin salve

"My mother used to put straight up oil in my hair. Olive oil, coconut oil, lanolin!" Anita Poree

Prickly pear salve

"We had prickly pear growin' in the yard, and Momma would take the prickly pear, pull the thorns out, skin it, and fry it. She always said it had to be in a cast iron skillet. She would fry the prickly pear in vaseline until it turned green and then she would strain that through three layers of cheese cloth. There'd be this film of very, very fine pricklies left in there. She would pour that in a jar and put it in the refrigerator and leave it there a certain period of time. And that was what she used to oil our scalp with." Luisah Teish

Sulfur

"A pure unadulterated sulfur salve is a wonderful healer. I would use this for sores, scratches and scars." Anita Poree

Treatments For Specific Conditions (continued)

Headaches and Migraines

Bay leaf tea

Make a tea using 1 whole dried bay leaf or 2 fresh bay leaves in 1 cup of hot water, cover and steep for 10 to 15 minutes. Drink 3 cups daily to treat headaches and migraines. Optional: add 1 teaspoon of turmeric[152] to increase effectiveness and reduce pain and inflammation.

Carmacrishan[153]

Soak rag in a solution with leaves and water, then wrap around head.

Flaxseed

Poultice for fever and headache

Crush or grind 2 to 4 tablespoons of flaxseeds with a mortar and pestle or coffee grinder. Place the ground flaxseeds in a long strip of gauze or cotton cloth that is long enough to wrap around your head 3 to 4 times. Fold the gauze lengthwise to cover the flaxseed. Pour hot water over the flaxseeds in the gauze. This releases the oil. Let poultice cool enough to wrap around forehead. The flaxseed part must touch the forehead. Tie the end of the gauze tight enough so it stays on your head. Lie down for 30 to 60 minutes.

Vinegar

"And then when we had headaches, [Mama] would put vinegar on a brown paper bag and put it across your forehead and we lie down and it would go away." Levatus Gillory

Yellow root (goldenseal)

Tea

Drink a cup of yellow root tea and then make the poultice below.

Poultice

Make a poultice for your head with yellow root. Put dried and chopped yellow root in a pot, cover with cold water to 1 inch above the root. Bring to boil and then slowly simmer for 5 minutes. Place a cotton, wool, or gauze headband in the pot and let it soak until broth is cool. Drain mixture. Wring the cloth and put the yellow root in the cloth and place on forehead while lying down for 30 to 60 minutes.

Hemmorhoids

Castor oil

Soak a cotton ball or tissue with castor oil and apply it to the hemorrhoid. Lie down to do this. Make sure the castor oil pack stays in place and you can walk around.

High Blood Pressure/Hypertension

High blood pressure is a chronic disease that disproportionately affects African Americans. It is called "the silent killer" because the symptoms are not physically visible. Many in the health profession believe that African Americans or people of African descent are genetically predisposed to having high blood pressure. I do not. The Masai people of Kenya have one of the lowest documented blood pressure

---

[152] While turmeric is often in use among African Americans today, it was not a staple in early African American healing tradition.

[153] No available reference for standard spelling, so this item is spelled phonetically.

levels in the world today. Research shows there is a direct correlation between a high sodium diet and high blood pressure. The traditional African American Southern diet is high in sodium and fat. Studies also show that high stress and a sedentary lifestyle contribute to high blood pressure.

African Americans living in the South and particularly before they moved to urban centers up North had a more physical lifestyle. This resembled nothing like working out at the gym or today's farmworking. They worked long hours, from, "can't see to can't see," as one elder shared. Most jobs available to African Americans after slavery and during Jim Crow were not sedentary. Life was better than being enslaved but was still hard and unjust! Having more than one job was common. Many maintained the farms they owned or sharecropped, working as field hands picking cotton and tobacco. Some chopped pulp wood and raked pine straw for a living, while others hired out for domestic work (difficult work but keeps the body moving). Job security did not exist and there was little support from non-profits, NGO's, and other social justice-focused programs and agencies of today. In the long years between the end of the Civil War and the establishment of Franklin Roosevelt's New Deal social security programs, if you did not work, you did not eat.

The continuing stressors of "living while Black in America," lack of exercise, and obesity all adversely affect blood pressure. These causes are not genetic but a reaction to long-standing inequitable social conditions that are byproducts of colonization and slavery.

I am the only one in my immediate family who is not on high blood pressure medication. I am not overweight, exercise regularly, and eat healthy. My blood pressure level is often on the high side of normal so I always incorporate herbs and natural minerals in my diet to maintain healthy blood levels.

My own personal regimen is:
*   Eat 3 cloves of garlic with my meal 3 to 5 times a week
*   Supplement my diet with 400 to 500 mg of magnesium (citrate or citrate blend) daily
*   Drink hawthorn berry tea weekly or take the tincture
*   20 minutes or more of exercise

Below are remedies and routines used in African American healing traditions to treat high blood pressure and maintain healthy blood pressure levels.

Widely used throughout Europe and recommended by many healers today to reduce blood pressure, support heart health, normalize irregular heartbeats and circulation.

Lavender tea

While lavender is often in use among African Americans today, it was not a staple in early African American healing tradition.

A hot or cold tea is made to lift your mood, reduce stress and anxiety.

Dark Chocolate

Cocoa beans are rich with flavonoids, which is a powerful antioxidant. Consuming dark chocolate, which is made up of cocoa beans, may lower blood pressure and support vascular health.

Dosage of dark chocolate was 1 oz. 3 to 5 times per week.

Epsom salt

Tonic

1 teaspoon of Epsom salt in 1/2 cup of water 3 to 4 times per week to thin blood and relax blood vessels.

Bath

Soak in Epsom salt (magnesium sulfate) 3 times or more weekly for a minimum of 20 minutes. Your body absorbs the medicinal benefits of this mineral.

Garlic

Consume at least three cloves of garlic daily. Crush the garlic clove first to release the medicinal agent, allicin, that aids in the reduction of blood pressure by relaxing the vessels.

Treatments For Specific Conditions - High Blood Pressure/Hypertension (continued)

Adding garlic to a meal: to get the medicinal benefits and full flavor of garlic, add raw garlic to the last 10 minutes of cooking your meal. This can be chopped, sliced or a whole crushed garlic clove. Crushing the whole clove releases the medicine and flavor. Alternatively, you can sprinkle raw chopped garlic on your meal after it is cooked or saute raw chopped garlic in olive oil for 3 to no more than 10 minutes and add as a garnish to your meal. As another alternative, you can cook the whole garlic clove or bulb by baking in a 300 degree oven until it is soft, or wrapping in foil and placing on a grill until it is soft. However you decide to prepare garlic separately from your meal, it can be eaten on the side like a relish or chow-chow or however to fit one's taste.

(*Note*: Cooking garlic on high heat for longer than 10 minutes reduces its medicinal benefits.)

Hawthorn berries

Widely used throughout Europe and recommended by many healers today to reduce blood pressure, support heart health, normalize irregular heartbeats and to normalize circulation.

Magnesium

The African American traditional diet included magnesium rich foods such as dark leafy greens, beans/lentils, bananas, whole grains, fish, yogurt or clabber, and dark chocolate.

Meditation, Prayer, Stillness

Physical and emotional stress play a large part on the overall health of the body. Stress releases adrenaline into the body which raises the heart rate and blood pressure. This is a natural response and solution to an immediate problem perceived by the body, but when it is maintained for prolonged periods, such stress-caused response takes its toll on the body and can lead to cardiovascular disease. Particularly in modern times, managing and eliminating stress is as important as making dietary changes.

Meditation and prayer have been used to reduce stress and improve the health of the body and mind. The connection of African Americans to religion and spirituality has helped to alleviate the daily stressors of "being Black while in America" for over 400 years.

This spiritual connection reduces anxiety and builds one's faith, strength, hope, resilience, and determination. Spirituality maintains a person's connection to an infinite love and a sense of greater and higher purpose. A study conducted in 2006 by the University of Mississippi Medical Center in Jackson confirmed that there is a correlation between regular prayer, attending church-related activities, and lowering one's blood pressure.

Meditation like prayer also supports lower blood pressure and heart health. Meditation can be done sitting down either in complete silence or by using such sounds as a chime or chanting, or with movement as in tai chi. A recent 2012 study conducted by the Medical College of Wisconsin in Milwaukee revealed that African Americans who meditated twice daily were 48% less likely to have a heart attack or stroke. Meditation reduces the stress hormone adrenaline, decreases blood pressure, and helps to dilate blood vessels supporting overall heart health. Like prayer, meditation allows the mind and body to relax and feel both secure and connected to a divine power.

Immune System Support

(see also "Blood Toxins" this chapter)

Echinacea tea

While echinacea is often in use among African Americans today, it was not a staple in early African American healing tradition. Drink 1 to 3 cups of echinacea tea per day for no more than 3 to 7 days. To make the tea, put 1 to 2 teaspoons of dried echinacea or 2 to 4 teaspoons of fresh echinacea in 1 cup of hot water, cover and steep for 10 to 15 minutes.

Sassafras root or leaf tea

If you harvest the roots yourself, make sure you choose the red roots from the sassafras, not the white ones. Prepare a tea using the standard tea with roots formula of 1 to 2 teaspoons of dried root to 1 cup of hot water, covered and steeped for 25 to 30 minutes.

Drink 1 cup daily in the morning for 1 week. [154]

Yellow root/goldenseal tea or extract

If your system is feeling weak, drink 3 cups daily for one week. Rest for one week and then start again until you feel better. For regular maintenance take a dose 1 to 3 times a week.

Apple cider vinegar tonics

Drink daily first thing in the morning on an empty stomach: 1 to 2 tablespoons of apple cider vinegar (ACV) mixed with 1 to 2 teaspoons honey in 1/2 cup of warm water. Optional: add 3 to 5 pieces of chopped ginger, cover and steep for 10 to 15 minutes before drinking. After drinking the first cup, pour hot water a second time in cup over the residue of ACV, honey, and ginger remaining at the bottom. The second pouring of hot water should fill the entire cup. Let steep the entire day, drink again.

Cod liver oil (omega-3 and omega-6 essential fatty acids)

Taken daily or several times a week to support immune system, reduce inflammation and maintain healthy functioning of the organs. It is also rich with essential fatty acids and vitamins A and D.

Garlic

Eat 3 garlic cloves daily by crushing or chopping and adding to meals.

Pot licker/liquor

Regularly drink the broth from your cooked/boiled greens or root vegetables that has absorbed most of the nutrients.

Impotency

(see "Erectile Dysfunction" this chapter)

Indigestion

(see also "Stomach Problems" and "Flatulence/Gas" this chapter)

The teas below were drunk to help aid digestion. The standard tea preparation was 1 to 2 teaspoons of dried herb to 1 cup of hot water, covered and steeped for 10 to 15 minutes.

Astifidity/Asafoetida. Put a pinch in 1/2 cup of warm water and drink.
Baking soda. Mix 1 teaspoon in 1/2 cup of water and drink.
Catnip tea
Ginger tea made from fresh ginger
Peppermint tea
Sage bush tea

---

[154] An important warning note about sassafras and safrole: Sassafras contains safrole, which is known to have harmful effects if ingested over a period of time in large and concentrated quantities. See warning and instructions in the Sassafras section on pages 319-320 before using.

<u>**Treatments For Specific Conditions (continued)**</u>

Infections

(for external infections see also "Cuts and Wounds" this chapter)

Topical applications for external infections

Apple cider vinegar
Camphor
Castor oil and turpentine
Cayenne pepper and garlic oil salve or poultice
Chimney soot
Epsom salt soak
Garlic poultice (the garlic was crushed to release the medicinal agent)
Honey and sulfur
Onion poultice
Yellow root poultice (goldenseal)
Internal infections

Eucalyptus tea

Make a tea from the leaves or oil and drink 3 times a day.

Garlic tea

Make a garlic-cayenne tea by crushing 3 cloves of garlic to release the medicine from the plant in 1 cup of hot water. Add 1 to 2 shakes of cayenne pepper. Sweeten with honey. Cover and steep for 10 to 15 minutes, then drink the tea and eat the crushed cloves that remain at the bottom of the cup. Repeat 1 to 3 times a day, one of them definitely right before bedtime. Repeat daily until symptoms reverse.

Yellow root (goldenseal) tea

Make a strong tea using 2 to 3 teaspoons of dried goldenseal root in 1 cup of hot water. Cover and steep for 10 to 15 minutes. Drink 3 cups daily for one week.

Apple cider vinegar tonics

Take apple cider vinegar (ACV) 3 times a day for 1 week or use the ACV-based tonic mixture of herbs below:

Put equal parts of chopped garlic, ginger root, onion, horseradish, and cayenne pepper in a mason jar. Cover the ingredients with ACV, filling the jar. Place jar in a paper bag and put in a cool, dark cabinet for 2 weeks. Shake once or twice daily. After 2 weeks, strain into a clean jar and store in a cool cabinet or refrigerator. Sweeten with honey.

* Take 1 tablespoon twice daily as a preventive during cold and flu season.
* At the onset of illness or full-blown cold or flu, take 2 tablespoons 3 to 5 times a day for one week or until symptoms subside.

Epsom salt

Soak in an Epsom salt bath twice daily. If you do not have a fever, the water can be at any temperature you desire. However, if you do have a fever, soak in luke warm to room temperature water only, not hot water, to allow the Epsom salt to be absorbed in your body through your skin without elevating the fever.

Echinacea

While echinacea is often in use among African Americans today, it was not a staple in early African American healing tradition. Drink the tea or take the tincture.

Liquid flush

Drink plenty of water with lemon juice and unsweetened cranberry juice. Eliminate dairy products and sweets. Eat minimal meat.

Vitamin C

Either the crystals or the tablets can be taken. Take between 5,000 to 10,000 mg per day, spread out throughout the day, for one week. The amount taken in crystal form is approximately 4500 to 5000 mg per teaspoon. Tablets may not come in either 5,000 or 10,000 mg units, so some figuring must be done with available tablet units in order to achieve the desired amount.

Inflammation

(see "Swelling" and "Arthritis And Rheumatism" this chapter)

Insect Bites and Stings

Aloe vera gel

Rub the gel from the leaf on affected area several times a day.

Apple cider vinegar

Soak a cotton swab in apple cider vinegar and rub on affected area often. Works well to reduce itching and pain.

Bay leaf

Make a wash from the leaves and wipe on affected area. Alternatively, bruise the leaves to release the medicine and rub leaves on affected area. Or alternatively, make a poultice from bruised leaves and apply to affected area, wrap and leave on. Change daily and continue until symptoms are gone.

Comfrey root

Make a salve from the root and leaves and rub on affected area 3 or more times a day to reduce itching, swelling, and pain, or make a poultice and apply to affected area.

Eucalyptus

Bruise the leaves to release the oil and rub on affected area. Also worked well as an insect repellent for bees, fleas, or mosquitoes.

Lavender oil

While lavender oil is often in use among African Americans today, it was not a staple in early African American healing tradition. Apply lavender oil to skin to prevent or treat insect bites. If the oil is too strong, dilute with a natural oil such as olive oil, coconut oil, or any vegetable oil.

Pokeberry

Rub the juice of the pokeberry on exposed skin to treat and prevent mosquito bites.

Tobacco/snuff

"You can also use tobacco for wasp stangs, bee stangs and stuff like that." Oscelena Harris

Insomnia

A tea was made from one of the herbs below and drunk 20 to 30 minutes before going to bed.
Catnip tea
Chamomile tea
Valerian root tea[155]

---

[155] While valerian root tea is often in use among African Americans today, it was not a staple in early African American healing tradition.

Treatments For Specific Conditions (continued)

Intestinal Worms/Parasites

Astifidity/Asafoetida

Add a pinch (1/8 to 1/4 teaspoon) of astifidity to 1/2 cup of warm water and drink once a day for 3 days to treat intestinal parasites.

Black gum tree

A tea made from the bark was used to expel intestinal worms. Put 1 teaspoon of the shaved bark in 1 cup of boiled water, cover and steep for 20 minutes. Drink.

Castor oil

To treat intestinal parasites, take 1 tablespoon of castor oil and allow your system to purge.

Dogwood bark

Dogwood bark was made into a strong tea to treat intestinal worms Use the dried bark only. To make a tea, put 1 teaspoon of dried bark in 2 cups of hot water, cover and steep for 20 minutes. For a strong decoction, cover and steep and 30 minutes. Drink 1 cup 4 to 6 times a day.

Garlic and pine rosin tea

Crush and chop 4 cloves of garlic in a glass bowl. Add 1 tablespoon of pine rosin and mix well. Take 1 teaspoon of the mixture and put in a cup, pour 1/2 cup of warm water into the cup and mix. Drink this mixture twice daily for 3 days or until worms are expelled. Discontinue if you experience any signs of discomfort.

Jerusalem weed

Jerusalem weed contains compounds that paralyze intestinal worms and expel them from your body. It is commonly made into a tea and drunk to expel intestinal worms such as hookworms or round worms. Alternatively, eat a mixture of 1 teaspoon of Jerusalem weed (leaves and flowers), 1 tablespoon of molasses, and 1 teaspoon of pumpkin seeds to expel such parasites.

Jerusalem weed is also commonly used as a wash to treat skin fungus such as ringworm or athlete's foot.

Peppergrass

To make a strong decoction of peppergrass, add 2 teaspoons of the dried leaves or 3 to 4 teaspoons of fresh chopped leaves to 1 cup of hot water. Cover and steep for 30 minutes. Drink 1 to 2 cups daily to treat intestinal parasites.

Pine tree needles

To make a strong decoction or tea to expel intestinal parasites, gather a handful of pine needles, rinse in cold water, put in the bottom of a pot or saucepan, cover with water and top. Bring to a boil, then simmer for 20 minutes. Let cool. Strain and then drink 3 cups daily. Sweeten with honey if desired.

Walnut tree

Drinking a tea from the bark and leaves kills and expels intestinal parasites. Add 1 oz of dried bark or leaves to 1 pint of water. Bring to boil, cover and let cool. Strain and drink 1 cup, 3 times per day. Place remaining mixture in a glass container and store in the refrigerator.

Wormwood

To make a tea, put 1 to 2 teaspoons of dried leaves and stems in 1 cup of boiled water. Cover and steep for 20 to 30 minutes. Drink tea at least 30 minutes before a meal to benefit from its medicinal properties. Drink 1 to 3 cups daily for 1 week, rest for 1 week, then resume if necessary to treat intestinal parasites.

Joint Pain

(see also "Arthritis" and "Muscle Strains and Cramps" this chapter)

Castor oil poultice

Rub a generous amount of warm castor oil on affected area right before bed and wrap with a cloth. Cover feet with a sock and hands with a glove.

Comfrey root and aloe salve

Grind up comfrey root so it is almost a powder. Place in a small jar and cover completely with approximately twice as much grain alcohol (80 proof or more) in jar. Place in a brown paper bag and store in a cool dry cupboard for 3 to 7 days. Shake once or twice a day. Strain and keep the liquid. Get aloe vera gel or scoop out the meat from an aloe vera leaf. Mix an equal amount of aloe in with the liquid. Add a natural oil to give the consistency of oatmeal or icing. Let the mixture sit for 24 hours and use. Apply to affected area at least twice daily.

Red clay and apple cider vinegar poultice

Mix apple cider vinegar (ACV) in red clay so it is like a thick paste and apply to affected area. Wrap with a cloth. Leave on for 30 to 60 minutes or longer. Change once daily.

Kidney Stones and Kidney Health

Dissolve kidney stones

Lemon and olive oil flush

Combine 1/4 cup each of lemon juice and olive oil. Mix well. Drink all and then flush down with 1 cup of water. Continue drinking plenty of water throughout the day. Make and drink this mixture 3 times daily for three days or until you pass the kidney stones.

Kidney health

Eat dark leafy greens or dandelion greens and drink dandelion root tea to support kidneys in eliminating waste.

Lethargy

(see "Low Energy" this chapter)

Liver Health

Dandelion root tea

Drink the tea and eat the leaves to support liver health.

Yellow root/goldenseal tea

Drink 2 cups of the tea daily. Take for 7 straight days, stop for 1 week, and then resume the treatment. As a preventive health regimen, drink 1 cup of yellow root tea 3 times a week or store the tea in a mason jar and sip on it several times a day 1 to 3 times a week.

Red sassafras tea

Drink one cup of red sassafras tea in the morning instead of coffee. [156]

---

[156] An important warning note about sassafras and safrole: Sassafras contains safrole, which is known to have harmful effects if ingested over a period of time in large and concentrated quantities. See warning and instructions in the Sassafras section on pages 319-320 before using.

Treatments For Specific Conditions - Liver Health (continued)

Beets

Incorporate beets into your diet, drink the beet liquor made from boiling beets, and eat the greens.

Milk thistle

While milk thistle is often in use among African Americans today, it was not a staple in early African American healing tradition. Milk thistle has been used for over 2,000 years to treat liver disorders and as a tonic to support a healthy liver.

The seed contains most of the medicine, silymarin, which is harvested and ground into a fine powder. Dosage amounts and length of usage vary depending on the need, which can range from simple health maintenance to treatment of severe health problems.

For general maintenance, put 1 to 2 teaspoons of ground milk thistle seeds in 1 cup of hot water, cover and steep for 15 to 20 minutes. Drink 1 to 2 cups daily. Alternatively, take 200 to 250 mg of milk thistle/silymarin tablets up to 3 times daily, or make a tea by adding a few drops of milk thistle extract in 1 cup of hot water and drink 1 to 3 cups daily. For more severe ailments consult your health care professional.

Low Energy

Cherry tree bark and sap

"We used the bark and the sap off of cherry trees for energy. Boil it and strain it off and set it where it won't sour. It's just like water, like medicine. See, a lot of people would put whiskey in it. But I didn't. I just set it in the frigidaire and kep it cool like that. When I want it, I get a drink and that would be about every mornin. I'd take me a good drink of that and I hadn't been to the doctor in over 20 years."
Sally McCloud

Lymph Nodes

Castor oil

Rub castor oil over swollen lymph nodes daily to cleanse the system.

Poke root

A tincture was made from the poke root and 1 to 3 drops was taken daily. The tincture was made by cutting off part of a root that was 4 to 5 years old and chopping into small pieces. The pieces were put in a glass jar and then filled with a 80 to 90 proof liquor. The glass jar was covered in a brown paper bag and stored in a dark, cool cupboard for 4 to 6 weeks, shaking daily. After this time, the liquid was strained into another jar and stored in the refrigerator or in a dark, cool place until needed. "If you felt a little queer" (i.e., dizzy or nausea), then the dosage was reduced or stopped all together.

Measles

Corn shuck tea

Put dried corn shuck leaves in a pot, cover with water. Bring to a boil and let sit for 15 minutes. Drink freely. Pour remainder in a jar and keep refrigerated.

Cottonseed tea

"We gave hot teas for measles and thangs like that. Mostly it would be ... cottonseed tea, from the regular cottonseed. We was separating that core from the hull and you could make tea out of that hull. ... It's a core in them and its yellow and we get that core out and make meal out of it and people ate it."
Ola B. Hunter Woods

Sassafras root tea

Drink one cup of the tea daily to help reduce fever and symptoms. Put 1 teaspoon of dried root in 1 cup of hot water, cover and steep for 10 to 15 minutes. [157]

Sheeps shallots tea or manure tea

1 cup of sheep manure was gathered and put in a white cotton cloth. Other ingredients such as lemon, peppermint tea, or candy were added to sweeten and mask the taste. This was placed in a small pot and covered with water. The solution was brought to a boil and simmered for 40 minutes then cooled and strained through another white cloth or cheesecloth. A large, warm cup was drunk up to 3 times per day, one of those times being right before bedtime.

Men's Health

Coon root tea

A tea was made and drunk 1 to 3 times daily for prostate health and a healthy sex life.

Horny goat weed

Taken by many men today to maintain a healthy sex life. While horny goat weed is often in use among African Americans today, it was not a staple in early African American healing tradition.

Raw oysters

Eaten to stimulate a man's "nature."

Saw palmetto

Taken by many men today to treat enlarged prostates.

Menstruation

(see "Female Health" this chapter)

Mosquito Repellent

(see also "Insect Bites And Stings" this chapter)

Eucalyptus oil

Rub the oil from the eucalyptus leaf on exposed skin.

Lavender oil

Rub the oil from the lavender plant on exposed skin.

Pokeberry juice

Rub the juice from the pokeberry on exposed skin.

Mumps

Hog maws

"They would take hog maws and rub us with that and that would be good for mumps. When you get the mumps you have hurting jaws and they would swell. We would always rub up our jaws with the hog maws and it would go down." Mr. Pete Smith

---

[157] An important warning note about sassafras and safrole: Sassafras contains safrole, which is known to have harmful effects if ingested over a period of time in large and concentrated quantities. See warning and instructions in the Sassafras section on pages 319-320 before using.

Treatments For Specific Conditions - Mumps - Hog maws (continued)

Hog maws are the lining from the stomach of a hog. It is very muscular and contains no fat. Besides being used for healing purposes, it is also a cuisine used in Southern soul food and many other cultures.

Mullein

Make a strong mullein wash and apply with a cotton ball to affected area. Drink mullein tea freely. Mullein helped to relieve swelling and inflammation associated with mumps.

Sardine juice

Rub affected areas with the juice, particularly under the chin.

"We had all of the normal sicknesses when we were young including mumps and measles. I used the home remedy of tying sardines to my cheeks. You put the sardines in a cloth and tie them to your cheeks and tie that over your head like rabbit ears. The sardines took the swelling out of your cheeks because your cheeks swelled when you had it. And if one of us got it, they put us all in the room so we all get it at the same time so they can treat it all at the same time and be done with it and get it over with." Mr. Pete Smith.

Muscle Strains and Cramps

Apple cider vinegar

Pour 2 cups of apple cider vinegar (ACV) in a very warm bath and soak for at least 20 minutes. Can also add 1 cup of Epsom salt.

Banana and rubbing alcohol

Add one peeled banana to a jar filled with green alcohol. Leave the banana in with the alcohol until the liquid clears. Rub liquid on cramp. Can also leave peel in jar along with banana. Bananas are high in potassium, which helped alleviate cramps.

Camphor

Rub camphor salve, oil, or cream on affected area.

Castor oil

"You can make poultices with castor oil, too. If you have a sore spot or you got something in your muscle that's not quite right, you take a wool rag, fold it over and pour some warm castor oil on it, and take it to the spot. That's why they call it Palma de Cristo[158] because it is very healing."
Anita Poree

Comfrey root and aloe salve

Grind up comfrey root so it is almost a powder. Place in a small jar and pour in twice as much grain alcohol (90 proof or more). Seal, place in a brown paper bag, and store in a cool, dry cupboard for 3 weeks. Shake once or twice a day. Strain and keep the liquid. Scoop out the meat of an aloe leaf. Mix an equal amount of aloe in with the liquid. Let the mixture sit for 24 hours then apply to affected area 2 to 3 times daily.

Epsom salt

Soak in a warm bath filled with 2 cups of Epsom salt for at least 20 minutes. Can add 1 cup of apple cider vinegar (ACV).

---

[158] Spanish for "Hand of Christ"

Lemon with rubbing alcohol for cramps

"This other bottle is alcohol with lemon juice in it. This for muscle cramps too. I used to get muscle cramps a lot and I just rub this on it." Ms. Oscelena Harris

Get a pint or quart sized jar. Cut a lemon in half or in quarters and squeeze the juice in the jar and then drop the lemon in. Fill with alcohol. Let sit for 24 hours before use. Rub it on affected area as needed.

Ms. Dot's red clay with apple cider vinegar for muscle strain

"[U]se this bottle, the red clay, for strained muscle or ankle. We get some red clay dirt and make a poultice out of it and put it on the strain." Oscelena Harris

Potassium/Banana

Eat a banana daily to get more potassium in your body.

Pain Relief

(see also "Arthritis and Rheumatism" this chapter)
(see also "Headaches and Migraines" this chapter)
(see also "Swelling" this chapter)

Bay leaves

Bay leaves and bay oil were often used in African American healing as an effective pain reliever. Some claimed it helped to stop the pain from arthritis, headaches, and migraines. Bay leaf wash or oil from the fresh leaf was applied and rubbed on the affected area to give immediate relief.

To make a bay leaf wash, bring 3 to 4 leaves to boil in 1 liter of water, cover, and let simmer for about 15 to 20 minutes. Add this medicated water to a bath or tub and soak for 20 to 30 mintues to help relieve pain. Leaves were also added directly to a tub of hot water, cooled to the point where one can soak in comfortably for 20 to 30 minutes.

Parasites

(see "Intestinal Worms/Parasites" this chapter)

Poison Oak or Poison Ivy

Rat vein tea

Make a tea (1 to 2 teaspoons of dried herb or 2 to 4 teaspoons of fresh herb to 1 cup of water). Cover and steep for 10 to 15 minutes. Do not drink, but apply to affected area with a cotton ball 2 to 3 times daily. Alternately, make a strong decoction (up to 6 teaspoons of herb to 1 cup of water), cover and steep for 20 minutes, and apply to affected area in the same manner as you would the tea.

Aloe vera

Rub the gel of the aloe vera plant on affected area 2 to 3 times daily. Wash area with water and soap prior to each application.

Apple cider vinegar

Dip a cotton ball in apple cider vinegar (ACV) and apply to affected area 2 times daily. Wash area with water and soap prior to each application.

Baking soda

Make a paste using baking soda and water so it is the consistency of Cream Of Wheat. Apply to affected area and leave on until dry and it flakes off. Optional: add aloe vera gel or apple cider vinegar (ACV) instead of water.

Treatments For Specific Conditions - Poison Oak or Poison Ivy (continued)

Black tar soap

Wash affected area with black tar soap immediately after contact with poison ivy or oak.

Lemon juice

Make a lemon juice wash or apply the lemon juice directly onto affected area 2 to 3 times daily.

Oatmeal

Make an oatmeal poultice or take an oatmeal bath by placing oatmeal in a stocking cap or cheesecloth and placing in tub. Soak for at least 20 minutes. For poultice, soak oatmeal in warm water first to soften then wrap in cheesecloth or in a stocking cap and place on affected area.

Rheumatism

(see "Arthritis/Rheumatism" this chapter)

Ringworm

(see "Fungus" this chapter)

Scars

Aloe vera gel

Apply 3 times a day or more on scarred area.

Cocoa Butter

Apply 3 times a day or more on scarred area.

Comfrey

Make a comfrey root salve and apply often to scarred area. Can also mix with aloe vera gel. Comfrey root contains allantoin, which helps with repairs of scarred tissue and speeds up healing.

Sulfur

"A pure unadulterated sulfur salve is a wonderful healer. I would use this for sores, scratches and scars." Anita Poree

Sciatica and Other Nerve Damage

Comfrey root salve

Used to help relieve the chronic pain and heal the damage. Rubbed on as needed.

Sexual Pleasure/Enhancement

Coon root tea

Drink coon root tea for both men and women.

Raw oysters

Raw oysters were eaten as an aphrodisiac.

Sinus Infections

(see also "Colds And Flu" and "Congestion" this chapter)

Eucalyptus inhalation

Put a handful of eucalyptus leaves (5 to 10), in a medium-sized pot of water that has been boiled. Cover and let steep for 3 to 5 minutes, uncover the pot and then inhale steam by putting your head close to the pot. Use a towel to make a tent that covers the head and the pot to enclose the steam. Inhale the medicinal stream for 15 to 20 minutes. This was done 2 to 4 times a day until relief.

Garlic

Eat 5 crushed garlic cloves daily to treat sinus infection. Take 3 or more crushed garlic cloves daily as a preventative.

Mullein

Make a strong tea and drink 3 times a day. Put dried mullein leaves in a pipe and inhale the smoke. Make an inhalant with mullein leaves (similar to eucalyptus above) and breathe through nostrils.

Rabbit tobacco

To open up sinuses, put 1 teaspoon of dried leaves in 1 cup of boiled water, cover and steep for 5 to 10 minutes. Drink 3 times a day. Also used to relieve chest congestion and as an expectorant.

Pack a pipe filled with dried rabbit tobacco and inhale through your lungs and blow out through your nostrils. The leaves were gathered in the fall after they turned silvery-green in color and at their strongest potency.

Sage (white)

Make a strong tea and drink 1 cup 3 times a day. Make a sage inhalant (similar to eucalyptus above) and breath in the medicinal steam. Burn white sage in your home and close to your nostrils, breathing in the smoke through your nostrils. Do 3 times a day.

Saline wash

Mix one teaspoon of saline (sodium chloride) in 1/2 to 1 cup of water. (*Note*: Use fine grain salt or let salt thoroughly dissolve prior to moving forward with the preparation. Using sea salt is best.) Fill a syringe dropper with the solution, tilt head back, and release into one nostril. Leave in there for 1 minute and then blow the nose, removing solution and mucous. Repeat on other nostril. This treatment was applied in both nostrils 3 times and hourly until condition improved.

Skin Conditions

Acne

Apple cider vinegar

Apply to affected area on skin twice daily after washing.

Pokeberry

Take 1 to 2 pokeberries 3 times per week.

Boils

(see "Boils and Cysts" section this chapter)

Burns

(see "Burns" section this chapter)

Treatments For Specific Conditions - Skin Conditions (continued)

Dry skin/moisturizer/good complexion

Aloe vera gel

Apply to your skin often to soften and smooth. Keeps your skin healthy by reducing bacteria and infection.

Baby Afterbirth

"I asked her how she kept her skin so nice and she said she was a baby delivery nurse and that when every baby is born, she'll lightly rinse the blood off 'em and then there's an oil that's on the baby and when she's cleanin the baby up, she'll take that and rub it on herself." Luisah Teish

Castor oil

Rub castor oil on feet and hands at night and cover with cotton socks or gloves. Also helps to cleanse your body by pulling out toxins and reducing inflammation.

Olive oil, coconut oil

"If [Mama] could eat it, she would use it on her skin. So, she used olive oil, coconut oil, anything that you could ingest because your skin has pores and whatever you put on it goes right into your body." Anita Poree

Prickly Pear Cactus

The insides of the prickly pear cactus leaf was applied to the skin to soothe, moisturize and regenerate the skin. Carefully peel back the skin of a leaf and scoop out the gel inside into a glass bowl. Use directly onto skin or mix with a little water. Apply in the same manner you would a cream moisturizer. Cover the remaining gel and store in the refrigerator for future use. Alternatively, prickly pear gel can be mixed with coconut oil or olive oil to make a more effective skin cream.

Tallow – mutton or calf

Massage tallow on tough and calloused hands and feet. This helped to soften the skin by penetrating deep into the dead and hard skin. It also helped to soak hardened skin in warm Epsom salt water and then scrape with a pumice stone or callus scraper.

Watermelon rind

Grate or pound a piece of watermelon rind and apply on face for 15 minutes. Wash with hot water, then splash with cold water. Watermelon rind contains vitamins, minerals, and collagen enhancing properties and Lycopene, an amino acid which helps protect skin from sun and aids the skin's healing and regenerative processes.

Rashes, Psoriasis, Eczema, and Impetigo

Aloe vera gel

Apply up to 3 times daily to affected area to reduce inflammation, itching, and dryness.

Apple cider vinegar

Take apple cider vinegar (ACV) with honey as an internal tonic. To make, pour 1 to 2 tablespoons of ACV in 1/2 cup of warm water. Add 1 teaspoon of honey. Drink 1 to 2 times a day on empty stomach.

Baking soda

Soak affected area in a tub with baking soda at least twice daily.

Banana peel

Make a banana peel poultice and place on affected area. If large area, rub the inside of the skin of the banana peel on affected area and keep on for 30 to 60 minutes. Wipe with warm water. Apply at least twice daily.

Carnation Milk

For rashes and itching, rub carnation milk on affected area.

Castor oil

Rub castor oil over area 3 times a day and put a patch or adhesive bandage on it.

Coal tar/black tar soap

Wash affected area twice daily with this soap. Apply a soothing and healing salve like aloe vera gel or castor oil after wash.

Poke Root salve

Make a salve from the poke root and apply to affected area once daily.

Pokeberry

Swallow 1 to 3 pokeberries daily or take a shot of pokeberry wine daily or 1 to 3 drops of pokeberry tincture daily. Take for 30 days, then stop for one week, then resume. People who took pokeberry as medicine first had to find out how much of the medicine their body could tolerate. They started by swallowing 1 pokeberry for 3 days and if they experienced no side effects, swallowed 2 poke berries daily for 3 days and, if no side effects, they took 3 daily. If side effects such as dizziness or nausea were experienced, they reduced dosage or stopped.

Stretch marks

Cocoa butter, aloe vera gel, shea butter, olive oil, or coconut oil worked best to prevent stretch marks when the skin expands, such as in the case of pregnancy or weight gain. Massage the oil into the skin one to two times daily.

Yellow root/goldenseal

Rub a yellow root or goldenseal wash or salve on affected area.

Snake Bite

Kerosene/coal oil

Soak a clean cloth in kerosene (aka coal oil) and place on snake bitten area until you reach a doctor. Purported to neutralize the poison and the infection.

Turpentine poultice (mixed with kerosene or tobacco)

Place several drops of turpentine on bite and wrap with a cloth. Sometimes kerosene and/or tobacco were mixed in the turpentine and then applied. Another option for application was to first soak a cloth in turpentine and then wrap on affected area. If bite was venomous, this remedy was purported to draw out and neutralize poison and infection until an antivenom could be taken.

Sore Throat

(see "Throat (Sore)" this chapter)

Splinters

Baking soda

Soak affected area in a tub of hot/warm water with baking soda for 20 minutes at least 2 times daily. Splinter will either work its way out completely or enough to easily remove with tweezers or a needle.

Treatments For Specific Conditions - Splinters (continued)

Banana peel

Place a banana peel poultice over the affected area and wrap with a bandage. Change 1 to 2 times daily and leave on until splinter has worked its way to the surface.

Epsom salt

Soak the area that has the splinter in a tub of hot/warm water with Epsom salt for 20 minutes. Use 1 to 2 cups of Epsom salt per tub of water. Splinter will either work its way out completely or enough to easily remove with tweezers or a needle.

Fatback

"I remember having deep splinters in your hand and in your foot and she would put some salt pork and fat back on it and draw it out. It would make the whole damn wound just pucker up and spread it out and everything else that was in it would come out. She would in a couple of days pull it out with a tweezer." Author unknown

Tallow poultice

Cover splintered area with tallow and cover that with an adhesive bandage or wrap area so the poultice is secure. Check and change poultice daily until splinter is close to the surface to pull out safely.

Stomach Problems (Digestion, Flatulence/Gas, Nausea)

(see also "Constipation" this chapter)

Digestive aids that also helped treat flatulence (gas) and indigestion

Ginger tea

Drink ginger tea or eat pickled ginger slices with and after your meal.

Peppermint tea

Drink one cup of peppermint tea twice daily.

Astifidty/Asafoetida

Put a pinch of astifidty/asafoetida in 1 cup of room temperature water and then drink the mixture.

Baking Soda

Mix 1 teaspoon of baking soda in water and then drink the mixture. Optional: add sweetner. The baking soda neutralizes the gas.

Bay leaf

Add bay leaf to your meals while cooking. Alternatively, make a tea by putting 1 dried bay leaf or 2 fresh bay leaves in 1 cup of hot water, covering and steeping for 3 to 5 minutes. Drink twice daily.

Castor oil

Massage stomach and abdomen with hand-warmed castor oil or use a hot pack with the oil.

Pickled vegetables

Eating pickled vegetables helped digestion by adding healthy bacteria to the gut. Pickled cabbage or beets, chow-chow, and pickles themselves were often eaten in African American cuisine.

Nausea or upset stomach

1 to 2 cups of the herbal teas below were drunk 15 to 30 minutes before and/or after a meal to relieve nausea and improve digestion: catnip, chamomile, ginger, horsemint, peppermint, or sage.

Probiotics for healthy stomach bacteria

Fermented foods have probiotic properties and help maintain healthy stomach bacteria. The fermented or pickled foods below are in the traditional African American diet and are eaten regularly as part of a health maintenance routine.

Apple cider vinegar

Drinking shots of apple cider vinegar (ACV) helped promote digestion by encouraging the growth of good bacteria—the probiotic.

Clabber or sour milk

". . . take the milk and let it sour deliberately in the refrigerator... take cornbread, crumble it up in there and eat it and make it pudding like. It gives you a little more substance so you're not just drinking the clabber (sour milk) straight down. Eat some sort of fermented; without question, the bacteria are good for you!" Anita Poree

Fermented or pickled vegetables

Beets, chow-chow, relish, okra, cucumbers/pickles, or sauerkraut.

There are numerous recipes that were used to ferment or pickle vegetables using brine (salt and water), vinegar, or a combination of both, and adding a little bit of sugar.

To ferment/pickle vegetables:

1. Chop, shred or use whole (i.e., okra or pickling cucumbers).
2. Pack vegetables along with pickling spices—mustard, red or black pepper, coriander, fennel, celery seeds, and chopped garlic or peppers—in a mason jar that is one pint or larger.
3. Make a fermenting/pickling liquid that is either brine (salt and water) or brine and vinegar combined.
    Brine: 2 cups of water to 1 tablespoon of salt/sea salt. Put in a pot and let the salt dissolve on a low heat. Let cool.
    Vinegar/brine solution: Mix 1 part vinegar with 1 part brine. Add 1 tablespoon of salt per solution. Optional: Add 1 teaspoon of cane sugar. Put in a pot and let the salt dissolve on a low heat, cool.
4. Cover vegetables with the brine or vinegar/brine solution, filling to the top of the jar.
5. Cover with the air-tight lid and let sit at room temperature in a safe area for 2 to 3 days. Open jar daily to let out gas.
6. After 2 to 3 days, place jar in the refrigerator on a shelf on the door (this is the warmest part of the refrigerator and will benefit the fermenting process). Ferment for 3 weeks or longer depending on the taste you want.

"Sugar"/"High Sugar"/Hyperglycemia

(see "Diabetes" this chapter)

Swelling

(see also "Arthritis" this chapter)

Black clay

"Black clay is good for swellin. You just take it and pack it on there where it swolt up and wrap it with a bandage." Ruth Patterson

Epsom salt

Soak the affected area in Epsom salt. Add 1/2 cup of Epsom salt to 1 gallon of hot water. Use 2 cups in a bath. Soak for at least 20 minutes.

<u>**Treatments For Specific Conditions - Swelling (continued)**</u>

Goldenrod

Drink goldenrod tea 2 to 3 times daily. Apply a poultice to affected area and leave on for 30 minutes. Soak affected area for 20 to 30 minutes in a bath or tub with 2 to 4 cups of goldenrod leaves/stems.

Heart leaves for foot swelling

"Boil them up in a pot and put your feet in there." Mr. Red (Luther Stelly Smith)
Add 2 to 4 cups of heart leaves per tub to soak affected area.

Mullet/mullein

Drink mullein tea 2 to 3 times daily or soak in a bath. For a hot soak, break and bruise 4 to 6 whole mullein leaves to release the medicine, add them to a tub of hot water, and soak affected area for 20 to 30 minutes.

Oak Bark

Salve

Crush the oak bark into a powder and mix in tallow, olive, or coconut oil. Add a little bit of whiskey or grain alcohol for preservation. Rub salve on 2 to 3 times daily.

Soak and poultice for swelling and joint pain

Shave the bark off with an ax and then tear off several smaller pieces from the shaved bark. Place 5 to 10 of these pieces in a pot and cover with water about 1 to 2 inches above bark. Simmer for approximately 1 hour then soak the affected area in the solution for 30 minutes. Alternative: Soak a cloth in the oak bark solution and wrap affected area with the cloth. Leave on for one hour.

Orange weed

Crush or bruise the leaves first to release the medicine, then rub directly on affected area several times a day. Alternative: make a poultice, salve, wash or bath with the leaves.

Tapeworms

(see "Intestinal Worms/Parasites" this chapter)

Teeth and Gums Care/Toothaches

Cleaning and whitening

Twigs were used from the Dogwood tree (*Cornus florida*) as a toothbrush and toothpick to clean the teeth. Small branches were taken from the Blackgum tree (*Nyssa sylvatica*) by twirling them until they broke off. The broken end was frayed and could then be used as a toothbrush.

Gum Health

Swollen or inflamed gums

Make an alum wash by mixing a pinch of alum grains in 1/4 cup of water. Let dissolve and then use as a mouth wash. Alternatively, put 1 to 4 grains of alum on your wet toothbrush and brush and massage your gums for 1 to 2 minutes, particularly the area that is swollen. Rinse mouth afterward. Do 1 to 2 times daily until gums are better. For maintenance, do 1 to 3 times per week.

Toothache

Note: Tooth pain is usually indicative of a problem that can become severe if left untreated. While some natural remedies can both allay the toothache pain and effectively treat the underlying problem causing that pain, others may leave that underlying cause untreated. Seek advice from a dental professional if the problem causing the toothache pain persists.

Buttonwillow or Buttonbush bark

The bark was chewed from this plant to relieve toothache pain and infection.

Clove oil

Rub clove oil mixed with olive or coconut oil on affected tooth and gum three times daily for pain and to reduce infection.

Garlic

Bite down on one garlic clove where the affected tooth is. Leave there for as long as possible. Rub affected gum and tooth with garlic oil.

Ms. Dot's rat vein (aka striped wintergreen) recipe

Dry out a bunch of rat vein leaves. Wrap in a paper and smoke as a cigarette. Rat vein may have reduced pain and has properties that may help reduce and prevent infection.

Pickash Tree

"If you had a toothache we went to the pickash tree. It's full of sticky stuff and my mother would go to the tree and just shave off the bark. If you had a tooth with a hole in it, she would put some of that stuff right in it. You would go to sleep and when you wake up, you don't have a toothache. You could feel it just working. You have to be very, very bad before they take you to a dentist." Lacy Patterson

Saltwater

Rinse mouth out with very warm salt water 3 times daily, using a salt concentrate of 1/2 to 1 teaspoon per 1 cup of water.

White mulberry leaf poultice

Grind up fresh or dried mulberry leaves in a little water so it is a paste-like consistency. Wrap in gauze and place on affected area for 30 to 60 minutes 2 to 3 times daily.

Yellow root/goldenseal

Rub the gum and tooth of affected area with yellow root/goldenseal powder or chew on the root. Make a strong decoction of yellow root and rinse mouth out.

Teething

Birdbill tea

"You got a baby that's teething, you give it birdbill. ... We brews it up and when you put it in the jar, you can go ahead and give him some of it. You can keep it for a long time, just keep adding fresh water to it. It will kill that diarrhea too." Oscelena Harris

Note: if keeping herb tea for more than 3 days in a jar, it is best to refrigerate to preserve.

Hornet's or Wasps Nest (empty)

This made a very effective object for babies to gnaw on to relieve their teething pains. Wasps make their nests out of pulped wood and bark, which they gnaw, chew up, and turn into a pulp by mixing it with their saliva.

Teethweed or Titiweed (Elder grass)

Teethweed or titiweed grass was used for babies to chew on for teething. It toughens gums.

Throat (Sore Throat)

Peach tree leaf tea

Use 2 teaspoons of the dried leaves to one cup of boiling water. This tree was drunk freely to relieve sore throats and to soothe mucous membranes.

Treatments For Specific Conditions - Throat (Sore Throat) (continued)

Apple cider vinegar

Mix 1 tablespoon of apple cider vinegar (ACV) to 1 cup of warm water and gargle and spit out.

Elderberry syrup

Make a syrup from berries and take 3 times a day (see "Standard Medical Preparations" at the beginning of this chapter for general instructions on how to prepare a syrup).

Horehound

To make a tea, use 1 teaspoon of horehound to 1 cup of hot water. Cover and steep for 10 to 15 minutes. Drink 2 to 3 times daily. To make a gargle solution, take 2 teaspoons of horehound to 1 cup of hot water. Cover and steep for 20 minutes or until cool. Gargle 2 to 3 times daily.

Mullein

To make a tea, use 1 teaspoon of mullein to 1 cup of hot water. Cover and steep for 10 to 15 minutes. Drink 2 to 3 times daily. To make a gargle solution, take 2 teaspoons of mullein to 1 cup of hot water. Cover and steep for 20 minutes or until cool, then gargle 2 to 3 times daily. For both tea and gargle, add honey to help soothe the membranes and fight infection.

Pine needle and honey

To make a tea, put a handful of pine needles in hot boiled water, cover and steep for 20 minutes, or until cool. Add honey or cane sugar to sweeten. Drink 2 to 3 times daily. Alternative: make a solution twice as strong to use as a gargle.

Sage

To make a tea, put 1 teaspoon of sage in 1 cup of hot water, cover and steep for 10 to 15 minutes. Add honey or cane sugar to sweeten. Drink twice daily. To make a gargle, use twice as much sage. Gargle 3 times daily.

Salt Water

Add 1 tablespoon salt to 1/2 cup of warm to hot water and gargle. Do this 3 times daily to relieve sore throat.

Yellow root

To make a tea, put 1 teaspoon of yellow root in 1 cup of hot water, cover and steep for 10 to 15 minutes. Add honey or cane sugar to sweeten. Drink twice daily. To make a gargle, use twice as much herb. Gargle 2 to 3 times daily.

Water Retention/Fluid Retention

(see "Edema/Water Retention/Fluid Retention this chapter)

Whooping Cough

Whooping cough is medically different from a normal cough. It's clinical name is *pertussis* and its common name is "the 100-day cough." It is caused by the bacterium Bordatella pertussis, and a person contracting it may have common cold symptoms with runny nose, fever, and severe coughing fits with a high-pitched "whoop."

Horehound tea

Make a strong tea or drops. See "Coughs" this chapter.

Hog hoof tea

"Would take hoofs offa pig and boil them and make a tea and boil it and drink that for whooping cough. It would stop that coughing." Author unknown

Horse milk for whooping cough

"We would actually milk the tit of a horse just like a cow and drink that for whooping cough. Can you believe that, horse titty milk!" Ms. Valena Noble

Worms

(see "Intestinal Worms/Parasites" or the ringworm entry in "Fungus," both this chapter)

Wounds

(see "Cuts And Wounds" this chapter)

Aromatherapy

Aromatherapy uses the natural oils and aroma from plants to affect the mind, body, and spirit. It is an aromatic medicine chest which can relieve physical and emotional symptoms. For example, eucalyptus oil or the natural aroma from the plant can alleviate sinus congestion, while lavender oil or its natural aroma has been used to treat anxiety and depression as well as bee stings.

Bay Leaf

Fragrant-smelling bay leaf branches and individual leaves are placed in the home and purported to absorb negativity and boost strength and confidence. Discard when the leaves shrivel and replace with fresh ones.

Eucalyptus

Having fresh eucalyptus in your home naturally acts as a flea/insect repellent as well as freshens the air, supports the immune system, and provides relief for respiratory issues.

Lavendar

Natural lavender is said to boost your mood and help relieve depression. Lavender tea may help to reduce blood pressure. While it is often in use among African Americans today, lavender was not a staple in early African American healing tradition.

Sage

"I like sage bush, too. It's good medicine. I burn it, too. It smell good. I tell you what, you can burn it in your house and you sho' give it a good smell. And then you can take it and make sausage with it. Yeah, it's good." Oscelena Harris

Burning sage is a custom traditionally done in Native American communities to cleanse the environment and individuals. Sage is often used prior to and during spiritual ceremonies performed by Native Americans.

Food Seasoning

Adding herbal spices to food while cooking helped maintain good health by strengthening immunity and preventing and treating chronic ailments like high blood pressure, inflammation, and congestion. Many herbs lose their medicinal potency when cooked too long. Add them to your foods during the last 10 minutes of cooking to retain potency.

Food Seasoning (continued)

Bay Leaf

Add 1 to 3 whole leaves when cooking stews, rice, beans, meats, or vegetable dishes. Bay is a good source of Vitamins A and C, iron and manganese. It supports good digestion, helps clear up flu, bronchitis, and congestion and has antiseptic and pain-relieving properties for such conditions as migraines and arthritis.

Garlic

Garlic's purported benefits are numerous and range from reducing blood pressure to warding off colds, flu, and infection. Crushing garlic releases its medicinal agent, allicin. Add crushed or chopped garlic during the last 10 minutes of cooking or bake garlic whole in its skin.

Onion

Like garlic, onion's health benefits are numerous. It is a rich source of allicin, antioxidants, and sulfur. Onion has antibiotic, antiviral, and anti-inflammatory properties.

Sage

"For medicine I make a tea and it cleans out your stomach real good. My mama used to drank it for coffee in the morning." Oscelena Harris

Among sage's purported health benefits are stimulation of the brain and reduction of inflammation inside your entire body.

Sassafras (leaves) as filé in filé gumbo

Filé is made from ground sassafras leaves and is used as a thickening agent in stews and soups. Filé was first used by people of the Choctaw Nation throughout Mississippi, Louisiana, and Alabama and later became an important ingredient in the Louisiana Creole cuisine, gumbo. Sassafras tea was drunk often in African American healing traditions to ward off colds.

A note about safrole: The active ingredient in sassafras is safrole. Safrole is a compound found in many plants besides sassafras, such as mace, nutmeg, rosemary, dill, black tea, tamarind, cinamon, witch hazel, and ginger.

The U.S. government regards safrole as a weak carcinogen. Safrole and sassafras were banned in the United States in the 1960s because research from a study found that when laboratory rats were fed large amounts of sassafras for an extended period of time, it resulted in the rats contracting cancer. The danger of over-ingestion of safrole was not unknown in traditional medicine and, therefore, people traditionally were sensible about ingesting sassafras and did not use it as a long-term medicine.

There is little to no health danger to using sassafras in the normal minimal amounts, such as in teas and seasonings. Sassafras leaves only contain minute to no traces of safrole. One cup of sassafras tea, for example is determined to be 1/14th as carcinogenic as a cup of beer. Therefore, filé containing sassafras is still sold without any restrictions, and many products can be bought today containing sassafras that is safrole-free altogether.

Turmeric

While turmeric is often in use among African Americans today, it was not a staple in early African American healing tradition. Some of turmeric's numerous health benefits are: anti-inflammatory, natural pain-reliever, relief from arthritis and rheumatism, liver detoxifier, and anti-cancer. Turmeric has been used as a medicine and food spice in Chinese and Ayurvedic (East Indian) medicine and cuisine for thousands of years. Many people around the world add this spice to their foods while cooking daily.

Chapter 7 – Animal Care

All Animals

Comfrey for external wounds, boils, cysts, and growths

Make a comfrey leaf and root poultice and apply to affected area. Hold in place by wrapping with gauze or cotton cloth. Change dressing once daily or every 2 days.

Eucalyptus leaf and oil for flea repellent

Rub and massage a large bunch of eucalyptus leaves on the fur and skin of your animal. Make sure you bruise the leaves prior to use so the oil is released. Place eucalyptus leaves under your couch, bed, and other furniture to rid your house of fleas and to prevent flea infestation. Keep fresh eucalyptus leaf in a vase in your house.

Dogs

Kerosene for snake bites on dogs

Wash affected area and apply kerosene with a cloth. Kerosene packs have been used in folk medicine since the 1800's to pull out infection, poison, toxins, and inflammation.

Sweet potato or yams

Give your dog a baked sweet potato or yam to treat constipation, trouble eliminating, and stomach discomfort.

Pigs/Hogs

Lion's tongue for health maintenance

"We used to feed lion's tongue to the hogs to help keep them healthy. We chop up the leaves and put it in the feed. You can take lion's tongue and boil it and drink it yo'self." Luther Stelly "Red" Smith

Strychnine

"I also remember my grandfather used to give his pigs strychnine for a couple of days before he would slaughter them. He said he would run it through their system to run out all the poison." Bonita Sizemore

Chapter 8 – The Medicines

Derived from Roots, Herbs, Minerals, Food, and Animals

This section lists the natural medicines—plants, roots, leaves, berries/fruit, bark, food, animal parts, and mineral—that were commonly used in African American healing to treat ailments and in preventive healthcare. Many of these medical practices crossed the Atlantic with the slave trade from Africa, and some had their origins deep into African history all the way back to ancient Egypt. Even though practitioners might use these medicines to treat one ailment, the medicine oftentimes also had numerous other benefits that contributed to overall good health. The "Health benefits" section under each listing offers different ways that the natural medicine had been traditionally used and is still being used today to treat a variety of ailments. Also listed are the medicinal properties of each plant and its preparation and application for treatment and healing.

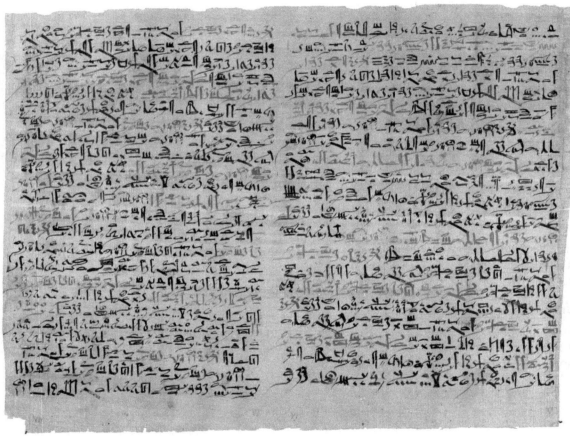

The Edwin Smith papyrus

The world's oldest surviving surgical document. Written in hieratic script in ancient Egypt around 1600 B.C., the text describes anatomical observations and the examination, diagnosis, treatment, and prognosis of 48 types of medical problems in exquisite detail. Among the treatments described are closing wounds with sutures, preventing and curing infection with honey and moldy bread, stopping bleeding with raw meat, and immobilization of head and spinal cord injuries. Translated in 1930, the document reveals the sophistication and practicality of ancient Egyptian medicine.

Image 8-a

IMPORTANT: Before taking any of these medications, you should consult the "Precautionary Note On Self-Treating, Recommended Dosages, and Regimens" at the beginning of Section II.

666

(see "Three Sixes" this chapter)

Aloe Vera

(cuts, burns, digestion, inflammation, skin conditions)

Botanical name

Aloe vera

Also known as

aloe

Medicinal properties

alterative, antibacterial, antifungal, anti-inflammatory, antioxidant, antiseptic, antiviral, astringent, cell proliferant, detoxifier, emollient, immune stimulant, vermifuge

Health benefits

This succulent has innumerable health benefits. Aloe vera nourishes the body with high amounts of antioxidants, minerals, vitamins A, C, and E, amino acids, enzymes, and fatty acids. When taken internally, aloe vera is a general tonic for overall health and treating digestion and gastrointestinal disorders. Aloe may alkalize the body and restore a balanced pH. Aloe may boost immunity, help lower cholesterol levels, support kidney health, relieve constipation, and reduce inflammation and pain.

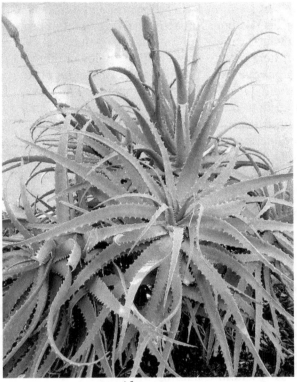

Aloe vera
Image 8-1

Description: succulent with green fleshly leaves; serrated edges and orange flowering top

When used topically, aloe helps speed the healing process in cuts, wounds, and burns and helps prevent infection. Aloe gel also helps to soothe many skin conditions and is an effective skin moisturizer.

Preparation and application

Most people cut a leaf directly from the plant and scooped out the inside—the gel—to use topically and internally for digestion.

Internally

The gel was extracted by cutting one medium-sized leaf from the plant, slicing it open, and scooping out the gel. The gel was mixed in a juice or added to a little water, honey, and lemon to make a tonic.

Poultice

Aloe gel was rubbed directly onto cuts, bruises, scrapes, burns, wounds, and other skin conditions 2 to 3 times daily. It was also used to treat sore muscles and arthritis pain, inflammation, to moisturize skin, and to treat acne, rashes, and other conditions.

Apple Cider Vinegar

(inflammation, digestion, gout, cuts, skin fungus, rashes, immune booster)

Medicinal properties

antiseptic, anti-inflammatory, digestive aid

Health benefits

Raw, unpasteurized, unfiltered apple cider vinegar (ACV) containing "the mother," a tiny, web-like ball of living enzymes and nutrients, makes this liquid an active healing agent. It has a wide variety of medicinal values. Raw unfiltered ACV may help help lower blood pressure and the risk of heart disease, regulate insulin levels, boost immunity, improve digestion, treat gout, reduce inflammation and pain from arthritis and rheumatism, treat cuts, reduce mucous, and generally detoxify the body. If used topically, raw unfiltered ACV has antibacterial, antiseptic, and antifungal properties and is often used to treat ringworm, rashes, acne, and minor cuts and scrapes. Raw unfiltered ACV also provides the minerals calcium, phosphorous, magnesium, copper, iron, and potassium.

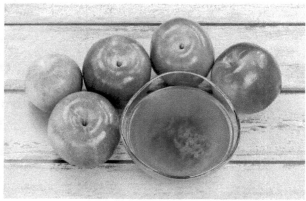

Apple cider vinegar
Image 8-2

Description: pale amber color with murky cobweb-like appearance

Preparation and application

Bath

Pour 2 cups ACV in a warm tub and soak your muscles.

Compress

Soak a washcloth in ACV mixed with hot water and place on sore muscles, joints, aches, and sprains.

Gargle

For sore throats, mix 1 tablespoon of ACV to 1 cup of warm water and gargle, then spit out.

Household Cleaning

To eliminate germs and odors, use 1 to 2 cups ACV to 1 gallon of water to create a cleaning solution.

Tonic

Mix 1 to 2 tablespoons of ACV with up to 1 teaspoon of honey in a glass of warm water. Drink 1 to 3 times a day.

Topically

Saturate a cotton ball with ACV and rub on affected area 3 to 5 times a day. Can be used to treat:
 * inflamed skin
 * fungus on nail and skin
 * bug bites
 * rashes and hives
 * allergies
 * warts
 * cuts and wounds to promote healing and prevent infection
 * vaginal yeast infections (mix 1/4 cup ACV to 2 cups of water and use as a douche 2 times daily for 3 days)
 * ear infections (mix 1 teaspoon of ACV in 2 tablespoons of water and put 2-3 drops in ear, cover with cotton cloth, do this for up to 3 days)

Asfidity, Astifidity, Asafoetida, Astifis, Acifidity

(colds, flu, congestion, coughs, whooping cough)

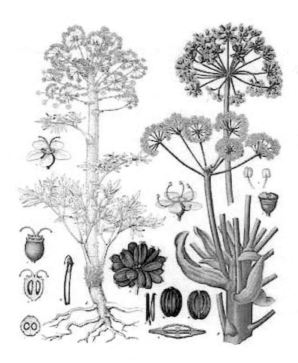

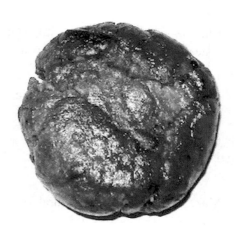

Astifidity resin
Image 8-3a

Description: dark amber-colored resin-like gum ball

Astifidity
Image 8-3

Description: fine green leaves at base; long stems with yellow flowers

Botanical name

Ferula scorodosma

Also known a

devil's dung, stinking gum, asant, food of the gods, giant fennel

Medicinal properties

abortifacent, antiepileptic, antimicrobial, antiviral

Health benefits

Many Southerners do not know the origins of the medicine they call astifidity, or even what is in it. Astifidity is a resin-like gum that comes from dried sap extracted from the stem and roots of the asafoetida plant, which is native to India and Iran/Persia. The resin is greyish-white when fresh but dries to a dark amber color. It is used as a spice in India and Iran and as a cold and flu prevention medicine in African American healing traditions. Asafoetida or astifidity has a pungent, unpleasant smell when raw, but in cooked dishes it delivers a smooth flavor similar to leeks.

Astifidity resin or powder was usually placed in a small bag and worn around the neck to fight off colds and flu during the winter season. Astifidity can also be made into a tea to aid digestion, reduce asthma, bronchitis, whooping cough, and flatulence.

Asfidity, Astifidity, Asafoetida, Astifis, Acifidity (continued)

Preparation and application

The asafoetida resin is hard and difficult to grate. It is traditionally crushed between stones or with a hammer to chip off pieces.

Tea

Chip or grate off a teaspoon full of the resin. Place it in 1 cup and pour hot water over it. Cover and let it steep for 10 to 15 minutes. Drink 1 to 3 times per day.

Cooking

Use as a seasoning similar to garlic to flavor foods and ingest the medicine as a spice.

Poultice

Using the resin or powder, make a small poultice bag and wear around your neck for protection against colds and flus.

Salve

Make a salve using a natural oil mixed with the powder and rub on chest or stomach for a decongestant or digestive aid.

Tincture

Take the entire resin ball and drop it in a bottle of whiskey, bourbon, or brandy. Let it sit for at least 3 days. Take a teaspoon full 1 to 3 times per day for ailments or as a preventive tonic during winter. Rub this tincture on the chest to relieve congestion or on the stomach to aid in digestion.

Tonic

Mix 1 teaspoon of the finely-grated powder in a shot of whiskey and drink to treat colds, coughs, flu, and digestion problems.

Baking Soda

(heartburn, indigestion, scalds, blisters, chicken pox, sore throat)

Also known as

bread soda, cooking soda, sodium bicarbonate

Medicinal properties

abrasive, acid neutralizer/antacid, anticaries (cavities), antifungal, antiseptic

Health benefits

Baking soda (or sodium bicarbonate) is a mineral found in many natural springs. It is a natural substance that helps regulate pH and prevents the body from becoming too acidic or too alkaline. It is often ingested as an antacid to balance body pH, detox, or

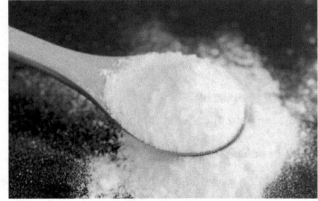

Baking soda
Image 8-4

Description: white odorless crystalline powder

treat infection, and is used topically to remove odors and stains. Baking soda is also used to treat multiple skin irritations such as poison oak, poison ivy, or skin fungus. Treat the affected area with a bath or a paste (see below for instructions) and apply directly to the skin.

In hoodoo medicine, baking soda is used in a "spiritual bath" to draw out negativity from the body.

Preparation and application

Heartburn Remedy

1. Dissolve 1/2 teaspoon of baking soda into 1 tablespoon of warm water
2. Add 1/2 cup of cold water
3. Add 1 tablespoon vinegar and 1/2 teaspoon of honey or cane sugar. Stir the mixture, then drink while it's fizzing.

Internal ailments due to high acid build-up (urinary tract infection, gout, kidney stones)

Mix 1/4 teaspoon of baking soda into an 8-ounce glass of water. Drink the remedy once per day for 2 weeks, then stop.

Skin conditions – itchy, burns, rashes, hives

Bath

Dissolve 1/2 to 1 cup of baking soda in a bath and soak for 20 minutes.

Paste

Mix baking soda with enough water to make a paste. Apply to chickenpox, shingles, blisters, or rashes. Repeat as needed.

Wash

Mix 1/2 to 1 cup of baking soda into 1 gallon of water and apply to your itchy patches with a washcloth soaked in the solution. Repeat several times as needed.

Toothpaste

Apply baking soda to a wet toothbrush and brush your teeth and gums. It will balance the pH in your mouth, helping to prevent caries and plaque build-up. Baking soda acts as an antiseptic and the abrasive texture will whiten teeth.

Banana Peel

(arthritis, warts, eczema, psoriasis, burns/scalds, acne)

Medicinal properties

antifungal, antibiotic, anti-inflammatory, high potassium

Health benefits

Banana peel contains natural antiseptic and cooling properties that can help reduce symptoms caused by skin conditions. Itching from insects and poison ivy may be relieved by rubbing the inside of the banana peel on affected area. Banana peel was also placed on the forehead to relieve headache pain. Bananas and the peel are high in vitamins and potassium which fight against arthritis and muscle cramps.

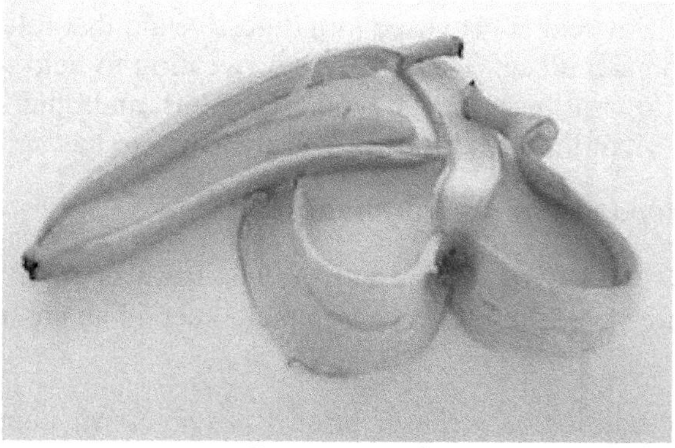

Banana peel
Image 8-5

Description: rubbery pale yellow skin with fleshy tan-colored inside

Preparation and application

For skin conditions such as psoriasis, eczema, acne, and itching, rub the inside of the banana peel on affected area and leave on for 20 to 30 minutes, allowing the skin to absorb the vitamins and nutrients. Leave on until the inside of the peel turns dark.

Banana Peel (continued)

Mix chopped/crushed banana peel and coal tar and make a paste. Rub on affected area 2 to 3 times a day.

For arthritis and muscle cramps, rub the inside of the banana peel on affected area and leave on overnight as a poultice. Hold the peel in place by wrapping with a cloth or bandage.

Bay Leaf

(headaches, colds and congestion)

Botanical names

Laurus nobilis or Umbellularia californica

Also known as

California laurel, California bay, Oregon myrtle, pepperwood

Medicinal properties

antibacterial, anti-cancer, antifungal, anti-inflammatory, antioxidant, antiseptic, appetite stimulant, astringent, carminative, diaphoretic, digestive, diuretic, emetic, insecticide, stomachic

Health benefits

The oil from the bay leaf makes this plant a powerful medicine. It was commonly used by both Native Americans and African Americans to treat colds, flu, headaches and migraines, congestion, bronchitis, arthritis, rheumatism, inflammation, and muscle pain.

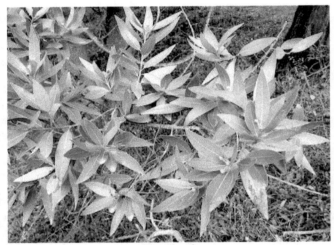

Bay leaf
Image 8-6

Description: dark green aromatic leaves

Bay leaf is also used as a digestive aid that relieves nausea and flatulence, upset stomach, colic, and stomach ulcers. It can promote sweating to help reduce fever and used topically as an insect repellent or to treat insect bites, wounds, rashes, and other skin conditions. Bay leaf is a rich source of vitamin C, vitamin A, and folic acid. Bay leaf also has antioxidants that give it anti-cancer properties.

Preparation and application

The leaves can be used either fresh or dried.[159] When cooking, they are best used dried so the bitterness is gone. Once you pick, keep in an air-tight jar or bag.

Tea

Add 1 to 3 fresh or dried bay leaves per cup of hot boiling water. Cover and steep for 10 to 15 minutes. Drink 1 to 3 cups daily to relieve ailments. Add 1 teaspoon of turmeric per cup of tea to help relieve headaches, migraines, arthritis, rheumatism, and inflammation.

Cooking

Add 2 to 3 dried leaves regularly to food dishes or make a tea from the leaves to help alleviate health ailments, maintain overall good health, or use as part of an excellent preventive health care regime.

---

[159] While fresh leaves are more potent, this does not make as much a difference with bay as it does with other herbs.

Inhalant-decongestant – Aromatheraphy

Add 2 to 3 fresh or dried bay leaves to a pot of boiling water or humidifier. For congestion and to relieve bronchitis, bring a pot of water to boil, then turn off. Place 7 to 10 fresh or dried leaves (or more, depending on the strength desired) in the water and place your head over the water and inhale the steam. Make sure you cover your head with a towel to contain the steam. You can place the pot on a table and sit in a chair or on a stool so you are comfortable. Inhale for 15 to 20 minutes or until steam has subsided. Repeat 2 to 3 times daily.

Poultice

Add several fresh or dried bay leaves to a pot of boiling water (2 to 3 bay leaves per cup of water), cover and let steep for 30 or more minutes. Soak a cloth in the warm bay leaf water, place several fresh or dried leaves in the cloth, and place it on your chest to help relieve respiratory infections, cold, cough, or flu. You can also place the cloth on affected areas to relieve headaches, muscle strains, sprains, and inflammation pain from arthritis and rheumatism.

Soak

Add several fresh or dried bay leaves to your bath or pan and soak affected areas to relieve muscle strains, sprains, and inflammation pain from arthritis and rheumatism.

Spiritual Alchemy and Cleansings

Use bay leaf to absorb negativity and to protect against bad energy. Take a branch filled with bay leaf from a tree and hang inside your dwelling from the ceiling, above doorways, or in front of windows. You can also line the entire perimeter of a windowsill with bay leaf. Once the leaves are dried and parched, take them outside to burn. The fire purifies and transforms the negativity into cleanliness and goodness.

Wash/Insecticide

Make a wash by placing several fresh or dried bay leaves (4 to 6 per cup of water) in a pot of hot water. Let cool and use topically to treat bee/wasp stings, other insect bites, and skin fungus. The leaf or branches with leaves are put in areas to keep moths, mosquitoes, bees, and other insects away.

Bee Shame

(good luck, attraction)

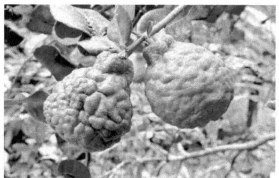

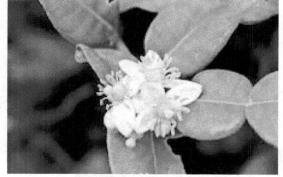

Bee Shame fruit on tree
Image 8-7

Bee Shame flower
Image 8-7a

Description: green leaves with reddish-purple on underside; flowers range from maroon to magenta to lilac

Botanical name

Citrus bergamia

<u>Bee Shame (continued)</u>

Also known as

bergamot, bergamot mint, bergamot orange, false lemon balm, lemon mint

Medicinal properties

carminative, rubefacient, stimulant

Spiritual properties for hoodoo medicine

good luck, good health, attracts money, attracts love, reverses a bad situation

Benefits

Used in African American hoodoo medicine as a tonic for good luck, prosperity, protection and positive attraction.

Preparation and application

Essential Oil

Rub the essential oil on your body.

Incense/smudge

Dry the leaves and flowers and burn as incense or smudge.

Medicine bag

Carry the herb in your medicine or mojo bag.

Wash or Bath

Make a wash using the herb and rub on your body or add 1 cup of the dried herb in your bath and soak.

Beet Root

(blood cleanser & fortifier)

Botanical name

Beta vulgaris

Also known as

garden beet, sea beet, spinach beet, sugar beet, white beet, mangel, wurzel

Medicinal properties

anticarcinogen, antioxidant, blood fortifier, immuno-stimulant, normalizes body pH

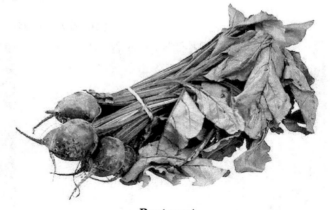

Beet root
Image 8-8

Description: deep purple root and stems; prominent veins on underside of green leaves are deep purple

Health benefits

The roots, greens, and juice of beets are good for your overall health. Beets strengthen your immunity, helping you resist sickness and disease. In African African American healing traditions, beet roots and juice are used as a "blood cleanser." Eating beets regularly may normalize your body's pH and build blood, lower blood pressure, lower cholesterol, strengthen nerves, tone the liver, and act as a laxative.

Beets are a mood enhancer and a stimulant (by bringing more oxygen to your blood). Beet greens are antioxidant-rich and have anti-cancer properties. In Africa, beet roots are used as an antidote to cyanide poisoning. Beets are rich in calcium, iron, potassium, magnesium, iron, phosphorous, folic acid, and fiber. They are an excellent source of vitamins A and C, and B vitamins such as B1, B2, B3 and B6.

Preparation and application

Cooking

Cook as green veggies or make into a salad by chopping up the stems and the leaves. The roots of the beets can be cooked whole: steamed, boiled, pickled, or baked. You can use them in salads either cooked or raw, or sprinkle vinegar on them.

In the late 1800s and early 1900s, beets were used as a blood cleanser by slicing them raw and leaving them out overnight in a bowl to catch the morning dew. Drink the juice and eat the beets.

Beet Salad Recipe
* Boil roots and let cool. Chop them so they are small and bite-sized
* Add chopped garlic and onions

Optional
* Add shredded carrots, chopped apples, walnuts, or sesame seeds
* Season with vinaigrette, apple cider vinegar (ACV), Spike, cumin, or sea salt

Bilberry

(eye health, sore throat, diabetes)

Botanical name

Vaccinium myrtillus

Also known as

dyeberry, huckleberry, whortleberry, wineberry

Medicinal properties

antioxidant, antifungal, antibacterial, anti-inflammatory, antihistamine, astringent

Health benefits

A tea was made from dried bilberry fruit to strengthen and improve eyesight and night vision and to prevent cataracts. Other uses for bilberry medicine have been to treat mouth sores, sore throats, diabetes, and diarrhea. The leaves and dried berries are used as medicine.

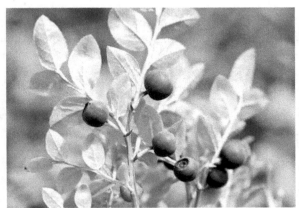

Bilberry
Image 8-9

Description: blue-black colored berries; medium-hued green leaves

Preparation and application

Put 1 teaspoon of the dried crushed berries in 1 cup of hot water, cover and steep for 20 minutes. Drink 1 to 3 cups daily. Sweeten to taste.

For sore throat and mouth sores, make a strong tea using dried bilberry leaves and drink or use as a gargle.

Birdbill Tea

(coughs, colds, congestion, tuberculosis)

Botanical name

Commelina dianthifolia

Also known as

birdbill dayflower

Medicinal properties

anti-inflammatory, demulcent, diuretic, mucilaginous

Health benefits

Birdbill tea was widely used among Native American tribes and in African American healing traditions to treat coughs and colds and to help strengthen patients with tuberculosis. The mucilaginous (sticky and moist) sap from the stem and flower are made into a tea to sooth irritations such as sore throats. The tea is also purported to relieve fevers and act as a diuretic to eliminate excess fluids. The stems, flowers, and leaves can be mashed or chopped up and used as a poultice to reduce inflammation on the skin. Leaves and shoots are edible and can be used in salads or lightly cooked with other greens.

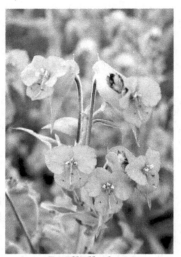

Birdbill plant
Image 8-10

Description: bright blue flower tops, medium green-hued leaves

Preparation and application

Tea

Use stems, roots, and leaves to make a tea by boiling for 5 minutes in hot water, covering and letting steep for 25 to 30 minutes. Strain, cool, and drink. Use 1 teaspoon birdbill to 1 cup of water. Drink 1 to 3 cups daily.

Poultice

Mash the stem, flower, and leaves with a mortar and pestle. Apply mixture to affected area and wrap with cheesecloth, muslin, or wool. Leave on for at least 1 hour or longer.

Black Cohosh

(menstruation disorders, PMS, hot flashes/menopause)

Botanical names

Cimicifuga racemosa or Actaea racemosa

Also known as

black snakeroot, bugbane, bugwort, rattleroot, rattletop, rattleweed

Medicinal properties

alterative, antibacterial, antifungal, anti-inflammatory, antispasmodic, diaphoretic, emmenogogue, estrogenic, mild sedative, stomach tonic

Health benefits

Black cohosh was commonly used to treat female disorders and has estrogen-like properties that may increase or decrease estrogen level in different individuals. It is well-known for it's purported ability to induce abortions and to regulate uterine contractions during childbirth. Each person responds differently to this herb. Black cohosh was taken to stimulate menstrual cycles and suppressed menstruation, treat uterine inflammation, relieve PMS, and to alleviate menstrual cramps and infertility. With menopause, black cohosh may help relieve hot flashes, irritability, and mood swings. Depending on the ailment, healers sometimes mixed this herb with blue cohosh (see discussion of blue cohosh below). Black cohosh roots have also been used to treat other ailments like colds, coughs, sore throats, constipation, kidney disorders, rheumatism, fever, and snake bites.

Preparation and application

Infuse 1 teaspoon of the dried root in one cup of hot water for 20 minutes and drink 1 to 2 times daily for 3 days.

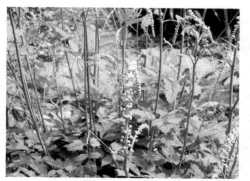

Black cohosh
Image 8-11

Description: glossy dark green leaves; feathery white flowers

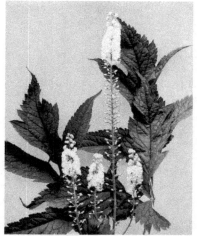

Black cohosh in bloom 1
Image 8-11a

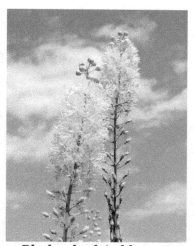

Black cohosh in bloom 2
Image 8-11b

Description: glossy dark green leaves; feathery white flowers

(**Caution**: Black cohosh is a very potent medicine and was not taken long-term (more than 5 days) or while pregnant. This medicine was used with caution or under the guidance of a health professional.)

Black Draught Tea

(constipation, colds)

Also known as

Black Draught laxative, Black Draught syrup, Thedford's Black Draught

Medicinal properties

purgative

Health benefits

Black Draught tea was commonly used in African American healing traditions to treat constipation and colds. Its history dates back to before the Civil War, when Dr. A.O. Simmons first introduced it as a laxative tea in 1840. Much like castor oil, Black Draught was used to treat many ailments. It was

Black Draught Tea (continued)

bought as a powder or liquid/syrup and then mixed in water, sometimes adding molasses, and then drunk 1 to 3 times a day depending on the ailment and age of the recipient. Lower doses were given to
children. Black Draught was also given to constipated horses and cattle. The early formula contained senna and magnesium. Versions of Black Draught sold today are in the form of a pill or syrup also contains other compounds that may or may not be natural.

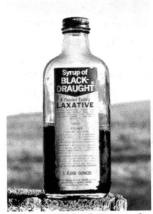

Syrup of Black Draught
(Image 8-12)

Preparation and application

Suggested dosage as prescribed on bottle.

Black Gum Tree

**(The black gum, dogwood, and pickash or prickly ash trees
are all commonly referred to as the toothbrush tree)**

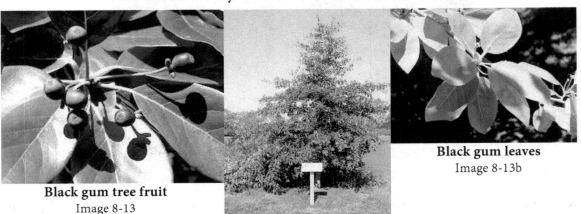

Black gum tree fruit
Image 8-13

Black gum tree
Image 8-13a

Black gum leaves
Image 8-13b

Description: green dark leaves, pale hairy underneath; bright scarlet or yellow colored leaves in autumn; light reddish-brown bark; yellowish green flowers, purpleish-blue fruit

Botanical name

Nyssa sylvatica

Also known as

black tupelo, gum, pepperide, sour gum, swamp tree, toothbrush tree, tupelo

Medicinal properties

emetic, ophthalmic, vermifuge

Health benefits

Known as the toothbrush tree, a twig or branch was broken from the tree and the bark was stripped at the top. The bark-stripped end was put in the mouth and chewed on until the ends frayed like toothbrush bristles, which were used to massage and clean the teeth and gums. A tea made from the bark was drunk to expel intestinal worms. The small fruit is edible.

Preparation and application

Put 1 teaspoon of the shaved bark in 1 cup of boiled water, cover and steep for 20 minutes.

Black Tar Soap

(rashes, eczema, psoriasis, skin fungus, head lice)

Also known as

coal tar soap, tar soap

Medicinal properties

antiparasitic, antiseptic, detoxifier

Health benefits

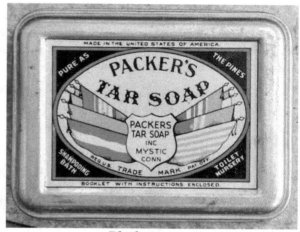

Black tar soap
Image 8-14

Black tar soap is a soap made from coal tar, a black liquid that is a byproduct of distilled coal. Black coal tar is also available as an ointment, salve, shampoo, cream, or gel. The antiseptic and detoxifying properties helped treat a variety of skin conditions such as psoriasis, eczema, acne, seborrheic dermatitis (dandruff), scabies, and ringworm. It reduced inflammation and itchiness from dry skin, slowed down rapid skin cell growth, and restored the natural appearance of the skin. As an anti-parasitic, black tar soap was used to treat head lice. It was used in small doses internally to help expel intestinal worms and parasites.

Preparation and application

Used as a wash applied to affected area and then rinsed, or as a medicinal ointment.

Blackberry Root and Leaves

(sore throat, diarrhea, bladder infections, inflammation)

Botanical name

Rubus fructicosis

Also known as

bramble, dewberry, goutberry

Medicinal properties

acerbic, antioxidant, astringent, diuretic, uterine tonic

Health benefits

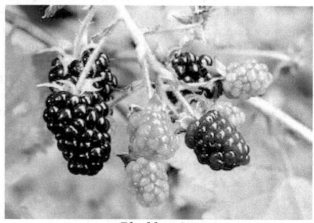

Blackberries
Image 8-15

Description: dark green leaves; purplish-blue fruit

The root, leaves, and berries are used as medicine. Blackberry root tea is a good treatment for intestinal disorders such as diarrhea and dysentery and to help relieve

Blackberry Root and Leaves (continued)

bladder infections, ulcers, and hemorrhoids.

Use as a gargle and wash for mouth and throat inflammation, thrush, sore throat, and gum inflammations. Blackberry medicine is an antioxidant that has high levels of anthocyanins, which may also help to maintain healthy blood pressure and healthy blood sugar levels, support the liver, and improve vision and mental acuity. Blackberry is also rich with vitamins C, E and the mineral selenium.

Preparation and application

Tea

Add 1 ounce of the dried leaves and/or root or bark to 1 pint of boiling water. Cover and steep 10 to 15 minutes if using leaves only, 20 minutes if using bark but not root, 30 minutes if using root. Let cool down, strain, and then drink. Drink warm or at room temperature. For diarrhea, sip about 1/4 cup of blackberry root tea per hour until symptoms subside.

Poultice – Medicinal Pack

Used on minor cuts and scrapes to help control bleeding. Gather the berries, crush and wrap in a piece of cheesecloth, and apply to affected area.

Blue Cohosh

(stimulates menstrual flow, uterine tonic)

Botanical name

Caulophyllum thalictroides

Also known as

blue ginseng, papoose root, squaw root

Medicinal properties

anti-cancer, anti-inflammatory, antirheumatic, antispasmodic, emmenagogue, diuretic, hyper-tensive, uterine tonic

Health benefits

Blue cohosh is best known as an herb to stimulate menstrual flow if it is suppressed and to induce labor in natural childbirth. It is also a tonic for decreasing menstrual cramps by improving the tone in uterine muscles, and is useful for regulating menstrual flow for women with irregular or spotty menstrual cycle. Blue cohosh is also helpful in alleviating breast tenderness and bloating. It has also been used to treat arthritis pain and inflammation. The herb was not taken by pregnant women because of its strong uterine contraction properties.

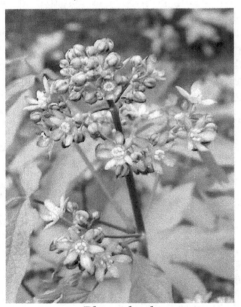

Blue cohosh
Image 8-16

Description: medium green leaves; yellowish green flower; dark blue fruit

Preparation and application

A tea or decoction was made by adding 1 to 2 teaspoons of the dried root to 1 to 2 cups of water, then slow boiling the mixture for 20 minutes. Drink 1 to 3 cups daily. May have been taken with black cohosh to strengthen and regulate uterine contraction during childbirth.

A note of caution: Blue and black cohosh are very potent medicines and were not taken long-term (more than 5 days) or while pregnant. These medicines were used with caution or under the guidance of a health professional.

Bloodroot

(see "Coon Root" this chapter)

Boneset

(swelling, colds, congestion, fever, muscle aches, immune booster)

Botanical name

Eupatorium perfoliatum

Also known as

agueweed, crosswort, eupatorium, feverwort, Indian sage, sweating plant, thoroughwort, tse-ian, vegetable antimony, wood boneset

Medicinal properties

anti-inflammatory, antispasmodic, aperient, astringent, bitter, diaphoretic, diuretic immune stimulant, laxative

Health benefits

Boneset got its name in the treatment of break bonefever (dengue), a viral infection that intense muscle pain that it feels like your bones will break. In general, boneset tea is used to treat colds and flu, break up chest congestion, induce sweating, and relieve aches and pains associated with arthritis, rheumatism, and muscle strains. It is also a bitter and astringent which is effective for loss of appetite, indigestion, and constipation. As a general tonic, boneset stimulates immunity.

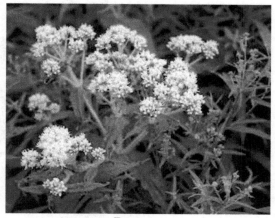

Boneset
Image 8-17
Description: medium green leaves, white flowers

Preparation and application

Use the leaves and flower tops. Collect the flowers as they open in late summer or early fall.

Tea

Pour 1 cup of boiling water over 2 to 3 teaspoons of dried herb, cover and let steep for 10 to 15 minutes. Drink as hot as possible. For flu or fever, drink 3 to 5 cups daily. Add honey and lemon to sweeten and flavor. Drink cold boneset tea thirty minutes before meals to aid digestion.

Buttongrass or Buttonweed

(for colds and flu)

Botanical name

Spermacoce glabra or Spermacoce laevis

Also known as

poorjoe

Medicinal properties

alterative, antibiotic, astringent, demulcent, muci-laginous

Buttongrass or Buttonweed (continued)

Health benefits

Buttonweed is often mistaken for what some people generalize as a pesky "wild weed" subject to be pulled up and thrown away rather than valued for medicinal use. Yet it is rich with calcium and phosphorous, and is used as medicine to treat a variety of ailments. A tea is made from the leaves or root to treat colds, coughs, and diarrhea, to reduce infections, to break fevers, and to treat colic and stomach aches. Buttonweed leaves and root are also used in Ayurvedic and Chinese medicine.

Preparation and application

Tea

Combine 1 teaspoon of the dried leaves or 2 teaspoons of the fresh leaves with 1 cup of hot water, cover and steep for 10 to 15 minutes and drink.

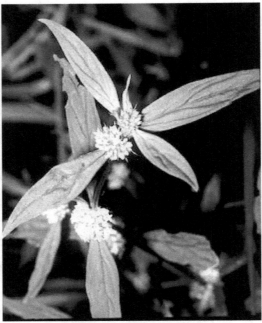

Buttongrass (weed)
Image 8-18
Description: green leaves with white, pink or reddish flowers

Buttonwillow or Buttonbush

(reduces fever, swelling, toothaches)

Botanical name

Cephalanthus occidentalis

Also known as

buttonbush, honeybells

Medicinal properties

anti-inflammatory, astringent, diaphoretic, diuretic, emetic, febrifuge, laxative, odontalgic, ophthalmic

Health benefits

The leaves, bark, and root are used medicinally to treat a number of ailments. A decoction made from the bark is used to treat fevers, diarrhea, stomach ailments, and hemorrhages. The bark is chewed to get relief from toothaches. A wash made from the bark can be used for eye inflammations. A decoction of the roots and leaves was made to treat fevers, constipation, toothaches, kidney stones, diarrhea, and dysentery, and to regulate menstrual flow.

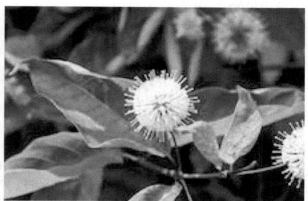

Buttonwillow bush (detail)
Image 8-19a

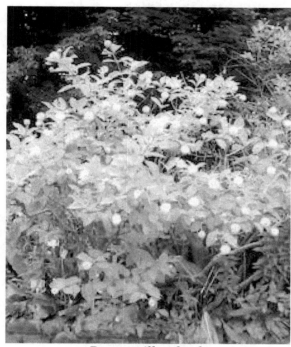

Buttonwillow bush
Image 8-19

Description: glossy dark green leaves with fuzzy white flowers

Preparation and application

Decoctions

Bark decoction

Bring to boil 1 teaspoon of bark to 1 cup of water, let simmer for 20 minutes, then cool. Strain and drink 1 to 3 cups.

Root and leaf decoction

Bring to boil in a pot of water 1 teaspoon of root and leaf to 1 cup of water, let simmer for 20 minutes, then cool. Strain and drink 1 to 3 cups daily until relief.

Tea

Use 1 teaspoon of dried buttonwillow, or 3 to 4 teaspoons of fresh leaves, to 1 cup of boiling water. Cover and steep for 10 to 15 minutes, cool and drink.

Buzzard Weed

(colds, swelling, general health tonic)

Botanical name

Porophyllum ruderale

Also known as

buzzard breath, buzzy weed, quinquilla, papalo, papaloquelite, polivian coriander, skunk weed

Medicinal properties

antioxidant, antibacterial, carminative, diuretic

Health benefits

A tea made from the leaves, or the leaves eaten raw, are used to reduce swelling from injuries, support liver function, and maintain a healthy blood pressure. Buzzard weed is native to the Americas and can be found growing wild in Texas and as far south as Argentina. The leaves of the plant are used as a garnish and in sauces similar to cilantro.[160]

Preparation and application

Tea

Fill a pot with the raw leaves, cover with water, bring to boil, turn off fire, and let cool. Strain and drink often. The leaves can be eaten as well.

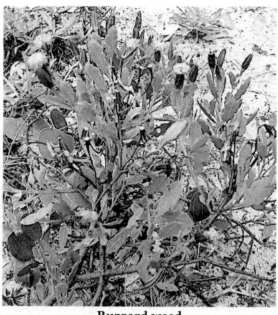

Buzzard weed
Image 8-20

Description: bluish green leaves with pale yellow dandelion-like puff balls emerging from a maroon base

Food

Buzzard weed is used in a variety of South American dishes. The leaves are chopped raw and sprinkled over a variety of traditional foods. Also used similarly to Mexican coriander and cilantro.

Calamus Root

(colds, flu, bronchitis, coughs)

Botanical name

Acorus calamus

Also known as

beewort, calmus, cinnamon sedge, flagroot, gladdon, myrtle grass, myrtle sledge, muskrat root, rat root, sweet calomel, sweet cane, sweet flag, sweet grass, sweet myrtle, sweet root, sweet rush, sweet sledge

Medicinal properties

abortifacient, analgesic, antibacterial, anti-cancer, antihistamine, antioxidant, aromatic, carminative, decongestant, diuretic, emmenagogue, expectorant, nervine, sedative, uterine tonic

---

[160] In a search for buzzard weed as a medicine used in African American healing traditions, that particular use for this plant was not found. The closest possible association was buzzy weed and buzzard breath, aka papaloquelite, that grows wild in Texas.

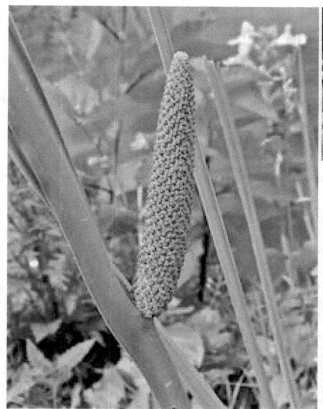

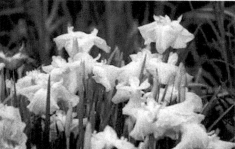

Calamus plant flowering
Image 8-21a

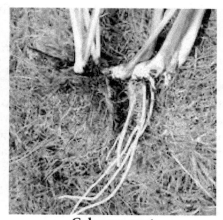

Calamus plant
Image 8-21

Calamus root
Image 8-21b

Description: greenish yellow leaves with tan-yellow cattail

Health benefits

Calamus root (or "sweet flag," as it is sometimes commonly called) has been used since ancient times for a variety of purposes that range from a medicine, an aphrodisiac, and as a spice. Practitioners of African American traditional medicine use Calamus root to treat lung and digestive system ailments and as an ingredient in conjuring and rootworking. Calamus root is used to treat colds, flu, and bronchitis by acting as an expectorant for coughs and eliminating phlegm. It is also an effective digestive aid treating flatulence, bloating, gastritis, heartburn, and nausea and as an appetite stimulant. Other medicinal uses have been for headaches, arthritis, sore throat, energy stimulant, asthma, allergies, regulating menstrual flow, and as an aphrodisiac and relaxant. It is also used in Ayurvedic and Chinese medicine.

Preparation and application

Medicine was made from the dried root in the form of a tea or powder or by chewing pieces of the dried root and then spitting it out when it was chewed up, much like tobacco or the powder form of snuff.

Tea

Use 1 tablespoon of dried cut, chopped, or shredded root per cup of hot water for tea. Cover and let steep for 25 to 30 minutes and drink.

Infusion

Cut pieces of the root and place in a mason jar. Pour lukewarm water over the root, using 1 tablespoon of root to 1 cup of water. Close the top. Let sit overnight and drink 1 to 3 cups a day. If using as a digestive aid, drink 1 cup of the mixture 20 minutes before a meal.

Calamus Root (continued)

Powder

Grind the dried root or pieces of the root into a powder. For a tea, mix 1 tablespoon of powder with 1 cup of hot water and sweeten with honey.

Place calamus root powder in corner of mouth or bottom lip (like snuff) until your saliva liquefies it. Then spit out the same way you would snuff or chewing tobacco. This treatment is purported to relieve congestion, coughing, and digestive problems.

Root

Chew a piece of the root until it is sufficiently broken down to be ready to swallow. Do not swallow, but instead spit out. Through the process of chewing, the medicine is mixed with your saliva and absorbed into your system. This is an effective way to alleviate digestive problems, to use as a relaxant, or for other treatments.

Spiritual-Hoodoo-Conjure

In the African American rootworking and conjuring tradition, Calamus root is used for control and domination of a person or a situation. This could be a love spell or controlling someone's decisions and actions to your benefit. Calamus root chips can be burned (like dry sage or on charcoal) in an area before the person you want it to affect enters, or while you are meditating on the situation you wish to affect. Calamus root can be put in the corners of the home of the person you want to affect or in an area they frequent. You can make a conjure bag containing calamus root in order to dominate a situation.

Camphor

(colds, congestion, infections, muscle/joint pains)

Botanical name

Cinnamomum camphora

Also known as

gum camphor, laurel camphor

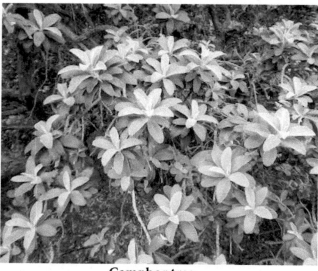

Camphor tree
Image 8-22

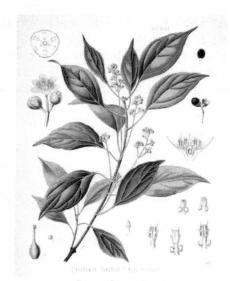

Camphor plant
Image 8-22a

Description: glossy waxy green leaves; in spring, bright-green leaves with white flowers and blackberry-like fruit

Medicinal properties

analgesic, antibacterial, anti-inflammatory, antimicrobial, antiseptic, antiviral, diaphoretic, expectorant, febrifuge, parasiticide, rubefacient, stimulant

Health benefits

Camphor was used as a topical salve or ointment that was rubbed on the chest and back to treat infections, colds that came with chest and nasal congestion, or as an inhalant. Camphor was used to treat cold sores, and was also used to treat aches and pains of joints and muscle due to strain, arthritis, back pain, tired feet, and other body stresses. Camphor is a medicinal ingredient in many healing salves like Vicks to treat colds, coughs, bronchitis, congestion, and other respiratory ailments. Camphor has been used as an insect repellent and in mothballs. The oil is toxic and potentially fatal when taken internally. Small doses were taken internally to treat diarrhea and colds. Camphor can be harvested from the wood of the camphor tree, an evergreen.

Preparation and application

Aches and pains, arthritis and strains

Rub camphor oil or salve on affected area 2 to 3 times daily.

For colds and congestion

Rub camphor oil or salve on chest and back. At night, wear a heavy shirt or long johns to help sweat out congestion.

Inhalant

* Put camphor oil drops in a humidifier.
* Put camphor drops in a pot of boiled water and allow the medicine to come up with the steam. Cover your head with a towel and put your head close to the pot and inhale the steam.

Cascara Sagrada

(constipation, digestive, bowel toner)

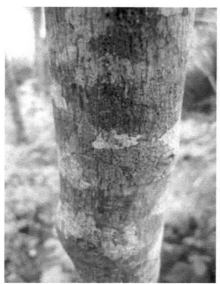

Cascara tree bark
Image 8-23

Description: gray-brown cascara sagarda bark

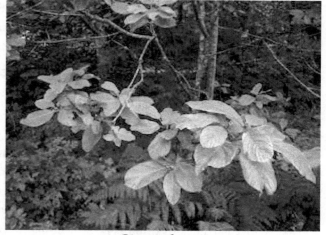

Cascara leaves
Image 8-23a

Description: green leaves, buds that give rise to small white flowers and small red berries (berries and flowers not shown)

Cascara Sagrada (continued)

Botanical name

Rhamnus purshianus

Also known as

bearberry, buckthorn, California buckthorn, chittam bark, chittam wood, pur-shiana bark, sacred bark

Medicinal properties

bitter, chittam bark, chittam wood, emetic, laxative, nervine, purgative, stomach tonic

Health benefits

Cascara sagrada medicine was used often by Native Americans in the Northwest who introduced it to European colonizers. The Spaniards were so impressed with its medicinal properties, mostly being its powerful laxative effects, that they called it sacred bark, cascara sagrada. Cascara medicine was used to treat mild to chronic constipation, gallstones, liver ailments, and digestive problems, and to tone the bowel muscles. Cascara medicine is rich with vitamin B complex, B2 and B6, calcium, flavonoids, manganese, and potassium. Cascara sagrada use is approved by the FDA.

Preparation and application

The cascara bark has the medicinal properties. The bark is most potent when harvested in spring or fall and allowed to dry for at least 12 months before using. Today cascara sagrada bark medicine is found in various forms including tablets, extracts, or the dried bark in tea bags or bulk. The dried bark can be cut into pieces, ground into powder, or made into an extract or tincture.

Tea

Hot infusion

* Put 1/2 to 1 teaspoon of the dried bark in hot water, cover and steep for 15 to 20 minutes. Drink 2 to 3 cups daily. Bowels should move within 6 to 12 hours.
* Put 1 tablespoon of bark in 1 cup of hot water 1 hour before bedtime. Cover and steep for 1 hour then drink immediately before going to bed.

Cold infusion

Put 1 tablespoon of the dried bark in cold water and let sit for 12 hours. Drink right before bedtime.

Tea bags

Steep 1 to 2 bags in hot water for 10 to 15 minutes and drink right before bedtime.

Tincture

Add 200 mg of the dried bark or 100 mg of powdered bark to 1/2 liter of 80 to 100 proof of denatured alcohol in a mason jar. Close the lid tightly and place in a cool dark area for 3 weeks. Shake vigorously daily. Strain through cheesecloth into a clean jar. Use 30 to 40 drops in warm water and drink 2 to 3 times daily.

Capsules

Take 1 to 2 capsules of dried bark at bedtime or at the start of the day with a full glass of water. Bowels should move within 6 to 12 hours.

Cautionary note: Cascarda sagrada should not be taken for more than 7 days, or by children or pregnant/lactating women.

Castor Oil, Castor Tree, Oil Bush Plant

(laxative, purgative, detoxifier, immune booster)

Botanical name

Ricinus communis

Also known as

castor, eranda

Medicinal properties

anti-inflammatory, antifungal, antioxidant, immune booster, purgative

Health benefits

Castor oil has many wonderful health benefits and has been used medicinally for thousands of years, although most people are only familiar with it as a strong laxative. Castor oil is a fatty acid that is 90% ricinoleic acid, which is known to prevent illness and strengthen the immune system. Castor oil medicine can be taken internally or applied externally in poultices and packs or rubbed directly on the affected area.

Castor oil's anti-inflammatory properties help treat pain associated with arthritis and rheumatism. Castor oil packs applied externally may help to detoxify the body, eliminate lymphatic congestion, increase white blood cells, and reduce inflammation. Castor oil has also been used to treat many everyday problems such as: yeast infections, constipation, gastrointestinal problems, menstrual disorders, migraines, acne, sunburn, athlete's foot, ringworm, skin abrasions, and inflammation. In pregnant women, castor oil has been used to induce labor.

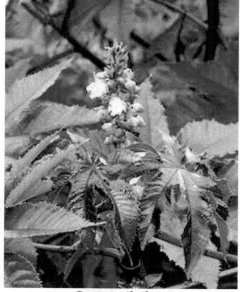

Castor oil plant
Image 8-24

Description: glossy dark green leaves that can be dark reddish purple or bronze when young, red, yellow or green pigmented flowers, greenish seed capsules

Preparation and application

Internal: as a laxative or purgative

Take 1 teaspoon in the morning. You can mix the oil with a juice such as orange, cranberry, or ginger to take away the taste. You should feel the effects in 6 to 12 hours. Do not take continuously for more than three days.

External

To treat a range of skin conditions, fungus, and inflammation:

Castor oil wrap for arthritis, rheumatism or joint pain

Massage castor oil on the affected area and cover (i.e., use a sock to cover feet), or wrap in a cloth soaked in castor oil at nighttime and let sit overnight. If the area is small enough, apply a castor oil soaked adhesive bandage. Cover with plastic or a towel to prevent oil transfer to clothes, furniture, or bedding.

Pack or poultice to treat a range of internal conditions:

Use a castor oil pack to increase circulation, promote elimination and healing of tissues and organs underneath the skin so as to stimulate liver, relieve pain, increase the production of white blood cells, stimulate lymphatic circulation, eliminate lymphatic congestion, reduce inflammation, improve digestion, and reduce menstrual discomfort such as cramps, cysts, and other irregularities. The castor oil medicine is absorbed into the skin to treat and detoxify the body.

Castor Oil, Castor Tree, Oil Bush Plant (continued)

Soak a piece of wool, cotton or natural flannel in castor oil and place it on the affected area. Cover the cloth with a thin piece of plastic (bag, Saran Wrap, etc.), and then place a heating pad or hot water bottle over the plastic to heat the pack. Leave on for 1 to 2 hours overnight. Place on right side of abdomen to detoxify the liver. Place on whole abdomen to treat constipation and digestive orders and to stimulate lymphatic system. Place on lower abdomen for menstrual discomfort. Place directly on area affected by muscle strains, arthritis, inflammation, or pain. Regrigerate and reuse pack for 2 months, saturating cloth with more oil with each use. Replace with a new cloth if continuing to use after 2 months.

Catnip

(menstrual cramps, insomnia, relaxation, colds, flu, fever, colic, digestion)

Botanical name

Nepta cataria

Also known as

catmint, catswort

Medicinal properties

antispasmodic, antitussive, astringent, antibacterial, carminative, diaphoretic, sedative, sudorific, slightly emmenagogue, slightly stimulant, stomachic and tonic

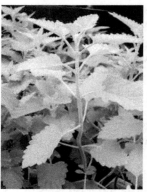

Catnip
Image 8-25

Health benefits

Catnip tea is widely used in African American healing traditions to promote relaxation and sleep and to relieve colic, headaches, migraines, and menstrual cramping. Catnip tea made from the leaves is also used to treat symptoms from flu, colds, fever, sore throat, nasal congestion, bladder inflammation, digestive disorders, diarrhea, and as a detoxifier. Catnip contains vitamins A, B, and C, calcium, iron, magnesium, manganese, phosphorus, potassium, selenium. and sodium. Drinking it as a tea is the best way to get the medicinal benefits.

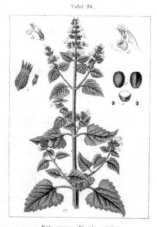

Catnip (Illustration)
Image 8-25a

Preparation and application

Tea

Use one teaspoon of dried catnip or three or four teaspoons of fresh catnip leaves to one cup of warm water. (Make sure the water is not too hot. Adding catnip to hot water decreases the medicinal benefits and flavor.) If using the fresh leaves, be sure to "bruise" the leaves by rubbing them together and slightly cracking them before infusing in warm water. Cover and let steep for 15 to 20 minutes. Drink 2 to 3 cups daily.

Description: green to green-gray leaves, flowers can be blue, white, pink, lilac, or lavender with purple dots

You can add lemon, honey or orange for added flavor. If you are harvesting catnip, cut the stem and hang in a dark, cool area to dry. When the leaves and flowering tops on the stem are fully dried it is ready for use. Store the dried catnip leaves and flowers in a glass jar or plastic bag. Store in a cool, dry place.

Cayenne Pepper

(circulation, colds, congestion)

Botanical name

Capsicum annum

Also known as

African bird, cow-horn, guinea spice

Medicinal properties

antifungal, carminative, increases circulation, cicatrizing, rubefacient, stimulant, stomachic that improves digestion

Health benefits

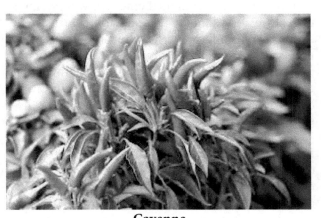

Cayenne
Image 8-26

Description: Green leaves with bright red peppers

Cayenne peppers are hot chili peppers related to bell and jalapeño peppers. There are many different types of cayenne (capsicum) peppers grown and used to spice and flavor the cuisine of many cultures such as Louisiana Creole, Thai, Mexican, East Indian, and African.

Cayenne peppers can be made into health tonics to ward off and treat illness and disease. Ingested regularly, cayenne helps to maintain good health and acts as a preventative. Cayenne pepper increases circulation and body temperature which helps expel toxins and congestion from the body. It also boosts metabolism and is an excellent digestive, as it stimulates the flow of stomach secretions and saliva.

Today, modern health advocates claim cayenne is a "super-herb" that can help treat everything from heart disease, sudden heart attacks, psoriasis, diabetes, and more.

Preparation and application

Tea

Make a tea using 1/4 teaspoon of cayenne or 1 teaspoon of chopped cayenne pepper to 1 cup of hot water, sweeten to taste. Lemon and other herbs optional. Drink in the morning as a stimulant and to rid body of toxins and congestion. Drink before or after a major meal to aid digestion.

Food

Add the chopped pepper or a few shakes of the powder/spice to your favorite foods and drinks.

Tonic

Add 1/4 to 1/2 teaspoon of cayenne in with other herbs used to treat a specific ailment.

Cedar (Eastern Red Cedar)

(colds, coughs)

Botanical name

Juniperous virginiana

Also known as

red cedar

Medicinal properties

antiseborrheic, antiseptic, antispasmodic, astringent, diuretic, emmenagogue, expectorant, fungicide, sedative, general health tonic

Cedar (Eastern Red Cedar) (continued)

Health benefits

Cedar is a powerful medicine rich with vitamin C. The leaves, bark, twigs, and fruit are used to extract the healing properties. Cedar medicine was used to treat a variety of ailments that included: respiratory and fungal infections, bronchitis, coughs, congestion, excess mucous, menstrual delay, uterine contraction, venereal warts, gonorrhea, kidney and urinary tract infection, headaches, rheumatism, arthritis, and inflammation. It also helps treat itchy skin rashes such as dermatitis, eczema, psoriasis, dandruff, acne, and oily skin conditions. Cedar medicine also acts as a diuretic and stimulates circulation. Many Native American tribes burn cedar wood in ceremony.

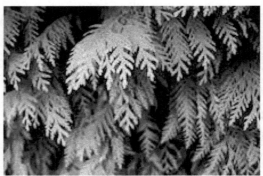

Cedar leaves
Image 8-27

Preparation and application

Cedar bark, twigs, leaves, and fruit were used as medicine in a decoction, tea, poultice, salve, powder, wash, and inhalant.

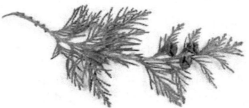

Cedar leaves with seeds
Image 8-27a

Decoction for internal use

Use 1 cup of fresh cedar green leaves (can also add twigs and berries) to 2 cups of water. Wash the leaves before you use them. Bruise leaves (rub together to break open) and put them in a pot, cover with water, and bring to boil. Pour out water, then cover again with 2 cups of water, bring to boil a second time, strain. Sweeten with honey if desired. Drink 1 cup daily for 3 days. The oil in cedar tea can be extremely toxic. Boiling once, and throwing out the water and then boiling a second time removes the toxicity, but it still must be used with caution.

Inhalant (congestion, respiratory ailments, coughs, bronchitis, etc.)

Put fresh cedar leaves and/or twigs and berries in a pot so it fills the pot half way. Fill the pot with water. Bring to a boil and then turn down to a low simmer. Put your head over the pot so you can inhale the steam while a towel or blanket covers your head to enclose the steam. Inhale for 15 to 30 minutes then rest.

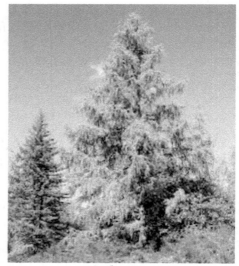

Cedar tree
Image 8-27b

Description: green leaves with green or yellow-brown flowers, sienna-colored cones with shiny brown seeds

Poultice for external use (arthritis, aches and pains, skin conditions)

Use berries, twigs or leaves externally as a poultice or salve to treat arthritis, rheumatism, warts, fungus, swelling, lesions, and skin conditions and as an antibacterial.

Place fresh leaves, twigs, and berries in a pot of hot water that has already been boiled. Use 1 cup of cedar matter to 1 cup of water. Let soak in the hot water until cool. Strain with cheesecloth so the leaves are in the cloth and the liquid is in a bowl. Place enough of the cedar matter in a clean cloth (muslin, cotton, gauze) so that it will cover the affected area. Wrap the cedar medicine in the cloth and place over affected area. Hold in place using another cloth or ace bandage as a wrap. Pour the liquid into a jar for use as a wash to apply to skin conditions like ringworm and rashes.

Salve for external use (skin conditions, arthritis, aches and pains, circulation)

Finely chop leaves and twigs or blend in a blender until they are like a powder. Use 1 cup of cedar matter to 2 cups of natural oil such as coconut, shea butter, or olive. Use beeswax to increase thickness as desired. Simmer in a pot for 1 hour. Let cool. No need to strain if the cedar matter used was similar to powder. If the matter is larger, strain mixture so matter is removed. What remains is the salve, which has absorbed the cedar medicine.

For a berry salve, follow the above, but crush or bruise the berries slightly either with a mortar and pestle or mashed in a bowl with a spoon or spatula. Place in a pot. Can mix with chopped or blended leaves.

Soak or Bath

In a bath or soak of hot water, place several cedar leaves and soak entire body or affected area for 20 to 30 minutes.

Wash for external use (preferred for skin conditions)

Follow directions in "Poultice" above except use 1 cup of the cedar matter to 2 cups of water. Apply the wash to affected areas.

Celery

(gout, blood cleaner, uric acid build-up)

Botanical name

Apium graveolens

Medicinal properties

antiasthmatic, carminative, digestive aid, diuretic, expectorant

Health benefits

In African American healing traditions, celery and celery broth were often used to cure and relieve gout. Celery medicine is a diuretic that promotes urination. This may reduce uric acid and excess water buildup, conditions that cause pain and inflammation in gout and arthritis. In Ayurvedic medicine, celery is used in treatments for colds, flu, water retention, poor digestion, arthritis, and liver and spleen ailments. Celery is also known to lower blood pressure by relaxing the arteries and dilating the blood vessels, which helps increase blood flow. Celery is a good source of potassium, calcium, and magnesium, vitamin K, folate, fiber, B vitamins, manganese, iron, and tryptophan (an essential amino acid).

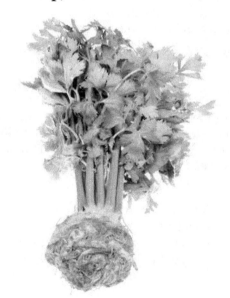

Celery
Image 8-28

Description: medium to light green leaves and stalk, white flowering tops

Preparation and application

Add celery to meals or eat plain.

Broth

Chop up the celery stalk, put it in a pot of water, bring to boil, cover pot and let steep for 30 minutes. Drink the broth and eat the celery, but mostly drink the broth, which has absorbed the nutrients.

Today, the power of celery medicine has been put into pill form or tincture and can be bought at a natural health and food store.

Chamomile

(insomnia, calming, anxiety, nervousness, cramps)

Botanical name

Maticaria recutita

Medicinal properties

anti-inflammatory, antiseptic, anti-anxiety/sedative, cicatrizer, decongestant, detoxifier, emollient

Health benefits

Chamomile tea has many health benefits, but is often used as a mild tranquilizer. It was commonly used in African American healing traditions for menstrual cramps, menstrual suppression, colic, stomach problems such as gas and nausea, anxiety, insomnia, and as a general calming tonic. Chamomile also has antiseptic, anti-inflammatory, and emollient properties, and has also been used to treat colds, flus, sinus problems, asthma, rheumatism, sore throats, mouth wounds such as abscesses and gingivitis, external wounds, burns rashes, and skin conditions. Chamomile is often used in cosmetics because of its emollient and anti-inflammatory properties. Chamomile is also rich in vitamins B1 and C, and minerals.

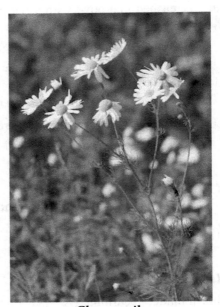

Chamomile
Image 8-29

Description: green leaves and stalk, flowering top with white petals and yellow center

Preparation and application

Tea

Use 2 teaspoons of dried chamomile flowers or 4 teaspoons of fresh chamomile flowers per 1 cup of hot water. Cover and steep for 10 to 15 minutes, strain if necessary, then drink freely to treat ailments. Add more herb and steep for twice as long for an infusion.

Gargle

For a gargle to treat mouth sores or sore throat, use 4 teaspoons of dried chamomile flowers or 8 teaspoons of fresh chamomile flowers per 1 cup of water (double the amount to be used to make a tea, below), cover and let steep for 20 minutes. Cool to a comfortable temperature to use as a mouthwash and gargle. Strain prior to use and pour remaining in a mason jar and refrigerate for future use.

Wash for external use

For a wash to treat irritating skin conditions or wounds, follow the tea recipe except double the ingredients per 1 cup of water, cover and let steep for 20 minutes. Cool to a comfortable temperature to use as an external skin wash. Strain the mixture and pour medicine into a mason jar and refrigerate for future use.

Chaste Tree Berry

(women's health, hormonal balance, PMS, perimenopause, menopause)

Botanical name

Vitex agnus-castus

Also known as

chasteberry, cloister pepper, monk's pepper, Vitex

Medicinal properties

hormone tonic for women

Health benefits

The chaste tree has many medicinal benefits but is most often used to support women's health and regulate hormones. The leaves, flowers, and berries of the chaste tree or vitex have medicinal properties. Chaste medicine has been used to support healthy hormone levels in women of all ages, relieve PMS, balance irregular menstrual cycles, and reduce symptoms of perimenopause and menopause.

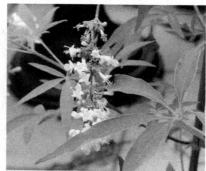

Chaste tree berry
Image 8-30

Traditional use

While chaste tree berry is often used today, it was not a staple in African American healing tradition.

Preparation and application

Tea

Pour boiled water over a teaspoon of fresh or dried chaste tree berries. Steep for 20 minutes and strain. Drink 1 to 2 cups daily.

Tablets and Capsules

Take up to 400 mg tablet or capsule daily, depending on individual need and response to the medicine.

Tincture

Take 30 to 40 drops in a cup of warm water 1 to 3 times daily.

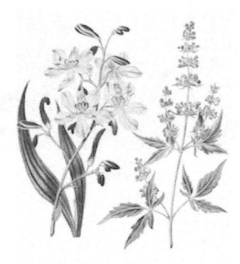

Chaste tree berry illustration
Image 8-30a

Description: medium-green leaves and stalk with lilac-lavender flowering top and pale maroon-colored fruit/berries

Cherry Tree Bark

(energy, digestive stimulant, coughs, colds, respiratory ailments)

Botanical name

Prunus avium or *Prunus serotina*

Medicinal properties

anti-inflammatory, astringent, digestion stimulant, demulcent, expectorant, sedative

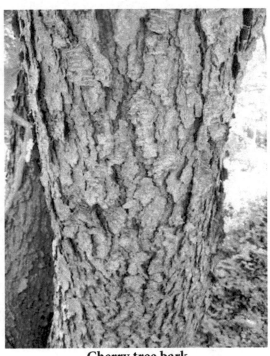

Cherry tree bark
Image 8-31

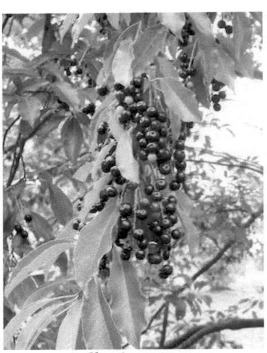

Cherries on tree
Image 8-31a

Description: reddish brown to gray bark, small soft round red or black fruit, green leaves

Health benefits

Cherry tree bark was drunk to aid digestion and to help alleviate colds and other related conditions such as coughs, respiratory ailments, and congestion.

Preparation and application

Peel a piece of the bark from a branch or the trunk using a knife. Make sure you leave the inner bark intact. Make a cold infusion by placing 1/2 to 1 cup of bark in a mason jar and cover with room temperature water so the water is about 1 inch above the bark. Close lid and let sit for 12 hours. Strain the liquid and sip on medicine directly from jar or pour small glasses, drinking 1 to 3 a day.

Chocolate (Dark)

(heart health)

Botanical name

Theobroma cacao

Also known as

cocoa

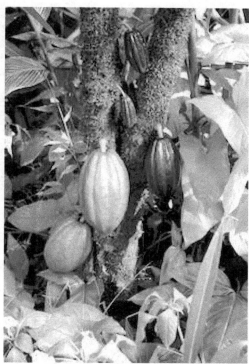

Chocolate (cacao) pods on tree
Image 8-32

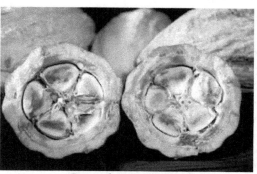

Cacao beans in pod
Image 8-32a

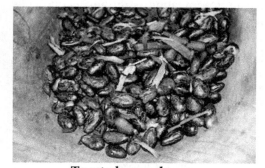

Toasted cacao beans
Image 8-32b

Description: green leaves, clusters of pale yellow flowers, cocoa pods can be green-white, yellow, purplish, or red, each containing 20 to 25 seeds

Medicinal properties

antioxidant

Health benefits

Dark chocolate has been used for its health benefits for centuries. It was traditionally used in Black folk medicine to support heart health. It is a powerful antioxidant which supports heart health and reduces body inflammation. When dark chocolate is eaten, the good bacteria in our stomach ferments it into anti-inflammatory compounds that are good for the heart and entire body. Consistently eating a small bar daily may help relax the arteries and control high blood pressure, prevent heart disease, stroke and heart attack. Eating dark chocolate also stimulates the pleasure center in our brains, making us feel better and strengthening the immune system. Dark chocolate is nutrient rich with the minerals: iron, magnesium, copper, manganese, potassium, phosphorus, zinc and selenium.

Preparation and application

Eat 1 to 2 small squares of 70% or higher cocoa content dark chocolate.

Clay or Chalk

Red or White

(Ingested and used as a poultice and salve)

Scientific name

Phyllosilicate

Also known as

bentonite, dirt, kaolin clay, Mississippi mud

Medicinal properties

absorption of toxins and heavy metals, antibiotic, anticarcinogenic, antidiarrheal, antiinflammatory, antimicrobial, antiseptic, cicatrizing, detoxifier, emollient, refrigerant (cools body), provides trace minerals

Health benefits

Clay has been used internally and externally as a healing medicine for thousands of years. In African American healing traditions, eating clay (geophagy) is a tradition brought directly from Africa. Pregnant women often had the urge to eat red and white clay, which provided the body with essential minerals such as calcium, iron, sodium, phosphorus, copper, magnesium, and zinc. Clay paddies were baked and eaten. Chalk or clay was also eaten to treat diarrhea, and the pharmaceutical kaopectate derives its name from the kaolinite found in clay.

Clay is a powerful detoxifier that absorbs certain heavy metals and toxins, which are then eliminated along with the clay during a bowel movement. As a result, ingesting clay may promote healthier digestion, bowel regularity, less toxicity in the body, alertness and more energy, tissue repair, reduction of pain, and a strong immune system.

As African Americans moved from the South to the urban North for a better life, many women replaced eating clay with eating starch, 'Argo' starch being the preferred type. Eating starch did not

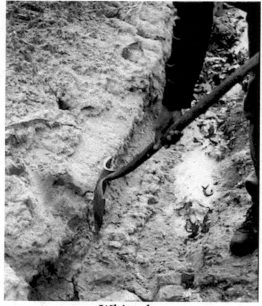

White clay
Image 8-33

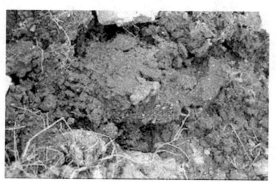

Red clay
Image 8-33a

Description: moist soil that can easily form a ball and is either red, yellow, white or brown in color

have the same benefits as eating clay and consuming large amounts led to anemia and other problems, as it blocked the body's absorption of iron. Health professionals call the craving for eating clay or dirt "pica," an appetite disorder caused by a deficiency of minerals such as iron.

Externally, clay has been used as a poultice or pack to reduce inflammation and pain due to arthritis, rheumatism, muscle strains, and sprains. A poultice can also draw out infection.

Things to consider while taking clay: Clay has both *adsorptive* properties (adheres metals, ions, atoms, gas, and liquids on surface) and *absorptive* properties (soaks in or sucks up like a sponge). Depending on the condition being treated, clay may cause constipation, as it may soak up too much water out of the stomach. If this happens, drink plenty of liquids while cutting back dosage or stopping clay consumption completely. Alternatively, while clay is pulling out bad "gut" bacteria, viruses, heavy metals, and toxins as intended, it may also pull out too much good "gut" bacteria needed by the body for proper functioning. Probotics are taken by some clay eaters to replace the lost good bacteria and rebalance digestion.

Preparation and application

Bath

Add 1/4 cup of clay to your bath. You can also add Epsom salt. This is excellent for muscle strains, pains, and inflammation.

Eating/Ingestion

In African American healing traditions, people ate clay from sites or mounds in their rural environment that they knew were safe from toxins and contamination. Some would harvest a bucketfull and make the clay into little cookie paddies to sell or give away to others. Today, most people buy ingestible clay (which is a liquid paste) from their natural medicine store in the form of bentonite, also used in many colon cleanser treatments.

For general health maintenance, take 1 tablespoon of clay on an empty stomach, preferably in the morning, with 8 ounces of water anywhere from once weekly to once per month. Drink plenty of water throughout the day during such treatment.

For digestion problems, take 1 tablespoon of clay with 8 oz of water twice daily at least 1 hour before meals. Treatment should be taken on an empty stomach.

To stop diarrhea, take 2 tablespoons of clay twice daily for 3 days. *If diarrhea condition worsens, seek help from your health care professional.*

Externally as a pack or poultice

Apply a thick and moist layer of clay and wrap with a gauze. Leave on for at least 60 minutes or until it dries, then wash off with cool water. Optional: add apple cider vinegar to clay for enhanced therapeutic results. Used for skin irritations such as insect bites, acne, burns, itching, chicken pox, and aches and pains due to arthritis, rheumatism, and muscle strain.

Toothpaste

Apply white clay to the toothbrush to combat gum disease and inflammation.

Cod Liver Oil

(preventative and general health maintenance)

Medicinal properties

anti-inflammatory, immune booster, lubricates joints

Health benefits

Cod liver oil is the one medicine in African American healing traditions that people remember taking on a daily basis and not knowing why. It is also a medicine that many people stopped taking in any dosage once they migrated out of the South.

Cod liver oil is rich with omega-3's and considered one of the "super-foods" because it is one of the most concentrated food sources for human health.[161] It is rich with four essential nutrients: DHA,

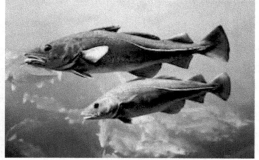

Cod

Image 8-34

Description: light brown fish with gold undertones swimming in blue-green ocean

---

[161] Other food sources besides cod liver oil that are rich in omega-3's: salmon, cod, tuna, halibut, algae, herring, sardines, walnuts, tofu, flaxseeds, clove, soybeans, kale, cauliflower, collards, and winter squash. It is recommended to eat fish 2 to 3 times per week.

Cod Liver Oil (continued)

EPA, vitamin A, and vitamin D. These four nutrients are needed for: healthy skin, strong bones and teeth, healthy joints, healthy cardiovascular system, healthy digestive tract, healthy immune system, healthy nervous system, and prevention of depression and other mood disorders. Taking regular doses of cod liver oil was a wise holistic health maintenance routine that may have strengthened immunity, thereby maintaining overall good health and preventing colds, flu, and chronic illnesses like heart disease, diabetes, and arthritis.

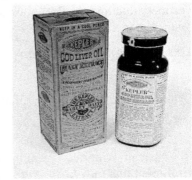

Cod liver oil
Image 8-34a

Description: pale yellowish oil derived from liver of cod fish

Cod liver oil and its medicinal properties may be effective in preventing and treating the following ailments: arthritis (rheumatoid arthritis and osteo arthritis), asthma, diabetes, heart disease, high blood pressure, high cholesterol, inflammatory bowel disease (IBD), macular degeneration, menstrual pain, osteoporosis, skin disorders, systemic lupus, breast cancer, colon cancer, prostate cancer, attention deficit/hyperactivity disorder (ADHD), bipolar disorder, cognitive decline, depression, and schizophrenia.

Preparation and application

A routine dose of cod liver oil ranged from 1 tablespoon weekly to 1 teaspoon daily. Today's daily supplement recommendation is 600 to 1,000 mg daily, usually 1 teaspoon to 1 tablespoon, depending on potency.

Cod liver oil packs can be placed on affected areas to treat conditions of inflammation and pain due to arthritis and rheumatism.

Cautionary warning: because high doses of omega-3 fatty acids may increase the risk of bleeding, care should be taken in not ingesting too much cod liver oil at one time.

Comfrey Root

(wounds, breaks/fractures, muscle strains, inflammation, skin conditions)

Botanical name

Symphytum officianle (meaning to knit together)

Also known as

all heal, gum plant, heal-herb, knitbone, woundwort

Medicinal properties

alterative, anodyne, antibiotic, anti-inflammatory, antioxidant, antiseptic, astringent, demulcent, emoillient, expectorant, general tonic, homeostatic, nutritive, pectoral, proliferant, styptic, vulnerary

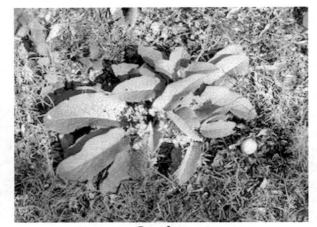

Comfrey
Image 8-35

Description: green leaves with cream or purplish flowers

Health benefits

Comfrey, often called knitbone and "the blood, bone and flesh builder," has excellent healing properties. The leaves and roots contain allantoin and tannins which speed up skin regeneration, promoting wound healing. The leaves and roots also contain rosmarinic acid, which reduces inflammation. Comfrey medicine assists the body to heal any part that is torn or broken by promoting the healing of broken bones, fractures, dislocations, strains, ligaments, and skin wounds. Comfrey was also used to treat any type of inflammation (and associated pain) externally and internally, including arthritis, tumors, acne, boils, bedsores, and more. Comfrey is rich in vitamins A, C, E, the B-complex, and many essential minerals.

Comfrey was used externally as a poultice, salve, or wash to speed up healing in humans and animals. Comfrey leaves were added to baths to promote youthful skin.

Internal application of comfrey has been used historically to treat a variety of conditions including stomach and bowel problems, menstrual problems, diarrhea, ulcers, coughs, lung conditions, tumors, joint inflammation, lupus, high blood pressure, high cholesterol, mouth and dental ailments such as gum disease, and digestive, respiratory, and urinary problems. Southern farmers would occasionally mix comfrey leaves in the food given to their livestock as a preventive measure to ensure good health.

Today, the internal use of comfrey as a medicinal herb is controversial. It is considered to be toxic at high dosages due to its high content of compounds called pyrrolizidine alkaloids, which can cause serious damage to the human liver and even lead to cancer. Consequently, oral use of comfrey is banned in North America and United Kingdom and is only sold for external purposes.

Preparation and application

Comfrey tea or wash

For sipping comfrey tea, use 1 teaspoon of dried leaves for each cup of hot water. Chop or cut leaves and infuse in hot water for 10 to 15 minutes. Drink 1 cup daily.

For making a comfrey wash, use 1 tablespoon of dried leaves or root or 2 tablespoons of fresh leaves or root per cup of water. Infuse leaves and/or root in hot water, cover, and let cool. Strain and pour medicine into a mason jar. Use 2 to 3 times per day as a wash over affected area for such ailments as acne, irritating skin conditions, cuts, wounds, burns, boils, etc.

Comfrey leaf poultice

Pick 3 to 5 comfrey leaves. Pound them to prepare a puree, chop them up really fine, or put in a blender. If the resulting mixture is too thick or sticky, add aloe gel, water, or a type of natural oil with healing properties such as olive, cod liver, or castor until you reach the consistency of thick oatmeal. Wrap this mixture in cheesecloth or muslin cloth and apply to affected area. Leave on for 1 hour or overnight. You can also apply or rub mixture directly to affected area and wrap with a cotton, cheese, muslin, or wool cloth to hold in place. This medicine was used on broken ribs or toes or hairline cracks in larger bones. Used 1 to 3 times daily.

Comfrey root poultice or salve recipe

Chop or grate the root into small pieces and put in a blender or use a mortar and pestle. Add a small amount of water and a natural oil or aloe gel and blend mixture until it is thick and creamy. Use more oil or gel to create a thicker salve. Apply mixture directly to affected area or wrap mixture in cheesecloth, muslin or wool cloth and apply to affected area. Leave on for 1 hour or overnight. Used to ease pain, inflammation, heal wounds, skin conditions and assist to mend bones, ligaments, joints, sprains, etc. Used 2 to 3 times per day.

Comfrey root tincture

Grind the dried root into small pieces using a grinder or mortar and pestel, or chop into small pieces with a knife. Place roots in a glass mason jar and cover with a grain alcohol that is minimum 90% proof. Close the jar with an air-tight lid and store in a cool, dry, and dark cupboard for 2 to 4 weeks, shaking at least once daily. Strain liquid through a cheesecloth into a clean glass container and discard the root. Rub tincture directly on affected area or use to make a salve adding other healing herbs and medicines like aloe. Use 2 to 3 times daily.

Coon Root

(good for your nature, colds, flu, congestion, and coughs)

Botanical names

Sanguinaria canadensis or *Sanguinaria minor*

Also known as

bloodroot, India plant, paucon, puccoon root, queen root, red paint root, red puccoon, redroot, she root, snake bite, sweet slumber, tetterwort or titiweed

Medicinal properties

anesthetic, antibacterial, anticholinesterase, antiedemic, antigingivitic, anti-inflammatory, antimicrobial antineoplastic, antioxidant, antiperiodontic, antiseptic, cathartic, diuretic, emetic, emmenagogue, expectorant, febrifuge, fungicide, gastrocontractant, hypertensive, pesticide, respiratory stimulant

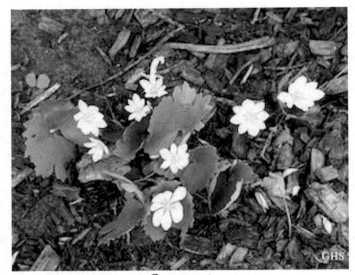

Coon root
Image 8-36

Description: green leaves with white blooms with yellow center

Health benefits

In African American healing traditions, coon root/bloodroot was used to treat coughs, colds, congestion, sore throats, and other bronchial problems. Coon root acts as an expectorant, promoting coughing and clearing mucus from the respiratory tract. Coon root paste is used externally for skin diseases, eczema, herpes, warts (hence the name tetterwort), ringworm, skin fungus, and also acts as a local anesthetic and repels insects.

Native Amerians called coon root by the name "bloodroot," and used it extensively as a medicinal and ceremonial herb. As a medicine, it was taken to treat fevers, reduce inflammation due to arthritis and rheumatism, and to induce vomiting when needed. In ceremonies, it was used as a ritual skin paint or war paint. The red juice from the root makes an excellent dye for cloth, yarn, and many other materials and can be used as a wood stain.

In England, coon root is the plant called tetterwort and was used as a remedy to treat tetter as well as a variety of skin conditions such as warts, herpes, eczema, and ringworm. It was also applied topically to the skin as a local anesthetic.

Like poke root, coon root was used carefully and not eaten, as it contains poisonous toxins and was not used by pregnant and lactating women.

Hoodoo medicine

Coon root has a colored root. In hoodoo medicine, the pink root is called "Queen" or "She" root, while the red root is called "King" or "He." Coon root was believed to help with family troubles and enhance sexual pleasure. When the root is cut open a red juice flows out that looks like blood.

Preparation and application

External use

Direct application

Often, the juice from the crushed root was used directly on affected area.

Dye

Bring to slow boil 4 tablespoons of fresh coon root juice in 1 gallon cold water. Let cool. Add 1 tablespoon of alum, which helps the dye hold onto the fabric. The end result is a reddish-orange hue. Wear gloves when handling Coon root/bloodroot.

Paste or salve

For the treatment of warts and other skin conditions, crush the root in a grinder or in a bowl with pestle. Mix with a natural vegetable oil until it is creamy. Add 1 tablespoon apple cider vinegar to mixture. For future use, put mixture in a glass jar and store in a cool, dark, dry place or put in paper bag and store in refrigerator. After washing apply a small amount to affected area 2 to 3 times daily.

Wash

Put 2 to 3 teaspoons of the root in 1 to 2 cups of hot water, cover and steep for 20 to 30 minutes. Allow to cool. Strain and add 2 tablespoons of vinegar (apple cider vinegar with "the mother" is preferred, but either ACV without "the mother" or white vinegar will suffice). Apply to affected area 2 to 3 times daily. For future use, put remaining mixture in a glass jar and store in a cool, dark place or put in paper bag and store in refrigerator.

Internal use

Tea

Gather the rootstock in spring, before the plant flowers. The dried plant is less potent than the fresh. Put 1 teaspoon of root in hot water, cover and steep for 25 to 30 minutes. Strain and let cool. Drink 1 cup daily.

Decoction

Add 1 teaspoonful of the root to a cup of cold water and slowly bring to a boil. Turn off the heat, cover, and let the root infuse for 10 minutes. Strain the liquid into a glass container. Drink 1 to 3 cups daily for 1 week. Store remaining liquid in the refrigerator.

Tincture

Gather fresh or dried coon root, chop and place 1/4 to 1/2 cup in a mason jar. Cover with grain alcohol that is at least 90 proof. Close with an air-tight lid and place in a cool, dry, and dark cabinet for 2 to 4 weeks. The longer the root tinctures, the stronger the potency. Strain and place liquid in a clean medicine bottle with an eye-dropper lid. Take 5 to 10 drops in a cup of warm water and drink 1 to 3 times a day. Discontinue use if you experience nausea, diarrhea, or vomiting.

Corn Shuck, Corn Husks, Corn Silk

(bladder infection, urinary tract infection)

Botanical name

Zea mays

Also known as

mother's hair

Medicinal properties

anti-inflammatory, demulcent, detoxifier, diuretic, mild stimulant

Health benefits

The corn silk inside of the husks contains the medicine. Corn silk medicine is often used to treat ailments associated with acute bladder and urinary tract infections, cystitis, kidney stones, prostate

Corn Shuck, Corn Husks, Corn Silk (continued)

disorders, water retention/edema, and bed-wetting. Corn silk is rich with potassium and vitamin K. Corn silk is also known to lower blood sugar, increase insulin, and lower blood pressure. Corn silk poultices were used to treat inflammation. Poultices prepared with the silk and cooked kernels have also helped to relieve sores, wounds, contusions, and rheumatic pains.

Note: Today, most corn is grown from GMO seeds that are specifically engineered so that the seeds themselves act as an insecticide to control pests. The result is a crop that may produce a different medicinal agency and corn than when the plant was popularly used in African American healing traditions before such modifications were implemented.

Preparation and application

Tea

Place the cornsilk in a pot of hot water, making sure the water covers 1 to 2 inches above the silk. Cover and steep for 10 to 15 minutes. Strain and drink. You may add lemon or honey for flavor.

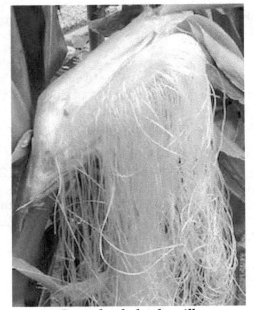

Corn shuck, husks, silk
Image 8-37

Description: pale greenish-yellow skin with silky-yellow pale strands

Cottonseed, Cotton Bark, Cotton Root

(female health and menstruation support)

Botanical name

Gossypium hirsutum

Also known as

American upland cotton, common cotton, upland cotton, wild cotton

Medicinal properties

abortifacient, antipyretic, aphrodisiac, emmenagogue

Health benefits

The cotton plant is regarded as female medicine and the seed, root, bark and oil have all been used as medicine mostly to treat female problems. Cotton medicine has been used for centuries within the Native American, African American, Chinese, and Ayurvedic healing traditions. Cottonseed tea was used to treat excessive menstrual bleeding, endometriosis, and colic in babies. The oil in the cottonseed contains the medicine.

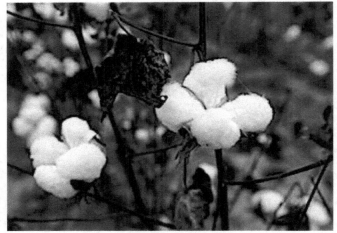

Cotton plant
Image 8-38

Description: soft fluffy fiber boll, brown seeds, green leaves

Cotton root tea is purported to help treat problems associated with childbirth and to help facilitate delivery. The bark of the cotton root was chewed or made into a tea to induce abortions, start menstruation, promote breast milk in nursing mothers, and is also purported to be an aphrodisiac. Enslaved African American women chewed on cotton root bark or drank the tea to induce abortions. Cotton root tea was also a remedy used to treat snake bite, dysentery, and fever.

Preparation and application

Cottonroot tea

Boil 1/2 cup of the inner root to 1 quart of water. Cover and let steep for 25 to 30 minutes or until cool. Strain. Drink 3 to 5 cups a day.

Cottonseed tea

Place the seeds in a large mortar bowl and crush with a pestle or other tool to crack open the outer husk of the seed and release the oil. Place the crushed seeds in a cup and cover with hot water. Cover cup and let steep for 20 minutes and strain. Drink the strained tea.

Cotton Bark

Chew on the bark to help start menstrual flow or to induce abortion. Make a tea by using 1 oz. of bark to 1 cup of water. Cover and steep for 20 minutes. Drink 1 to 3 cups daily.

Cow Chip Tea

(colds, flu, coughs, congestion, pneumonia)

Also known as

cow pat, many-weed tea

Medicinal properties

antiviral, expectorant, immune stimulant

Health benefits

Cow chip tea was used to treat colds, flu, coughs, chest and sinus congestion, and to protect against viruses. The cow chips (manure paddies) were gathered from the field and placed in a natural cloth bag, often with other ingredients such as lemon, peppermint candy, Vicks lozenge, rabbit tobacco, etc., to mask the taste. This bag was boiled in hot water and after cooling, the bag was removed and

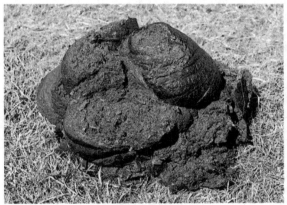

Cow chip
Image 8-39
Description: dark brown paddie intertwined with grass

the tea was ready to drink. Cow chip tea is also called many-weed tea because the paddies contain grasses and weedy growths from the cow grazing.

Preparation and application

Tea

A dried cow patty from a cow that had been grazing a lot of fresh green grass was scooped up and put in a white cloth or natural cloth bag free from dye. Other ingredients such as lemon, peppermint tea or candy, rabbit tobacco, or Vicks cough lozenges were added to sweeten or mask the taste. This was

Cow Chip Tea (continued)

placed in a small pot and covered with fresh water, brought to a boil, and then simmered for 40 minutes. Mixture was cooled and then strained. A large, warm cup was drunk up to 3 times per day, one of those times being right before bedtime.

Dandelion

(water retention, kidney and liver support)

Botanical name

Taraxacum officinale

Also known as

lion's tooth, monk's head

Medicinal properties

diuretic, digestive, appetite stimulant

Health benefits

Dandelion is a hardy plant that grows voraciously. Most people see it as a weed. Dandelion root and leaf have been used in healing practices across the globe for centuries. It was used in Native American and African American healing traditions to treat kidney and liver problems and swelling due to excess fluid (edema). Its diuretic action expels excess water without your body losing necessary minerals. Dandelion is nutrient-rich with the minerals potassium, iron, and zinc and vitamins A, B, C, and D. The leaves are good for detoxifying and toning the kidneys and expelling excess water (edema). The roots are usually steeped into a tea and drunk to support liver and bladder health.

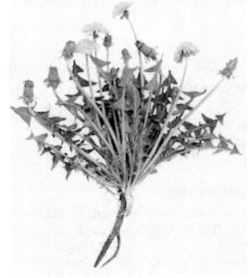

Dandelion root
Image 8-40

Description: green leaves and stem that produce yellow flowers, tan colored root

Preparation and application

Leaf tea

Use 1 teaspoon of dried leaves or 2 teaspoons of fresh leaves to 1 cup of hot water. Cover and steep for 10 to 15 minutes. Drink up to 3 cups daily.

Root tea

Harvest a bunch of roots and rinse them well, getting the dirt off. You can let them air dry or chop them, spread on a cookie sheet, and roast them in the oven at 300 degrees until brown. Use 1 teaspoon of the dried root to 1 cup of hot water. Cover and steep for 10 to 15 minutes. Drink 1 to 3 times daily.

Food

Harvest the leaves, wash, and add to your salad or greens. Today, many people blend in a smoothie or juice.

Devil's Shoestring

(menstrual cramps, uterine tonic, protection, good luck)

Devil's shoestring is the common name for several plants in the honeysuckle family that grow in North American woods. Devil's shoestring usually refers to various species of Viburnum: *alnifolium* (hobblebush), *opulus* (cramp bark), or *prunifolium* (black haw).

Botanical names

Viburnum alnifolium, Viburnum opulus, Viburnum prunifolium, Viburnum lantanoides

Also known as

black haw, cramp bark, hobblebush, witch hobble

Medicinal properties

astringent, antispasmodic, gynecological support, relaxant

Health benefits

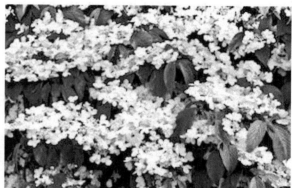

Devil's shoestring flowering plant
(*Viburnum opulus*)
Image 8-41

Description: dark-green leaves; yellow, orange, red or maroon fall foliage; white flower with red to black berries in summer

The whole long roots are commonly used in African American conjuring/spirit work. The bark is used medicinally to treat menstrual cramps, prevent miscarriages, and to boost fertility. The berries from the black haw species are eaten to prevent miscarraiges and support pregnancy. In the 19th century, American slave owners forced enslaved African American women to eat the berries and drink a tea made from the bark for the purpose of preventing miscarriages and having them bear more children, who the slave owners viewed as commodities.

Spiritual properties

protection, good luck

Spiritual benefits

In hoodoo medicine, Devil's shoestring was used to protect your home from the Devil, to "trip up the Devil." People also carried the roots around for luck in gambling, job hunting and protection from gossip.

Preparation and application

Tea

Make a medicinal tea by placing 1 teaspoon of the dried of the dried root bark in 1 cup of hot water, covering and steeping for 10 to 15 minutes. Drink 1 cup up to 3 times daily to relieve menstrual cramps.

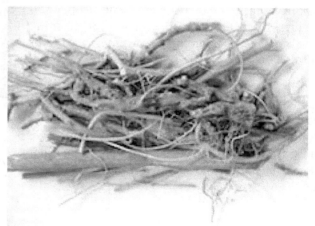

Devil's shoestring root
Image 8-41a

Description: light-brown colored bark

Spiritual

Carry seven Devil's shoestrings in a medicine bag for good luck and protection.

Dogwood

**(The black gum, dogwood, and pickash or prickly ash trees
are all commonly referred to as the toothbrush tree)**

Botanical name

Cornus florida

Also known as

dogtree, toothbrush tree

Medicinal properties

astringent, febrifuge, stimulant, general health
tonic

Health benefits

Many used twigs from the dogwood tree to
clean their teeth and maintain healthy gums. The
twig was used as a toothpick and chewing stick and
the frayed ends as a toothbrush. The astringent
property in dogwood helped to keep gums and
teeth healthy. Dogwood bark was made into a
strong tea to treat intestinal worms, measles, and
diarrhea, and into a poultice to treat cuts and other
skin disorders. Dogwood medicine was used often
during the Civil War.

Preparation and application

Tea/decoction

Use the dried bark only. Put 1 teaspon of dried
bark in 2 cups of hot water. Cover and steep for 20
minutes for a tea and 30 minutes for a strong
decoction. Drink 1 cup 4 to 6 times a day for
worms.

Toothbrush/teeth cleaning

Pick a fresh twig about 5 to 7 inches long. Use
the end as a toothpick to clean teeth, then put in
mouth as a chew stick, letting your saliva soften
and fray the ends. When the ends are fanned out
and become brush-like, gently brush your teeth and
gums.

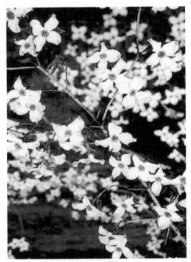

Dogwood flowers
Image 8-42

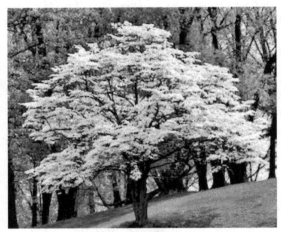

Dogwood tree
Image 8-42a

*Description: dark green leaves, turns red in fall;
white-yellowish green flowers blooms early spring;
bright red fruits mature summer to fall*

Ear Wax

(cold sores, canker sores)

Scientific name

Cerumen

Medicinal properties

antibacterial, lubricant

Health benefits

Earwax is a self-cleaning lubricant for the inner ear that has antibacterial properties. Earwax helps to maintain the pH balance in your ear and protects against the penetration of water into the inner ear, both of which are important for inhibiting the growth of bacteria. It can serve that same function for cold sores, but it must be applied manually. At the first sign of cold sores, rub *your own* earwax on the cold sore several times a day until the cold sore is gone.

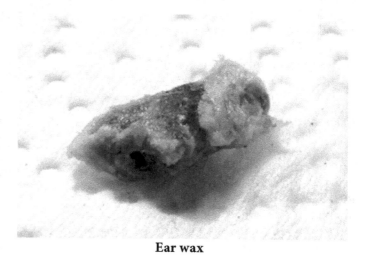

Ear wax
Image 8-43

Description: brownish red to yellow waxy substance

Preparation and application

Use your finger or a cotton swab to remove excess wax from your ear. Apply to affected cold sore area 2 to 3 times daily until gone.

Ear wax removal

Too much earwax can make your ears feel clogged. To help remove or dissolve, use the following solution and it should clear up in one day:

Make a 1:1 solution of apple cider vinegar (ACV) and hydrogen peroxide, or ACV and water, or peroxide and water. Put 2 drops in the ear, and cover with a piece of cotton. Best results if you lie down with the ear side up where the solution was placed for at least 1 hour or to do right before bed.

Elderberry

(coughs, colds, flu, bronchitis)

Botanical name

Sambucus

Also known as

blackberry elder, elder, red-berry elder

Medicinal properties

antioxidant, antiviral, diaphoretic, diuretic, expectorant, immune stimulant

Health benefits

Elderberry medicine is made from the berries, leaves, and root of the elderberry tree. It can be used to treat a variety of ailments, including colds, coughs, flu, fever, bronchitis, asthma, nervous conditions,

Elderberry (continued)

inflammation, rheumatism, diabetes, infections, and constipation. It can also be taken regularly to strengthen immunity and as a general health tonic. Elderberries are rich with vitamin C, A, B, amino acids, and other necessary nutrients the body cannot produce. Elderberry medicine acts as a mild laxative and is diaphoretic (promotes sweating).

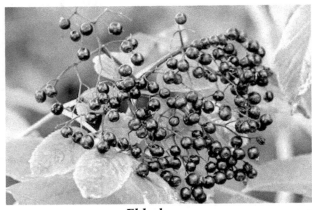

Elderberry
Image 8-44

Description: green foliage; small white flowers; abundant fruit/berries green, red then black when ripe

Preparation and application

Berry and/or flower tea

Add 1 teaspoon of dried berries and/or flowers to 1 cup of boiling water. Cover and let steep for 10 to 15 minutes if using flowers only, 20 minutes if using berries, strain, and drink 3 times per day. Add peppermint or lemon, sweeten with honey.

Fresh bark and root tea

Put 1 tablespoon in 1 cup boiling water, cover and steep for 20 minutes. Drink no more than one cup at a time.

Elderberry cough syrup

Pour 1 cup of dried berries into 3 cups of boiling water. Add ginger, 1 clove, and 1/2 to 1 teaspoon cinnamon powder or 1 stick of cinammon to pot. Reduce heat and simmer for approximately 45 minutes. Remove from heat, let cool, and strain into a glass bowl. Discard the berries and other ingredients. Sweeten with honey to taste. Pour mixture into a mason jar and use to treat colds and flu. Dosage: Adults - 1 tablespoon every 2 to 3 hours. Children - 1 teaspoon every 2 to 3 hours.

Elderberry tonic

To use as immune booster, expectorant, and for colds/flu
  * Fill one pint mason jar with fresh elderberries
  * Pour in 1/3 cup of raw honey
  * Fill the jar with brandy
  * Shake vigorously and make sure the lid is closed tightly
  * Place in a cool, dark place for 4 to 6 weeks, shaking daily
  * Strain and store liquid in an airtight container in a cool, dark place
  * Take 1/4 to 1/2 dropper of elixir every 2 to 3 hours at first sign of illness
  * For preventive health care, take 1 dropper full 3 to 5 times per week

Epsom Salt - Magnesium Sulfate

(swelling, muscle and joint strain, inflammation, relaxant for arteries)

Medicinal properties

antifungal, anti-inflammatory, antiseptic, emollient, nutritive, sedative

Health benefits

Magnesium sulfate, better known as Epsom salt, is another multi-purpose medicine that is a staple in African American healing traditions. Epsom salt was used to relieve aches and pains, swelling, and inflammation, as well as to relax muscles, sedate the nervous system to relieve stress, reduce blood pressure, prevent strokes, treat constipation, kill fungus and bacteria (athlete's foot), heal cuts faster, soften skin, pull out toxins from the body, and more.

Epsom salt really isn't salt. It's a mineral compound of magnesium and sulfate that got its name from a bitter spring at the village of Epsom that is located in Surrey, England. Magnesium is one of the most important of the essential minerals in the body, responsible for over 350 chemical processes. It is commonly deficient in the American diet.

Excess adrenaline and stress drain magnesium from the body. Magnesium is necessary for the body to have a feeling of well-being and relaxation. By replacing magnesium levels in your body that are depleted by stress, Epsom salt can help to elevate your mood.

Both sulfates and magnesium in Epsom salt are difficult to absorb from food but are readily absorbed through the skin. When magnesium sulfate is absorbed through the skin, such as in a bath, it is both medicinal and therapeutic. Soaking in Epsom salt will help improve your body's absorption of nutrients and use of oxygen.

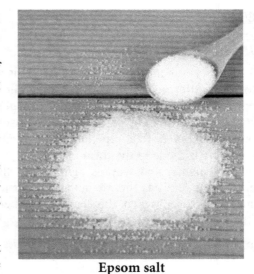

Epsom salt
Image 8-45

Description: small white crystalline mineral

Preparation and application

<u>External use</u>

Bath

Add 2 cups of Epsom salt to a bath and soak whole body for aches and pains.

Foot soak

Put 1/2 cup Epsom salt in a pan of hot water. Let your feet soak to relieve aches.

<u>Internal use</u>

Laxative

Mix 2 to 4 teaspoons in 1 cup of water and drink. You should eliminate after 30 minutes. If not, take another dose in 4 hours.

Protect arteries/prevent stroke

Put 1 teaspoon of Epsom salt in 1 cup of water. Stir and make sure the Epsom salt dissolves. Drink 1 to 3 times per week to help prevent hardening of arteries, improve blood circulation, and to reduce risk of sudden heart attach deaths.

Eucalyptus

(colds, congestion, respiratory ailments, flea repellent, insect bites)

Botanical name
Eucalyptus globules (clove family)

Also known as
blue gum, red gum

Medicinal properties
antiseptic, decongestant

Eucalyptus (continued)

Health benefits

Eucalyptus medicine is most often used to treat allergies, colds, sinus and chest congestion,respiratory problems, coughs, sore throat, minor cuts, muscle strains, insect bites, and as a flea repellent. Eucalyptus medicine is made in the form of teas, salves, oils, inhalants, and washes. The oil in the eucalyptus leaf has the medicinal properties and is released when the leaf is steamed, steeped, boiled, bruised, or crushed.

Preparation and application

Tea

Use 1/4 to 1/2 teaspoon of dried leaves or 1 teaspoon of fresh leaves per cup of hot water. Cover and steep for 10 to 15 minutes, then strain. Drink up to 3 cups per day. Add lemon and honey for additional flavor and healing properties.

Eucalyptus oil or salve

Use as an insect repellent or antiseptic for sores, cuts and wounds, or to treat boils, alleviate arthritis and aching joints. For direct immediate use, crush or bruise the leaves to release the oil and then rub the leaf on affected area.

How to make eucalyptus oil

Fill a glass jar with eucalyptus leaves and pour olive, sesame, almond, or jojoba oil to the top of the jar. Let the mixture sit on a windowsill where it will get sun exposure for a minimum of 2 weeks. Strain the leaves and bottle the oil.

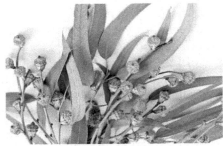

Eucalyptus leaves
Image 8-46

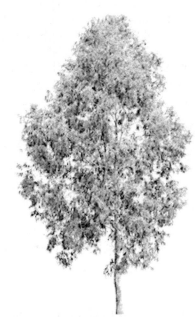

Eucalyptus tree
Image 8-46a

Description: dark to pale greenish-blue leaves; cream, yellow, pink or red stamens that flower out of a bud; smooth to rough bark that is shiny or satiny

How to make eucalyptus salve/linament

Make the eucalyptus oil above. In a small pot, gently melt an equal amount of natural oil. Stir in the eucalyptus oil. While still liquid, pour into a glass jar. Add more salve base like beeswax or shea butter if you need to thicken.

Flea and insect repellent

Take several branches of eucalyptus with the leaves on them and place under your couch, bed, in the dog house, or in any area with flea infestation. Replace after one month.

Inhalant for congestion, colds, bronchitis

Bring to boil a big pot of hot water. Remove from heat and add two handfuls of eucalyptus leaves. Cover the pot. Steep in the covered pot for 3 minutes. Uncover pot and bend over the pot with a towel covering your head and the pot and inhale the steam with the vapors for up to 15 minute. Do up to 3 times a day.

Soak/bath for congestion, muscle strain, respiratory and cold relief

Fill a tub or basin with hot water and add 1 to 2 bunches of bruised eucalyptus leaves. Let soak for 10 minutes, then fill the remainder of the tub or basin with hot water and soak affected area or whole body for 20 minutes or more.

Fig (Juice)

(ringworm, warts, fungal skin conditions)

Botanical name

Ficus carica

Medicinal properties

antipyretic, aperient, demulcent, diuretic, emollient, expectorant, nutritive, purgative

Health benefits

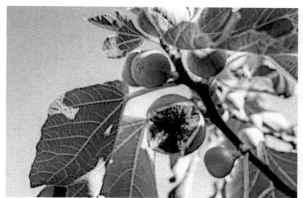

Figs
Image 8-47

Description: green leaves, smooth green fruit with dark brown pulp-like insides

Fig milk, or sap, is commonly used to treat ringworm, skin irritations, warts, and insect bites. Figs are also made into a syrup or tonic to treat coughs, colds, and upper respiratory problems.

Figs are high in fiber and when eaten, they act as a natural laxative, encouraging regular bowel movements while strengthening the intestines. Fig medicine and regular consumption of figs has been used to treat and help prevent a variety of chronic health conditions, including high cholesterol, hypertension, heart disease, cancer and more. Fig leaves have been used to treat diabetes. Figs are rich with potassium, magnesium, calcium, iron, omega-3 and omega-6 fatty acids, and vitamins A, B1, B2, and K.

Preparation and application

Fig leaf tea for bronchitis, coughs and respiratory ailments

Use 1 tablespoon dried leaves or 2 tablespoons fresh leaves to 1 cup of hot water. Cover and let steep or slow simmer for 10 to 15 minutes and strain. Drink 2 to 3 times per day. Can also add chopped figs to this mixture.

Laxative

Eat 1/2 cup of figs daily to relieve constipation and maintain regularity.

Milk or sap to treat ringworms, fungus and skin irritations

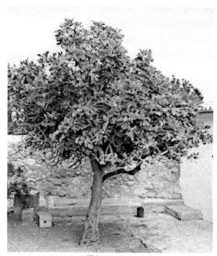

Fig tree
Image 8-47a

Description: green leaves; smooth grayish-brown bark; purplish red or green fig fruit

Apply the juice (which is white and has the appearance of milk) from an unripe or green fig to the affected area to treat skin fungus such a ringworms and other irritations. The juice from a bruised fig leaf can also be applied directly to the ringworm or affected area. Drink the fig milk or fig

Fig (Juice) (continued)

leaf tea to cure warts or make a wash from the leaves and apply to warts, poison oak and other similar skin conditions.

Wash for poison oak, warts and skin irritations

Use 1/2 cup of fig leaves to 1 cup of water. Bring fig leaf and water to boil in a pot and turn off heat. Let cool and strain. Pour the liquid in a jar and use as a wash 2 times or more per day on affected area.

Flaxseed

(headaches, digestion)

Botanical name

Linum usitatissimum
Also known as flachs, flax, flax fignans, flax meal

Medicinal properties

anti-cancer, anticholesterol, anti-inflammatory, hormone balancer for menopause and PMS, laxative

Health benefits

Flaxseed is the richest source of omega-3's in the plant kingdom. It also contains an abundance of three essential nutrients that our bodies do not produce but need for optimal health: omega-3 essential fatty acids, omega-6 essential fatty acids, and lignans. Flaxseed also contains both soluble and insoluble fiber, which is necessary for healthy digestion, absorption of nutrients, and regular elimination.

One of the ways flaxseed was used in traditional Black folk medicine was to make a poultice and apply it to the forehead to treat headaches and migraines. Flaxseed medicine taken regularly in the form of flaxseed oil or meal may also help prevent and treat many chronic health conditions such as high cholesterol, heart disease, menopausal symptoms (hot flashes), diabetes, arthritis, rheumatism, inflammation, high blood pressure, irritable bowel syndrome, digestion disorders, anxiety and nervous disorders, headaches, migraines, and more.

It's difficult to digest the whole flaxseed seed because of its hard shell, which will pass through you undigested, so the best way to benefit from flaxseed medicine is by ingesting the oil or meal. Flaxseed meal isprepared by grinding the seed in a grinder or with a mortar and pestel.

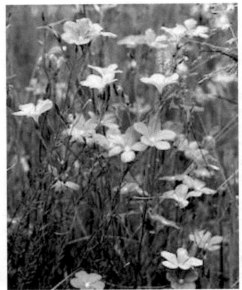

Flax plant
Image 8-48

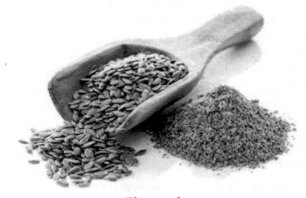

Flax seeds
Image 8-48a

Description: pale green leaves and stem; flowers are pale blue, white, yellow or red

Preparation and application

Daily health maintenance

Take 1 to 2 tablespoons of flaxseed oil, or 1 to 3 tablespoons of ground flaxseed, per day. Add the meal or oil to cereal, oatmeal, drinks, baking recipes, vegetables, soups, casseroles, salads, and more.

For baking, substitute 1/4 to 1/2 cup of flour with ground flaxseed meal if the recipe calls for 2 or more cups of flour.

Flaxseed poultice for headaches, sores, boils, inflammation, and skin conditions

Take 2 tablespoons of ground flaxseed and stir in 1/2 to 1 cup of hot water. A gel mixture will form. Put this mixture into a cloth and put on affected area. Rub flaxseed oil or castor oil on the area prior to applying the poultice.

Flaxseed tea for inflammation, headaches, migraines, congestion, and constipation

Mix a tablespoon of flaxseed meal in 1 cup of warm water. Let dissolve and drink 1 cup 2 times daily. Drink plenty of water because flaxseed meal expands when you eat it.

Storing flaxseed oil

Buy in bulk or already bottled. Make sure it is stored in a glass bottle. Store in refrigerator to keep it fresh. Do not use for cooking.

Storing seeds or meal

Put the seeds or meal in an air-tight bag or glass jar and store in freezer or refrigerator.

Note: Flaxseed oil and omega-3's can interfere with certain medications, especially blood thinners.

Garlic "The Wonder Drug"

(high blood pressure, infections, colds, flu, circulation, warts)

Botanical name

Allium sativa (onion family)

Also known as

garlic bulb, garlic clove

Medicinal properties

antibiotic, anti-inflammatory, antimicrobial, antioxidant, antiviral

Health benefits

Garlic has been used for thousands of years as medicine and to enhance food. The main healing agent in garlic is allicin, a sulfur compound released by crushing or chewing fresh garlic. Allicin has a range of strong healing properties that may effectively treat

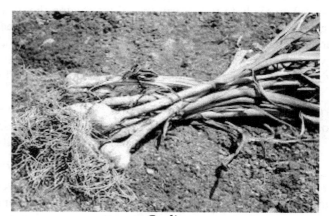

Garlic
Image 8-49

Description: Light to medium green narrow leaves; cream and rose flowering bulb heads

and prevent numerous ailments. This is why garlic is called "the wonder drug." Garlic also has selenium, vitamin C and B6.

Eating garlic regularly, ingesting the oil, or using the oil in teas and healing tonics may help boost immunity, lower blood pressure, control blood sugar, lower cholesterol, prevent heart disease, kill worms, parasites and harmful bacteria, stimulate digestion, reduce inflammation associated with

Garlic "The Wonder Drug" (continued)

arthritis and rheumatism, act as an anti-cancer agent, and generally detoxify the body. Garlic medicine may also be effective in treating yeast infections, strep throat, ear infections, bladder infections, respiratory ailments (coughs and congestion), allergies, toothaches, warts, and as a mosquito repellent.

Preparation and application

Garlic medicine is most effective when crushed or chopped and when raw. Eat a minimum of 3 cloves daily for preventive health care or to treat ailments.

Tea/tonic for colds, flu, pulmonary infections and general health

Use 1 to 2 crushed garlic cloves per 1 cup of hot water. Put crushed garlic clove or cloves in a cup and fill with hot water. Cover and steep for 20 minutes. Add honey, lemon, cayenne, or other healing herbs and drink freely. Eat garlic after you have finished tea.

Cooking/In food and drink

Cooking garlic for longer than 10 minutes will reduce its effectiveness. Wait until the last 10 minutes of cooking to add in the chopped or crushed garlic. Add raw, chopped garlic to your food or bake a bulb whole in the oven until soft. Peel and eat the cloves.

Garlic-mullein-honey cough syrup and decongestant

Garlic has antibacterial and antiviral properties and the mullein is an expectorant. In a small pot, boil 2 cups of water and turn off the heat. Add 1/4 to 1/2 cup of chopped or crushed garlic and 1/4 to 1/2 cup of mullein. Cover and let cool. After 30 minutes, add 1 tablespoon of honey, 1 tsp. of cayenne pepper, and squeeze the juice of 1 lemon in mixture. Drop the lemon rind in the mixture and stir. Cover and let sit for 12 hours. Strain and pour mixture into a glass container, cover, and refrigerate. Take 1 tablespoon of mixture 3 times per day for cough.

Garlic oil for ear and topical fungal infections

Chop or crush 1/2 cup of garlic. Place in small pot and cover the garlic with olive oil or sweet oil. Slow simmer for 10 minutes. Let cool and pour the mixture into a glass jar or bottle (straining the garlic out is optional). Place in refrigerator.

When ready to use, warm the oil by placing the glass container in hot water. Use an ear dropper to suction up the garlic oil and place 1 to 2 drops in the ear. Cover the ear hole with a cotton ball and go to bed, making sure the affected ear is up, not down. In the morning, use the ear dropper to rinse the ear with a solution of hydrogen peroxide and water (1:3) and place a small piece of cotton over the ear for the entire day. If symptoms persist, repeat the garlic oil treatment at night.

If using this treatment during the day, put warm garlic oil in the ear and put a cotton ball over the ear and lie down for 20 to 30 minutes with the affected ear side up. Leave the cotton ball in for the rest of the day and rinse with hydrogen peroxide at end of day.

You can also rub this oil on your skin to treat fungal infections, insect bites and as a repellent.

Paste/Salve

Place 6 to 10 crushed or finely chopped garlic cloves in a small saucepan. Add a natural vegetable oil and slow simmer for 10 minutes. Add shea butter or beeswax to thicken. Turn off heat and let cool. Scoop paste from pot and place in a glass jar. Refrigerate and use as necessary on affected areas.

Poultice

Use garlic as a topical medicine for warts, cuts, fungal infections, insect bites, and as a mosquito repellent. Crush the garlic clove and rub directly on the affected area. It will probably sting. For warts and more sustained application, place the crushed garlic on the affected area and wrap with a bandage or band aid. Leave on for 8 hours, wash the area gently with warm water, and repeat treatment with fresh garlic until ailment is gone. For toothaches, place the crushed garlic clove on the affected area and leave there for 20 minutes.

Vaginal wash for yeast infections

Boil 2 cups of water and remove from heat. Place 6 to 10 crushed garlic cloves in the water and cover. Let stand for at least 8 hours before using. Strain garlic water into a glass jar or bowl. Douche with this solution in a tub.

Optional: Add 1 tablespoon of apple cider vinegar (ACV) containing "the mother," the tiny, web-like ball of living enzymes and nutrients that makes this liquid an active healing agent. Repeat every other day for one week. Sugar, alcohol, and caffeine feed the yeast, so eliminate eating sugar or processed foods, and eliminate drinking coffee, alcohol, and sodas.

Ginger

(gas, nausea, indigestion, colic, inflammation, thins blood, health tonic)

Botanical name

Zingibar officinale

Also known as

black ginger, cochin ginger, gingembre, Jamaican ginger

Medicinal properties

analgesic, antibacterial, antiemetic, antiflatulent, anti-inflammatory, anti-microbial, antispasmodic, antipyretic, anti-viral, blood-thinner, carminative, stimulant, detoxifying, diaphoretic, digestive aid, lymph-cleansing, mild laxative, perspiration-inducing, sedative, warming, general health tonic

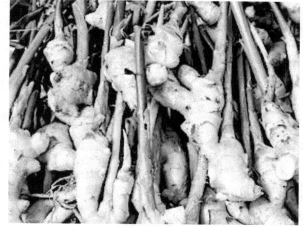

Ginger root
Image 8-50

Description: tan colored root with green stalk

Health benefits

Ginger root is a powerful medicine. It is commonly used to treat digestive ailments like nausea, indigestion, bloating, heartburn, nausea, and flatulence. Ginger root medicine has also been used to treat diarrhea, constipation, menstrual cramps, toothaches, colic, irritable bowel, to stimulate appetite and circulation, to reduce pain and inflammation, and to thin blood. It may even help to reduce blood sugar levels and cholesterol levels. Ginger is often used in remedies treating colds, flu, chills, fevers, coughs, and bronchitis. Ginger is rich with vitamins B6 and B5, potassium, manganese, copper and magnesium.

Traditional use

While ginger is used today to great benefit, it was not a staple in African American healing tradition.

Preparation and application

Fresh or powdered ginger root is added to drinks and food in both sweet and savory dishes.

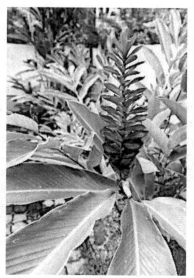

Ginger plant flowering top
Image 8-50a

Description: narrow green leaves; red flower tops

Ginger (continued)

Tea

A cup of warm ginger tea after a meal helps aid digestion. Cut slices of fresh ginger root (approximately 1/4 to 1/2 cup), place in pot with 2 cups of water, bring to boil, cover and steep for 25 to 30 minutes. Add honey, lemon, or orange to taste. Drink 1 cup after meals.

Fermented ginger

Including and eating fermented ginger as a garnish to meals will aid in digestion and also add beneficial bacteria to your stomach.

Food

Add ginger slices to sautéed vegetable dishes or to casserole.

Smoothies

Add chopped ginger as one of the ingredients for smoothies. Blend well.

Goldenrod

(inflammation and swelling)

Botanical name

Soldiago

Also known as

Aaron's rod, blue mountain tea, liberty tea , mountain tea, sweet goldenrod, woundwort

Medicinal properties

anti-inflammatory, antifungal, antiseptic, antispasmodic, aquaretic agent, expectorant, relaxant, stimulates liver and kidney

Health benefits

Goldenrod is a bitter medicine that has been used to treat a wide range of ailments externally and internally. African American healing traditions used goldenrod to help treat and prevent colds, flu, and coughs and to support healthy liver and kidneys (helping to treat and prevent kidney stones and urinary track infections). Goldenrod medicine has also been used to treat inflammation, asthma, hemorrhoids, muscle spasms, inflammation, diabetes, hemorrhoids, internal bleeding, colic and digestion problems.

Topically, goldenrod is used as an antiseptic and antifungal to treat wounds, eczema, rashes and other skin irritations and to treat pain and inflammation associated with arthritis and rheumatism. As a gargle it is effective in treating mouth inflammations, sore throat and laryngitis.

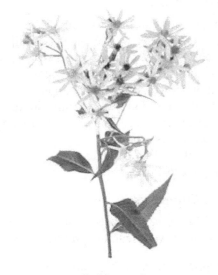

Goldenrod
Image 8-51

Description: green wood stems; yellow flowers in August and September

Preparation and application

Tea

Drink the tea to help prevent and relieve allergies, colds, flu, internal inflammation and pain, urinary tract infections, and water retention.

Use fresh or dried leaves and flowers to make a tea by putting in 1 to 2 teaspoons of dried leaves—or 2 to 4 teaspoons of fresh leaves—per 1 cup of boiled water and covering and steeping for 10 to 15 minutes. Strain and add honey or another tea such as mint. For stronger medicine, use 2 times as much goldenrod per cup of water. Place in a pot and bring to a slow boil and then simmer for 30 minutes.

Goldenrod root medicine

Use this medicine for slow-to-heal wounds and sore joints. Dig up the root and rinse off. Let roots dry on a rack or hang them in a safe dry place. After about 1 week, when the root is dry, store in a glass jar. Brew a strong tea or make a decoction with pieces of the dried root and apply the mixture directly to the affected area. Wrap with gauze or cheesecloth. Change the cloth and medicine daily until ailment is better.

Soak the dried root for 30 minutes then grind the root, flowers, and leaves into a powder and mix with a natural vegetable oil until you get a thick paste. Store in a glass jar. Apply to affected area 1 to 3 times per day.

To treat any of the ailments internally that are listed in the "Health benefits" section above, use 1 teaspoon of dried root to 1 cup of water. Alternatively, cover the bottom of a pot or saucepan with root and cover that with 1 to 2 inches of water, bring to slow boil, and then simmer for 30 minutes. Drink 1 cup daily of either preparation.

Poultice or direct application

Bruise the leaves by crushing and rubbing them on the skin and affected area. Place a handful of the leaves on the affected area and then wrap the area with gauze or cheesecloth that has been wet with warm water.

As a food

Goldenrod leaves can be eaten raw in a salad. They can also be cooked like greens and eaten as a side dish, or added to soups, stews or used in other creative culinary ways. Eating the leaves raw or cooked offers the same health benefits as making a tea.

Wash and gargle

Prepare the standard tea, adding 2 to 3 times as much herb to 1 cup of water. Strain the mixture and keep medicine in an air-tight jar to use as needed. Apply the wash to the affected area for skin conditions and to clean and treat wounds. Can also be applied to treat areas affected by rheumatism and arthritis. Gargle with the solution to treat throat and mouth conditions that would benefit from goldenrod's antiseptic, antifungal, and anti-inflammatory properties. Drink the tea also so the healing can work inside and out.

Goldenseal

(see "Yellow root" this chapter)

Hawthorn Berry

(promotes heart health and lowers blood pressure)

Botanical name

Crataegus oxyacantha

Also known as

mayflower

Medicinal properties

anti-inflammatory, antimicrobial, antioxidant, astringent, bitter, heart tonic, sedative

Hawthorn Berry (continued)

Health benefits

Hawthorn berry is a powerful antioxidant that is often used to promote heart health and reduce blood pressure. Hawthorn berry may also reduce cholesterol levels and treat a variety of other conditions, including hardening of arteries, irregular heart beat, stomach ulcers, indigestion, insomnia, stress, hot flashes, inflammation, and poor circulation.

Preparation and application

Tea

Add 1 tablespoon of dried hawthorn berries to 2 cups of boiling water. Cover and steep for 20 minutes and strain. Drink 1 to 2 cups daily. Alternatively, put 1 teaspoon of dried leaves and flowers in 1 cup of hot water, cover and steep for 10 to 15 minutes. Drink 1 to 3 cups daily.

Decoction

Add 1 cup of hawthorn berries to 4 cups of water. Bring to boil and slow simmer for 30 minutes. Cool and strain. Drink 1 to 2 cups daily. Place remaining mixture in glass jar and refrigerate to preserve for future use.

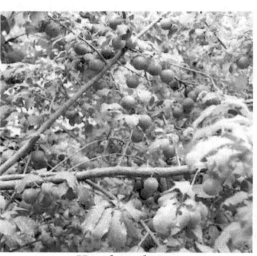

Hawthorn berry
Image 8-52

Hawthorn berry tincture

If you gather fresh hawthorn berries, let them dry before using. After they are dried, de-stem and crush the berries, place them in a mason jar. Cover with at least 80 proof grain alcohol, leaving about 1 inch space from the top of the jar. Close the jar with an air-tight lid and let sit for 4 weeks in a cool, dark cabinet. Shake vigorously once daily. After 4 weeks, strain liquid into a clean glass jar. Discard the berries. Take 1 dropper full of the tincture once daily. Can add to a 1/2 glass of warm water and drink.

Description: green leaves and stem; white, red or pink flower clusters bloom in May; red or black berries called haws sprout after flowers

Heart Leaves, Hart Leaves

(colds, chest congestion, coughs, decongestant, swelling)

Botanical name

Anemone hepatica

Also known as

common hepatica, kidneywort, liverwort, pennywort

Medicinal properties

anti-inflammatory, astringent, demulcent, mucilaginous, immune booster, vulnerary

Health benefits

Used in the African American healing traditions to treat colds, flu, coughs, leaves

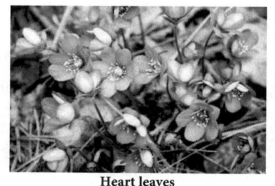

Heart leaves
Image 8-53

Description: waxy green leaves that are burgundy and brown in winter; white, lavender or pink flowers in spring

congestion, and swelling. A tonic of heart helps relieve chest congestion. Heart leaves or liverwort was also widely used to remedy indigestion and disorders of the liver.

Preparation and application

Place 1 ounce of dried leaves in 2 cups of boiling water. Turn off heat, cover and let steep until cool. Strain and drink frequently.

High John The Conqueror

(command of a situation, good luck, protection, and sexual potency)

Botanical name

Ipomoea jalapa

Also known as

bindweed, jalap root, John the Conqueror, moon flower, morning glory, sweet potato

Medicinal properties

cathartic (agent for purging bowels)

Health benefits

In hoodoo medicine, High John the Conqueror is employed to bring good luck, increase wealth, command a situation, draw love to you, win a court case, and to strengthen male potency and attraction.

Preparation and application

Carry the whole root in a medicine bag. Alternately, wrap a symbol of your desired outcome around the root in a manner such as wrapping money around the root, putting the root in a medicine bag with cards or dice, or writing the name of a desired love on a piecdeof paper and wrapping it around the root. Some have chewed the root right before a court case and spit out the juice before entering court to bring a favorable outcome.

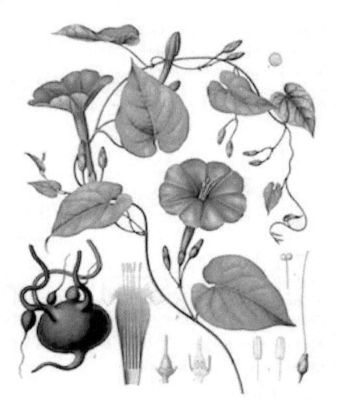

High John the Conquerer
Image 8-54

Description: brownish twisting stems; purplish-red flower; green leaves

High John in fiction

"There is no established picture of what sort of looking-man this John de Conquer was. To some, he was a big, physical-looking man like John Henry ... he lived on the plantation where, their old folks were slaves. He is not so well known to the present generation of colored people in the same way that he was in slavery time. Like King Arthur of England, he has served his people, and gone back into mystery again. High John de Conquer went back: to Africa, but he left his power here, and placed his American dwelling in the root of a certain plant. Only possess that root, and he can be summoned at any time."

From the short story "High John de Conquer" by Zora Neale Hurston

Hog Hoof Tea

(colds, flu, coughs, whooping cough, bronchitis)

Also known as

hoof tea

Medicinal properties

antiviral, germicide

Health benefits

Used to remedy very bad colds, flu and coughs, whooping cough, and bronchitis.

Preparation and application

Put crushed particles of a hog's hoof in a pot, fill with water, and boil for 15 to 20 minutes. Let cool, strain, and drink. Alternative: Boil hog's hoof in whiskey and drink.

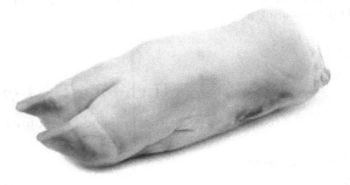

Hog hoof
Image 8-55

Description: pale, pink rubber-like flesh

Hog Maws

(mumps, fever reducer)

Also known as

buche (Mexico) , cuajos (Puerto Rico), gog maws, seimagge (Pennsylvania Dutch)

Medicinal properties

febrifuge

Health benefits and use

Hog maw is the lining of a pig's stomach. It was used to treat mumps and as a fever reducer by placing the hog maw on the jaws or forehead and wrapping with a bandage to keep in place.

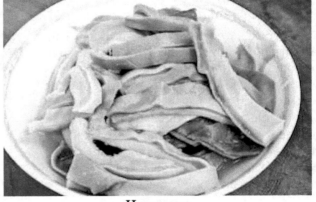

Hog maws
Image 8-56

Description: pale pinkish color, stomach of the pig

Honey

(inflammation, pain, infections)

Medicinal properties

antibacterial, anti-inflammatory, anti-microbial, antioxidant, antiseptic, demulcent, emollient, nutritive

Health benefits

Like castor oil, cod liver oil and other staple medicines in African American healing traditions, honey is a powerful healing agent with numerous benefits that go far beyond its sweet taste and it's intended use. Honey's antimicrobial and antibacterial properties kill viruses, bacteria, and fungus, and its anti-inflammatory properties help treat pain and inflammation.

In African American healing traditions, honey was most often used to

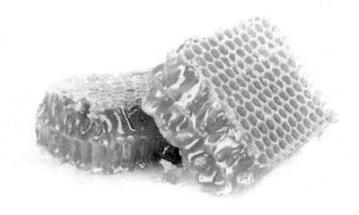

Honey comb
Image 8-57

Description: golden brown in color, thick and sticky consistency

sweeten terrible tasting medicine and make it easier to go down, especially for children. When added in remedies to treat colds and flu, honey's medicinal properties help treat hacking coughs, sore throats, sinus, lung and chest infections, and pain. Some practitioners also used honey to treat wounds, cuts, and burns. When applied directly to the affected area, honey acts as an agent that accelerates wound healing and prevents infection. Honey's anti-inflammatory properties may help in treating arthritis, rheumatism, and the associated pain.

Honey's other health benefits are: immediate energy booster, stimulates the immune system, and may have anti-cancer properties. Honey is a food and medicine rich with minerals like magnesium, potassium, calcium, sodium chlorine, sulfur, iron, and phosphate. It also expels mucous. Honey contains vitamins B1, B2, C, B6, B5 and B3, and several kinds of hormones.

Preparation and application

Tea/tonic

All-purpose detox and preventive health tonic for colds, flu, arthritis, rheumatism, pain, and inflammation:

2 tablespoons of apple cider vinegar (ACV), 1 tablespoon of honey, 1/2 cup of warm water. Drink twice a day, once in the morning and again before bed. Can add 1/4 to 1/2 teaspoon of cinnamon.

Add 1 tablespoon of honey to any of your natural healing remedies to treat ailments. Only add honey to warm remedies (not hot) to retain the nutritional and medicinal properties.

Sore throats

Swallow 1 teaspoon of honey by first letting it sit in your mouth until it melts and then let the honey go down your throat. The antibacterial, antimicrobial, and antiseptic properties will begin to treat the ailment. Do not drink any liquids for 15 minutes after swallowing to allow the medicine to work.

Wounds, burns, cuts

Apply a generous amount of honey to a dressing first and then apply the dressing to the affected area. Change the dressing 2 to 3 times a day depending on wound seepage.

Note: Cooking honey or adding to high degree temperatures destroys the nutritional and medicinal benefits.

Cautions: Many health professionals suggest not giving honey to children under 12 months of age because it may contain spores of bacteria that cause botulism.

Horehound

(whooping cough, expectorant)

Botanical name

Marrubium vulgare

Also known as

adorn, bull's blood, eye of the star, grand bonhomme, haran haran, houndsbane, seed of horus, white horehound

Medicinal properties

anti-inflammatory, antioxidant, bitter, bowel and uterine stimulant, diuretic, expectorant, vasodilator

Health benefits

Horehound was widely used in African American healing traditions to treat coughs, bronchitis, whooping cough, asthma, and other respiratory ailments. Horehound is an expectorant that loosens phlegm to produce a more effective cough that expels mucous

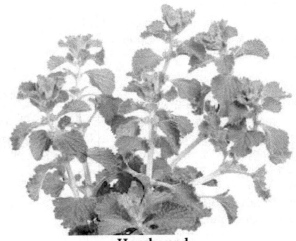

Horehound
Image 8-58

Description: dark green wrinkled leaves on top, white hairs on underside; small white flowers bloom from June-August

with ease. Its anti-inflammatory properties were also used to relieve pain and treat sprains, swelling, muscle cramps, toothaches, and headaches. Drinking horehound tea may also aid the digestive system by stimulating the liver and the spleen, thereby reducing indigestion, heartburn, bloating and other gastrointestinal problems.

Preparation and application

Best to use the horehound leaves shortly after you harvest them. The longer you store them, the less potent they become. Store unused leaves in an airtight glass jar.

Tea

Use 1 tablespoon of dried leaves or 3 tablespoons of fresh leaves per 1 cup of water. Pour 1 cup of boiling water on the herb, cover and let steep for 10 to 15 minutes. Strain and drink 3 to 4 cups a day for no more than 7 days.

Cough and congestion syrup

Add 1 ounce of leaves to 2 cups of boiling water, remove from heat, cover and let steep until cool. Strain into a glass jar or bowl and add honey and lemon. Mix well and store in an airtight glass jar. Take 1 teaspoon as needed 3 to 4 times daily. Take for no more than 7 consecutive days.

Food use

Leaves can be chewed or chopped and added to other foods like salads.

Horny Goat Weed

(male potency, sexual tonic)

Botanical names

Epimedium grandiflorum or Epimedium sagittatum

Also known as

epimedium, yin yang huo

Medicinal properties

aphrodisiac

Health benefits

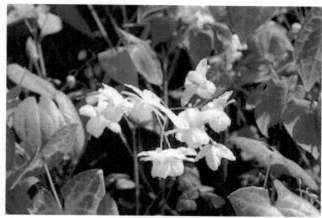

Horny goat weed
Image 8-59

Description: green leaves; yellow flowers

The traditional Chinese herb called horny goat weed got its name because it treats male erectile dysfunction, low libido, and acts as a sexual tonic for both men and women. Epimedium, or horny goat weed, may also aid conditions of fatigue, rheumatism, back pain, muscle spasms, arthralgia, and osteoporosis. It is also a general kidney tonic.

Traditional use

While horny goat weed is often used today, it was not a staple in African American healing tradition.

Suggested use

Best prepared as tea, tincture, or capsule.

Horse Milk

(whooping cough, colds, congestion)

Medicinal properties

antibacterial, anti-inflammatory, antiviral

Health benefits

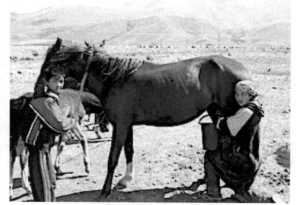

Horse milking
Image 8-60

Description: a mare being milked in Kyrgyzstan (Central Asia)

Horse milk was used as medicine for its antibacterial and antiviral properties and also as an alternative to cow's milk. Horse milk resembles human milk more than any other animal and is an important food for people of Central Asia. It has less fat and caesin than cow's milk, more whey proteins, and about 40% more lactose until it is fermented. The people of the Central Asian steppes (e.g., Mongolia, Kazakhstan, and Tajikistan) make a mildly alcoholic drink from fermented horse milk called Kumis. The fermentation process reduces the lactose content and makes it more digestible and nutritious for people who are lactose intolerant.

Horse Milk (continued)

Kumis was a popular treatment for tuberculosis, bronchitis and anemia toward the end of the 19th century in Russia.

In African American healing, horse milk (probably fermented) was drunk to treat whooping cough and other infections of the chest and lungs, and also to increase immunity and resistance to colds. Due to its antibacterial components, horse milk lasts longer than cow's milk and it stimulates the increase of good bacteria in the bowel, promoting healthy digestion.

Drinking horse milk and using it as a topical cream may also help treat and relieve skin conditions like psoriasis or eczema. Horse milk is nutrient-rich with calcium, potassium, magnesium, iron, and vitamins A, B2, B6, B12, C, E, carbohydrates, proteins, lactose, and fat.

Preparation and application

People drank 1 to 2 cups of horse milk daily for ailments.

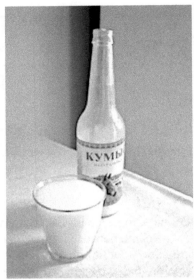

Horse milk
Image 8-60a

Description: kumis, fermented horse milk; creamy-white, similar in appearance to cow milk

Horsemint

(nausea, upset stomach, vomiting, digestive ailments)

Botanical name

Monarda punctata L.

Also known as

bee balm, monarda, wild bergamont, wild oswego

Medicinal properties

aromatic, calmative, cardiac, carminative, diaphoretic, diuretic, emmenagogue, mild alterative, stomachic, sudorific

Health benefits

Horsemint tea was used often in Native American and African American healing traditions. A mild tea can made to promote sweating to treat colds and flu and to treat digestive and stomach problems such as flatulence, colic, nausea, vomiting, diarrhea, and suppressed urine. Horsemint can also be used to treat rheumatism, expel worms, and stimulate heart action.

The leaves are rich in the medicinal oil thymol, an antiseptic. When rubbed on the body or made

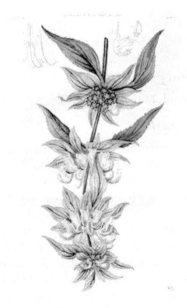

Horsemint
Image 8-61

Description: light to medium green stalk and leaves; red, pink, lavender flowers

into a poultice, horsemint medicine helps relieve pain from arthritic joints and reduce inflammation, and eases backache pain.

Preparation and application

Tea

Put 1 teaspoon of leaves or tops in 1 cup of water, cover and steep for 10 to 15 minutes. Drink 1 to 2 cups a day for no more than 1 week. Was not used long term.

Salve for aching joints and pain

Rinse 2 cups of harvested horsemint leaves. Bring 2 cups of water to boil in a pot, turn off the heat, and add the leaves. Cover and let steep approximately 20 minutes. Melt 1 cup of natural vegetable oil in a small pot. Add 1/2 cup of strained horsemint tea and leaves to the oil and stir well, mixing until creamy. Add beeswax or shea butter for thickening. Let cool and place in an airtight glass container. Rub the salve on arthritic joints and on areas suffering from aches pains, and inflammation.

Huckleberry

(diabetes, "high sugar")

Botanical name

Vaccinium parvifolium

Also known as

bilberries, European blueberries, whortle-berries

Medicinal properties

antibiotic, anti-inflammatory, antioxidant, antiseptic, astringent

Health benefits

Huckleberry leaves and berries were traditionally used in African American healing traditions to treat diabetes or "high sugar." The berries were eaten or dried and made into a powder that was used in a tea. Some say drinking the brewed leaves acted as

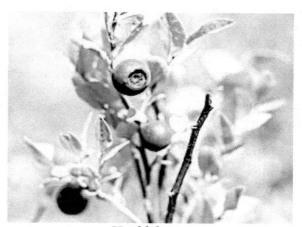

Huckleberry
Image 8-62

Description: green leaves; purple, dark purple or black fruit

natural insulin in the body. Huckleberry is rich with antioxidants and high in vitamin C, which helps strengthen the immune system and the body's ability to fight chronic diseases. Eating huckleberry reduces inflammation and may also lower cholesterol levels. Other uses for huckleberry are as a mouthwash and gargle to treat sore throat and mouth infections and as a tea to strengthen eyesight.

Preparation and application

Tea

Put 1 teaspoon of dried huckleberry leaves—or 2 teaspoons of fresh leaves—in 1 cup of boiled water, cover and steep for 10 to 15 minutes. Drink 1 to 3 times daily. Add honey to sweeten.

Berries

Eat the fresh berries or add to a drink, cereal, or salad. Grind the dried berries and make a tea using 1 teaspoon of powdered berries to 1 cup of water. Drink 3 cups daily.

Jerusalem Weed

(expel intestinal worms and parasites, treat ringworm)

Botanical name

Chenopodium ambrosiodes

Also known as

goosefoot, jerusalem oak, Mexican tea, wormseed

Medicinal properties

anthelmintic, antifungal, antispasmodic, carminative, digestive, expectorant, insecticide

Health benefits

Commonly used as a wash to treat skin fungus such as ringworm or athlete's foot, or made into a tea and drunk to expel intestinal worms (hookworms, round worms). Jerusalem weed is an expectorant that contains compounds that paralyze intestinal worms and expel them from your body. Also used to treat a wide range of ailments, including digestive disorders, coughs, colds, congestion, diarrhea, fevers, gout, and cramps. It is also used as an organic insecticide. Jerusalem weed is native to Mexico and the American Southwest. The leaves have been used in Mexico and Central and South America since pre-Columbian times to garnish food. A few sprinkles of leaves may be used to season, which aids digestion.

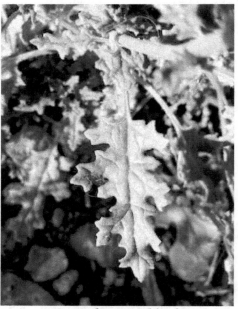

Jerusalem weed leaf
Image 8-63

Preparation and application

Caution: The oil extracted from Jerusalem weed and seed can be highly toxic.

Tea

Make a tea using 1/2 to 1 teaspoon of dried leaves and flowers to 1 cup of hot water. Cover and steep for 10 to 15 minutes and drink 1 cup daily.

Purgative

To expel intestinal worms and parasites, eat a mixture of 1 teaspoon Jerusalem weed (leaves and flowers), 1 tablespoon molasses, and 1 teaspoon pumpkin seeds.

Wash

Make a wash to treat skin fungus by adding 3 teaspoons of leaves and flowers to hot water. Cover and steep until cool, then drain. Pour liquid into a glass jar. Use as a wash on affected area 2 to 3 times daily. Store in refrigerator when not using.

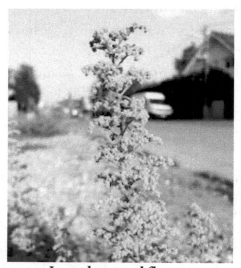

Jerusalem weed flowers
Image 8-63a

Description: green leaves; yellowish flowering top

Lavender

(depression/mood enhancer, relaxant, bee stings, insect bites)

Botanical name

Lavandula

Also known as

English lavender, French lavender, garden lavender, Spanish lavender, true lavender

Medicinal properties

analgesic, antianxiety, anticholinergic, anticonvulsive, antidepressive, antihistamine, antinflammatory, antimicrobial, antineoplastic, antioxidant, antiseptic, antispasmodic, antithrombotic, anxiolytic, mood stabilizer, neuroprotective, rubefacient

Health benefits

Lavender is renowned for its use as a calming medicine. In African American healing traditions, lavender would be used to treat bee stings and insect bites because of its calming, anti-inflammatory properties. Lavender can also be used to treat burns and headaches, aid in sleep and relaxation, and to reduce symptoms of anxiety and insomnia.

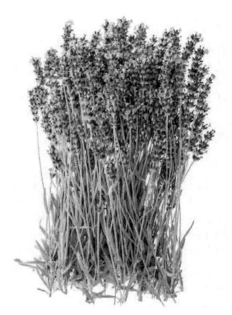

Lavender
Image 8-64

Description: green-gray narrow leaves; blue-violet flowers

Preparation and application

Tea

Prepare an infusion of the lavender flowers and leaves to soothe nerves and to decrease distress, anxiety, and insomnia. Use 1 teaspoon of dried leaves to 1 cup of hot water.

Bath – Aromatherapy

Add lavender leaves and flowers or drops of lavender oil to a bath to aid calming and relaxation.

Lavender oil

Rub oil from the flowers and leaves onto skin to soothe inflammation from bee stings and insect bites. Alternatively, make your own lavender oil and rub on affected area.

How to make lavender oil

Strip 1 to 2 cups of flowers from their stems and spread them out on a white paper towel, paper bag, or white cotton cloth. Let air dry for 2 to 3 hours. Pack flowers in a small glass jar and then fill with olive oil, packing in more flowers so there is no space left. Close jar with an air-tight lid or cover with plastic wrap and hold in place with a rubber band. Place in a cool, dark location for 1 to 2 weeks, shaking vigorously daily. (Put in a paper bag if area is not dark enough.) Strain mixture into cheesecloth, pressing all the oil out into a glass container. Cover the container and store oil in a cool, shaded place or in the refrigerator door for future use.

Lemon

(colds, infection, detoxifier, oily skin, gout, kidney stones)

Botanical name

Citrus limonum

Also known as

citrus

Medicinal properties

antiseptic, astringent, coagulent, cooling agent, diuretic

Health benefits

Lemon has been used for centuries for its medicinal properties. Lemon's overall medicinal power may treat and protect against colds, flu, inflammation, indigestion, constipation, skin problems such as acne and

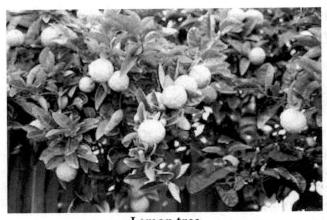

Lemon tree
Image 8-65

Description: dark green leaves; white purplish flowers; yellow fruit

oily skin, dandruff, respiratory disorders, throat infections, minor burns, and internal bleeding. It is also a general detoxifier, blood cleanser and immune enhancer. Lemon tonics may also help eliminate uric acid build-up which can lead to kidney stones and gout.

Adding 1/2 to 1 whole lemon to your daily diet may effectively prevent and treat many health related problems. This can be as simple as making and drinking lemon tea with honey (made by adding 1/2 to 1 whole lemon in 1 cup of warm water), making and drinking lemonade (made with lemons and a natural sweetener like cane sugar, honey, or stevia), or squeezing the juice from a lemon into your favorite drink.

Lemons are acidic but they are alkaline-forming when they come in contact with body fluids and help the body maintain a healthy pH level. Lemon is nutrient-rich with vitamins C and B, copper, calcium, iron, potassium, magnesium, phosphorus, carbohydrates, proteins, fiber, and cancer-fighting flavanoids.

Preparation and application

Tea

Squeeze all of the juice out of 1/2 to 1 whole lemon into a cup, drop the remainder of the lemon in, and fill with hot water. Add honey to sweeten and cayenne (optional) for extra medicine. This tonic was used daily to flush kidneys and detoxify the body.

Food

Squeeze lemon juice on salads, fish, and on other foods any time you want a tart taste.

Life-Everlasting

(see "Rabbit Tobacco" this chapter)

Liniment or Linton

(chest colds, joint pain, muscle strain)

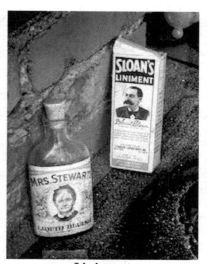

Liniment
Image 8-66

Many Southerners, due to their colloquial accents, used the term "linton" when referring to "liniment." A liniment is an oil or alcohol-based medicine made with herbs and rubbed on affected areas to alleviate chest colds and aches and pains from arthritis, rheumatism, and muscle strains.

Some herbs used to make a liniment included menthol, camphor, pine tar, pine needles, eucalyptus, and garlic. This medicine was intended for external use only.

Lion's Tongue (Wintergreen)

(diabetes, asthma/coughs, fevers, digestion, inflammation, pain, arthritis)

Botanical name

Gaultheria procumbens

Also known as

checkerberry, deer berry, winterberry

Medicinal properties

alterative, analgesic, anaphrodisiac, anodyne, anti-inflammatory, antirheumatic, antiseptic, antispasmodic, aromatic, astringent, carminative, diuretic, emmenagogue, galactagogue, stimulant

Health benefits

Lion's tongue is used as both a food and medicine in Native American and African American healing traditions. Medicinally, it is used to increase general health and well-being and to treat a wide range of ailments. The benefit from using a medicine that has numerous medicinal properties is that it may beused initially to treat one ailment and the patient also benefits from its other useful properties. The leaves contain methyl salicylates, the active pain-killler in aspirin.

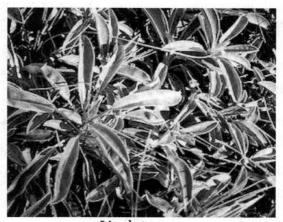

Lion's tongue
Image 8-67

Description: light to medium green leaves; bell-shaped white flowers bloom June-July with edible red berries

Lion's tongue medicine has been used to treat the following conditions: digestive disorders (diarrhea, flatulence, constipation, colic, congestion, hemorrhoids); diabetes and endocrine system support; urinary tract and kidney problems (inflammation and infection); lung and respiratory ailments (asthma, coughs, bronchitis); arthritis, rheumatism and associated pain; nervous conditions (used as a nerve tonic and to relieve sciatica); headaches and migraine; skin conditions such as boils, swellings and sores; colds, flu, and fevers; and irregular menstruation.

Lion's Tongue (Wintergreen) (continued)

Preparation and application

Tea

Use 1 teaspoon of leaves per 1 cup of hot water. Cover and steep for 10 to 15 minutes. Drink 1 to 2 cups daily to treat ailment.

Mouth wash or gargle

Make a strong infusion with the leaves, using 2 teaspoons of leaves to 1 cup of hot water. Cover and let steep covered for 20 to 30 minutes until cool. Use 2 to 3 times per day as a gargle or mouthwash to treat sore throat or mouth sores.

Poultice

Soak a cloth in a strong solution of the tea using 3 teaspoons of herb to 1 cup of water. Place the cloth in the mixture, cover the water and let steep for at least 30 minutes, soaking in the active ingredient. Remove the cloth and wring, removing as much water as possible. Strain the mixture. Take some of the leaves and place on the affected area and wrap with the cloth. Leave on for 30 to 60 minutes and then remove. Repeat twice daily. Used to treat joint pain, boils, swellings, ulcers, and hard to heal wounds.

Steam inhalant for coughs, bronchitis, congestion, respiratory ailments

Place two handfuls of lion's tongue leaves in a big pot of water. Bring to boil and use as a steam inhalant by covering your head with a towel, bending over close to the pot, and breathing in the steam from the boiled water infused with the medicinal agent. (For relief of these ailments, drink lion's tongue tea as well. See instructions above for brewing tea.)

Lydia E. Pinkham's Herb Medicine

(women's health tonic)

A 19th century herbal tonic that was developed by Lydia E. Pinkham in 1875. The tonic was specifically formulated with herbs traditionally found to aid in relieving menstrual and menopausal discomfort. It was popular and used amongst women of all races and cultures.

The original tonic included 5 herbs:

Unicorn root – estrogenic properties, supports female reproductive system, taken for suppressed menstruation/amenorrhea.

Life root – known as the "female regulator" and used in many Native American healing traditions; uterine tonic, relieves menopausal and menstrual discomfort.

Black cohosh – reduces menopause and menstrual discomfort; possible alternative to HRT (hormone replacement) therapy.

Pleurisy root – reduces inflammation, treats respiratory infections, promotes moderate perspiration, and aids expectoration.

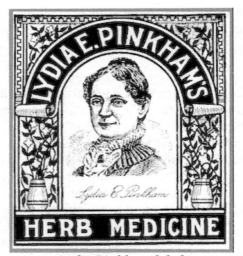

Lydia Pinkham label
Image 8-68

Fenugreek seed – has properties that mimic estrogen and helps relieve menopausal symptoms, possible alternative to HRT (hormone replacement therapy)

A later version of the tonic called Lydia Pinkham Herbal Compound is available today and is formulated with these 7 natural herbs:

Motherwort – eases menstrual discomfort and serves as a digestive aid, nerve tonic, and treatment for endometriosis; may have estrogen-like effect that relieves menopausal symptoms.

Gentian – improves appetite and digestion.

Jamaican dogwood – a sedative used to treat insomnia, nervous excitement, and migraine.

Black cohosh – reduces menopause and menstrual discomfort; possible alternative to HRT (hormone replacement) therapy.

Pleurisy root – reduces inflammation, treats respiratory infections, reduces inflammation, promotes moderate perspiration and aids expectoration.

Licorice – may be estrogenic and help relieve menopausal symptoms.

Dandelion – stimulates digestion, has a diuretic and mild laxative effect. Liver tonic that is rich in vitamins and minerals; leaves sometimes used in salads and teas.

Other Ingredients – vitamins C and E and 10% ethyl alcohol as a preservative.

Lydia Pinkham Herbal Compound is marketed by Numark Laboratories and can be bought online or at selected Walgreens, CVS, Rite Aid, and other drug stores across the country.

Caution – Today, many medicines that affect and mimic hormone levels should be used with caution as they may increase risk of breast and uterine cancer in women.

Maypop Vine

(anxiety, upset stomach, constipation, sciatica, insomnia)

Botanical name

Passiflora incarnata

Also known as

passion flower, purple passion-flower, true passionflower, wild apricot, wild passion vine

Medicinal properties

anodyne, antispasmodic, anxiolytic, aphrodisiac, aromatic, sedative

Health benefits

Maypop tea was used for its calming effect to treat pain, muscle spasms, nervousness, insomnia, and stomach problems such as irritable bowel syndrome, constipation, diarrhea, cramps and more.

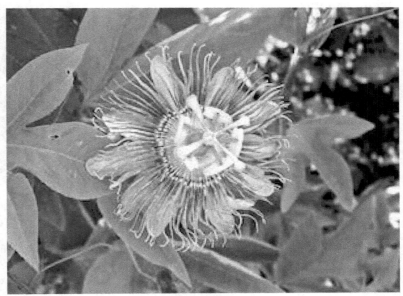

Maypop vine
Image 8-69

Description: dark green leaves; flowers with white petals and pink-purple crown bloom in summer; yellowish maypop fruits appear July through fall

Preparation and application

Tea

Use 1 teaspoon to 1 tablespoon of the dried herb (include stems and flowers) to 1 cup boiling water. Cover and steep for 10 to 15 minutes. Drink at bedtime or drink 1 to 2 cups during the day to calm nervousness.

Food

Add flowers to a salad or eat them whole.

Maypop Vine (continued)

Tincture

Fill a jar with chopped, fresh or dried herb and cover with a minimum 80 proof grain alcohol. Keep the jar in a cool, dark cabinet and shake daily for two weeks, then strain. Take one full dropper (30 to 40 drops) 1 to 3 times daily.

Milk Thistle

(supports liver health)

Botanical name

Silybum marianum

Also known as

holy thistle, St. Mary thistle, wild artichoke

Medicinal properties

antioxidant, anti-inflammatory, anticarcinogenic, hepato-protective, immuno-stimulating, mild estrogenic

Health benefits

Milk thistle is a time-honored treatment that maintains, supports, restores, and protects the liver. The active ingredient, silymarin, may help repair damaged liver cells from alcohol and other toxic substances and prevent liver toxicity. Milk thistle may encourage liver cell growth, reduce inflammation, and have antioxidant effects. It has been used to treat alcohol-related liver diseases, liver poisoning, and also to protect the liver against harmful medications such as the pain-reliever acetaminophen. It is a prescribed medication in Europe.

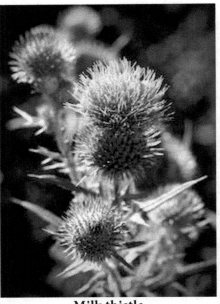

Milk thistle

Image 8-70

Description: spiny green leaves with white marbling; 2nd year flower stalk rises with purple-pink heads, followed by seed; leaves and stem exude milky sap when cut

Traditional use

While milk thistle is often used today, it was not a staple in African American healing tradition.

Preparation and application

Tea

Prepare a tea by putting 1 teaspoon of crushed milk thistle seeds or 1 1/2 teaspoons of milk thistle leaves and seeds in 1 cup of hot water. Cover and steep for 10 to 15 minutes. Drink 1 to 3 times daily. Alternately, purchase milk thistle tincture and add the suggested dosage of drops to 1 cup of hot water and drink as a tea.

Supplement

Today, many people take the supplement in a pill form with the active ingredient silymarin.

Tablets

Purchase milk thistle tablets or silymarin tablets (sylymarin is the medicinal agent in milk thistle) and take the recommended dose.

Tincture

Using either a mortar and pestle or a grinder, crush enough milk thistle seeds to fill a half-pint mason jar. Be sure to crush the seeds only slightly, just enough to activate but not so much that the seeds are turned into a powder. Place the crushed seeds in the mason jar and then fill the jar to the rim with either 80 to 100 proof grain alcohol or clear vodka. Close lid tightly and store in a cool, dark place (put in a brown paper bag to create more darkness, if necessary). Let sit for 4-6 weeks. The longer the tincture sits, the more potent it will be when taken. Shake jar vigorously every other day during the first week after preparation, then let it sit undisturbed for the remaining weeks until ready to use. When tincture is ready, strain liquid through a cheesecloth into a dark glass container. Keep in a cool, dark cabinet to preserve.

Molasses/Blackstrap Molasses

(nutritional tonic, antioxidant, laxative, energy booster, anemia)

Also known as

black treacle, golden syrup, syrup

Medicinal properties

anti-inflammatory, antioxidant, laxative

Health benefits

Molasses, especially blackstrap molasses, is a nutrient-rich food that has been used for a variety of ailments including arthritis, joint pain, gout, constipation, menstrual cramps, high blood sugar, intestinal worms, colds, and more. It is also used as a tonic for health maintenance and as an immune booster. Molasses contains antioxidants and essential nutrients that our bodies need to maintain optimal health, including iron, calcium,

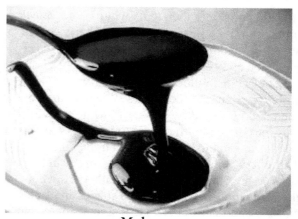

Molasses
Image 8-71

Description: thick brownish-black in color

copper, manganese, magnesium, potassium, selenium, phosphorous, chromium, cobalt, sodium, and vitamins B6, niacin, thiamin and riboflavin.

Molasses is produced after the first or second boiling of cane sugar. Blackstrap molasses is the product after the third boiling and it has the most health benefits and nutrition. In African American healing traditions, blackstrap molasses tonics were drunk first thing in the morning to start the day and for health maintenance. As a food, biscuits or corn pones were used to sop up molasses.

Preparation and application

Morning tonic

Mix 1 tablespoon of blackstrap molasses in a cup of warm water with vinegar or lemon and drink.

Mix 1 tablespoon of blackstrap molasses in a cup of warm milk. Today, one may substitute cow's milk with rice, almond, coconut, or soy milk.

To expel intestinal parasites and worms

Eat a mixture of blackstrap molasses with Jerusalem weed and pumpkin seeds.

Mulberry Tree (Mulberry Leaf Tea)

(diabetes, blood sugar balancer, coughs, colds, ringworm, gout)

Botanical name

Morus alba (white), Morus rubra (red), Morus nigra (black)

Also known as

black mulberry, red mulberry, sang (Chinese), white mulberry

Health benefits

All parts of the red, white, and black mulberry tree—leaf, bark, root bark, twigs, sap/milk, and fruit/berries—have been used as medicine and food.

The white mulberry is not native to North America. Because the mulberry leaf is the sole food source for silk worms, the white mulberry was introduced by the early American colonists hoping to establish a silk crop on the continent. The effort failed because the worms could not survive the North American weather. However, the white mulberry tree thrived so well in its new North American home that it is considered an "invasive" species in many states.

For centuries in Asia, a tea made from the leaves of the white mulberry tree has been drunk to treat diabetes. More recently in the United States, drinking mulberry leaf tea from the white mulberry has become a popular and effective treatment for Type 2 diabetes. Many African Americans, Native Americans, and other populations who have disproportionately high rates of this chronic disease are drinking mulberry leaf tea and noticing positive effects. Drinking the tea helps to prevent post-meal blood sugar spikes and helps to stabilize blood sugar and energy levels throughout the day.

The medicinal agent in the tea helps to prevent sugars from entering the bloodstream. Instead, the sugar is expelled through bowel movements.

White mulberry leaf tea was also drunk to treat colds, flu, fevers, and coughs. A poultice was made from the white mulberry leaves to treat toothaches and snake bites. The branches or small twigs were used to make a tea to treat pain from arthritis and rheumatism, high blood pressure, headaches, and to balance the concentration of sugar in the body. A tea made

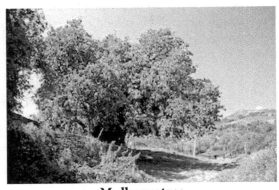

Mulberry tree

Image 8-72

Description: green leaves, brown bark

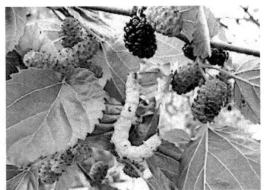

Mulberries on tree with silkworm

Image 8-72a

Description: close-up of white mulberry green leaves, dark purple and red fruit, white silkworm

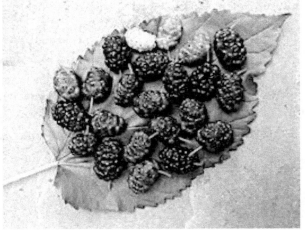

Mulberries

Image 8-72b

Description: deep purple, pink and white mulberries on a green mulberry leaf

from the white mulberry root bark treated coughs, bronchitis, and supported the lungs. The fruit is made into a blood tonic.

Unlike the white mulberry, the red mulberry tree is native to eastern and central North America and particularly flourishes in Virginia's Piedmont region. Native Americans used the red mulberry tree for medicine and food. The berries were eaten when ripe and/or dried and also used in drinks. A boiled stew was made with the corn, squash, beans, wild onion, mulberries, garlic, and greens. A milky juice similar to fig milk can be found in parts of the red mulberry and was used to treat ringworms and other fungal skin conditions.

A tea made from the red mulberry root bark was drunk as a urinary aid or laxative as well as to lower fevers or expel worms and as a stimulant to treat low energy. A cough syrup made from the red mulberry berry or a tea from the root was drunk to allay coughs, colds, and gout.

Black mulberry trees are native to Europe and Asia and are also cultivated in California and the southern region of the United States. A strong tea made from the black mulberry bark is drunk to expel worms. A syrup made from the fruit was used as an expectorant, laxative, and as a gargle to soothe sore throats. The berries, which are really a fruit, were used to make wine and jam.

The fruit or berries on all varieties of the mulberry tree are often made into a tonic to support blood, liver, and kidney functions. This tonic has been used in herbal medicine for thousands of years. Mulberries are also a rich source of vitamins C, B1, B2, K1, E, and the minerals iron and potassium.

Preparation and application

Leaves

White mulberry leaves can be made into a medicinal tea or poultice.

Tea

(for treatment of diabetes, blood sugar reducer, colds, fever coughs)

Fresh leaves: Gather 3 to 4 fresh mulberry leaves, rinse and cut into 1/4 inch strips. Place strips in 2 cups of boiling water. Simmer until water turns greenish colored. Strain leaves and drink 1 cup right before your meal to reduce blood sugar levels. Pour remaining tea in a glass jar and store in the refrigerator.

Dry leaves: Gather fresh mulberry leaves, rinse with cool water and let dry for 2 to 3 days. Crush 1 leaf with your hand and break into small pieces. Cover and steep in hot water for 15 to 20 minutes. Drink 1 cup right before your meal to reduce blood sugar levels.

Alternatively: purchase the mulberry leaf tea from a natural health store or order online.

Poultice

(for treatment of toothache, mouth sores, snake bites)

Grind up fresh or dried leaves in warm water so it has a paste-like consistency. Place mixture in between gauze and place on affected area 2 to 3 times daily for 30 to 60 minutes.

Fruit/Berries

Pick fruit when fully ripened and are dark purple to black in color. The fruit/berries can be eaten raw, juiced, preserved, cooked in a stew, or made into a syrup.

Juice/tonic

(for treatment of blood, liver, kidney, tonic, colds, coughs, sore throat)

Gather fresh ripe mulberries, rinse with cold water and place in a blender. Mix until it is a puree. Strain mixture into a glass jar. Take 2 tablespoons daily. Store remainder in refrigerator.

For a thicker mixture, add a little water and/or other ingredients you put in your favorite blended drinks along with the mulberry. Mix well. Drink as a smoothie.

To use as a tonic, gather 1 or more pounds of fruit. Place in a bowl and mash with a mortar and pestel or spatula to squeeze out the juice. Strain into a mesh sieve or cloth, pressing as much liquid through the strainer material as possible. Drink 2 to 3 tablespoons daily.

Mulberry Tree (Mulberry Leaf Tea) (continued)

Syrup/tonic

(for treatment of blood, liver, kidney, tonic, colds, coughs, sore throat)

Slowly boil 1 cup or more of mulberries in a pot until the juice is extracted, stirring and mashing occasionally. Remove the pot from heat and let sit overnight until cool. Slowly heat up again the next day. Strain the liquid into a glass jar using mesh cloth or sieve. Discard the remains. Store in the refrigerator. Take 1–2 teaspoons daily for a blood tonic to treat colds and to support good health.

White mulberry root bark

Prepare as a decoction to expel worms, reduce fever, as a laxative, stimulant, and to treat gout. Place 1 ounce of dried root or 2 ounces of fresh root in 2 cups of water in a pot. Heat up slowly. Bring to boil, then simmer for 20 minutes. Strain and drink throughout the day.

Mullet or Mullein

(respiratory ailments, colds, congestion, inflammation, arthritis, rheumatism)

Botanical name

Verbascum thapsus

Also known as

beggar's blanket, cowboy toilet paper, flannel leaf, velvet plant

Medicinal properties

analgesic, antiseptic, antibiotic, anti-inflammatory, astringent, bitter, demulcent, diuretic, emollient, expectorant

Health benefits

Mullein has numerous medicinal properties that make it effective in treating many ailments. In African American healing traditions, mullein is often used to treat colds, cough, congestion, respiratory and pulmonary ailments including chronic bronchitis, asthmatic coughs, whooping cough, hoarsness, and excessive mucous. Its anti-inflammatory and pain relieving properties may help to reduce swelling and pain associated with arthritis, bursitis, rheumatism, and gout. When mullein is applied externally as a poultice, its antiseptic and astringent properties may help treat boils, carbuncles, rashes, skin ulcers, and hemorrhoids. Mullein is also used to treat headaches, nervousness, muscle spasms, constipation, and is generally used as an antiviral.

Mullein is rich with minerals, vitamins and essential nutrients including iron, magnesium, sulfur, potassium vitamins B-2, B-5, B-12, and D, choline, hesperidin, PABA, mucilage, and saponins.

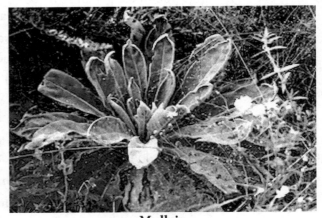

Mullein
Image 8-73

Description: grayish-green wooly leaves; yellow flower stock with purplish stamens; rises from leaves; blooms spring-summer

Preparation and application

Mullein leaf tea for respiratory ailments, coughs and congestion

Pour 1 cup of boiling water over 1 to 2 teaspoons of dried mullein flowers and leaves. Cover and steep for 10 to 15 minutes. Strain and drink up to 3 cups daily. Sweeten with honey if desired.

Mullein and garlic oil for ear infections/aches

In a glass jar, combine 1 teaspoon of chopped garlic with 1 teaspoon of finely-chopped dried or fresh mullein leaves. Cover with olive oil, pouring enough oil to cover 1 inch above the mixture. For 3 days, let mixture sit in a lighted area or on a windowsill to get direct sun. Remove and keep in a dark closet or cabinet for 24 hours, then strain oil into a dropper jar for easy access. Place in refrigerator. Keeps up to 1 year.

Warm the dropper of mullein and garlic oil in a cup of hot water. Place 3 drops of the oil in the affected ear 2 times daily. Do this once at night, sleeping with the affected ear up and covered with a cotton ball. When standing or sitting after applying during the day, make sure to cover the ear with a cotton ball. Use for up to 3 days on affected ear.

Mullein leaf bath or soak for arthritis and joint pain

Cut 4 to 6 dried leaves per 5 cups of water. Boil in a pot and soak your feet or whole body in a bath for at least 20 minutes.

Mullein leaf poultice

In a big pot, mix 4 parts dried and chopped mullein leaf to 1 part water to 1 part apple cider vinegar (ACV). Heat up and put in a cotton cloth and place on affected area.

Mullein leaf smoke for pulmonary congestion

Pack a pipe or make a cigarette out of dried cut-up mullein leaves. Smoke and inhale 3 times to relieve pulmonary congestion. Repeat twice daily.

Mullein leaf wrap

Take a large leaf, soak in warm water, and apply to affected area. Wrap with cheesecloth to keep in place.

Mustard Plant

(mustard salve or plaster for colds, congestion, bronchitis, pneumonia, and flus)

Botanical name

Brassica juncea

Also known as

yellow mustard

Medicinal properties

anti-inflammatory, decongestant, expectorant, hyperemic, stimulant

Health benefits

Mustard plaster and salve were rubbed on the chest to relieve congestion and coughs due to colds, flu, bronchitis, and pneumonia. Mustard medicine may stimulate and increase blood circulation and dilation of the capillaries to

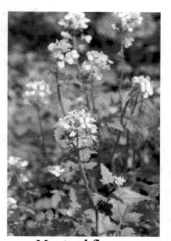

Mustard flower
Image 8-74

Description: yellow flowers

Mustard Plant (continued)

encourage coughing, expel mucous, and rid the body of respiratory toxins. Mustard, both the seed and in powder form, may also have anti-inflammatory properties. The salve or plaster was also used to treat rheumatic pains, joint pains, headaches, toothaches, and neuralgia. However, mustard plasters may easily irritate the skin if made too strong. Eating mustard is an excellent source of protein, calcium, magnesium and potassium.

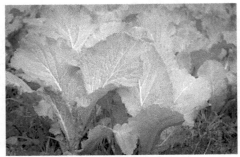

Mustard leaf
Image 8-74a
Description: medium to light green leaves

Preparation and application

Salve or Plaster

(for chest congestion, coughs, rheumatism, joint pain)

Recipe 1 (mixing with a fat)

Grind mustard seeds into a powder or purchase an organic grade of mustard powder. Make a thick salve or plaster with the consistency of icing by mixing with castor oil, olive oil, or another natural vegetable oil. The oil or butter helps protect your skin from irritations the mustard may cause. Thin by adding a little water. Rub mixture over the affected area: chest, back, joints. If using over chest area, cover nipples with an adhesive bandage to protect from sensitivity to mustard. Place a cloth (wool, flannel, or linen)

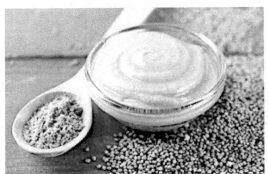

Mustard seed, powder, paste
Image 8-74b
Description: yellow-ochre in color

over the rubbed area or wrap with cheesecloth or fleece. Wear an old shirt or sweater to cover chest area if that is where the plaster has been rubbed. Leave on for no more than 20 minutes. Clean the treated area with cool water. If irritation or burning occurs at any time during treatment, remove and clean immediately, then dust area with baby powder or cornstarch to soothe the skin and relieve irritation.

Recipe 2 (mixing with flour and water)

Mix 1 part powdered mustard to 8 to 10 parts flour. Add enough warm water to make a paste. Keep adding water and mixing until you get a paste similar in consistency to pancake batter. Apply to affected area, wrap with cotton cloth, gauze or wool, and leave on for no more than 20 minutes. Wash off plaster with cool water.

Oak Bark

(inflammation, swelling, tooth decay, gum disease)

Botanical name

Quercus robor

Also known as

white oak bark

Medicinal properties

antibacterial, anti-inflammatory, antiseptic, antiviral, astringent, anthelmintic, antihemorrhagic

Health benefits

Oak bark medicine is often used to reduce swelling and inflammation, both internally and externally, and as a general health tonic. Native Americans used oak bark to treat dental conditions such as tooth decay and gum disease by chewing on the bark. The tannins in the bark help fight bacteria and prevent cavities or gum infection. Oak bark tea has been used to aid digestion, treat uclers as well as spleen and gallbladder problems, and to reduce kidney stones. Oak bark's antiseptic properties are useful in preventing infection and treating minor cuts, burns, insect bites, and other skin irritations.

Preparation and application

Tea/Decoction

Brew oak bark in a pot to drink as a tea by making a solution of 1 teaspoon of oak bark (with a bit of tree flesh still attached) to 1 cup of water. Bring to boil and simmer covered for 30 minutes. The longer you simmer oak bark, the stronger the medicine. Strain and drink. Drink 1 to 3 cups daily. Oak bark may dehydrate you so drink one cup of water to each cup of tea you drink.

Use same formula to brew a strong decoction to use as an astringent, to use in baths, douches, skin washes, and to use on boils, cuts, or burns.

Poultice

Make the wash/antiseptic mixture above, using small/chopped pieces of oak bark. Soak a cotton cloth in the mixture for 10 minutes. Wring out. Take a few pieces of the oak bark that was simmered in the wash and/or use new pieces or a combination of both. Put pieces in the cloth and wrap into a bundle that can be placed on the affected area. Keep poultice in place by wrapping with another cloth. Leave on for 2 to 3 hours or overnight. May be effective treating boils, sores, and inflammation.

Salve

Grind oak bark and some white oak tree flesh into a powder. Heat an equal amount of natural vegetable oil in a small pot and slowly mix in the mixed powder. Let cool and place in a glass jar. Apply to affected area twice daily. Store in a cool, dark area.

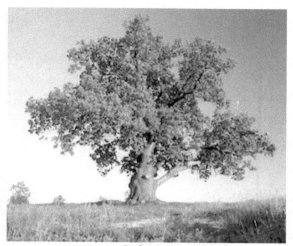

Oak tree
Image 8-75

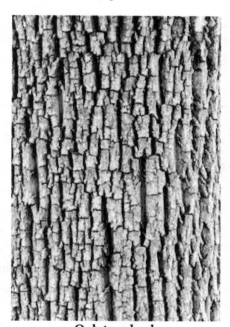

Oak tree bark
Image 8-75a

Description: brown to grayish brown bark; dark green leaves; light to dark brown acorn fruit

Wash/Antiseptic (use externally)

Brew a tea using 3 to 4 teaspoons of oak bark to 1 cup of water and let simmer for 1 hour. Let cool and apply the liquid to the affected area with a cotton ball, or soak a cloth in the mixture and wrap the cloth around the affected area.

Oil Bush Plant

(see "Castor Oil, Castor Tree, Oil Bush Plant" this chapter)

Okra

(constipation, gas, bloating, digestive problems)

Botanical name

Abelmoschus esculentus

Medicinal properties

demulcent, laxative, probiotic

Health benefits

Okra is a culturally important and staple vegetable for African Americans and most everyone who has Southern roots. Many Southerners say they eat okra when they need to be "cleaned out" (i.e., cleans intestinal tract so you have healthy bowel movements).

Okra is a hearty vegetable that is indigenous to Africa and travelled to North America on ships with enslaved Africans. It

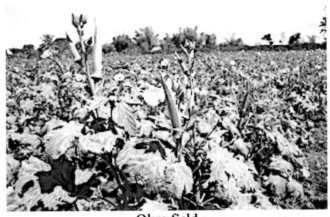

Okra field
Image 8-76

Description: hairy dark green leaves; light green pods (okra); hibiscus-yellowish flowers that flower in full sun

is rich with vitamins A, B6, C, thiamin, folic acid, riboflavin, calcium, and zinc, and is also a mucilaginous dietary fiber. Including okra in your diet may help maintain healthy blood sugar levels, prevents constipation, gas, and bloating, and helps soothe the gastrointestinal tract.

Preparation and application

There are numerous ways to prepare okra and add to your diet. Below are a few of my favorites.

Fried okra

Slice okra. Chop onions and garlic and sauté in olive oil for about 2 mintues. Add the okra and cook on medium heat, stirring frequently until cooked.

Okra and black-eyed peas

Cook black-eyed peas, season. Add whole, small okra during the last 10 to 15 minutes of cooking until they are soft.

Okra gumbo

(See Gumbo recipe in Sassafras entry in this chapter, with the special instructions for adding okra to the mix)

Okra succotash

Ingredients include okra, corn, tomatoes, onions, garlic, peppers, bay leaves, (optional: bacon, sausage, shrimp, celery, green onions). If using meat, first sauté bacon or sausage, add onions and garlic, add peppers (and other optional vegetables), and sauté all on low heat for approximately 5 minutes. Add okra and turn fire up to medium, sautéing for 1 to 2 minutes. Add cut-up tomatoes and continue cooking. Add salt, garlic powder, onion powder, bay leaf, cayenne and other seasoning as desired and continue to stir and cook. Add fresh corn. Cook an additional 2 to 3 minutes. If using shrimp, add fresh shrimp last. Optional: add tomato paste for more texture and flavor.

Pickled okra

Use small okra. Pickle okra the way you would any other vegetable, adding seasonings and vinegar.

Okra water

Add 2 okra pods to an 8 ounce glass of room temperature water. Cover and soak overnight. Drink first thing in the morning.

Onion

(colds, flu, congestion, coughs, cuts, toxicity)

Botanical name

Allium cepa

Medicinal properties

antibacterial, antifungal, antimicrobial, antioxidant, antiparasitic, antiseptic, antiviral, diuretic

Health benefits

Onions have been used as medicine and food for thousands of years in global healing traditions. Onions contain many medicinal agents that are beneficial in treating numerous ailments, making it an excellent immune booster and preventive health treatment.

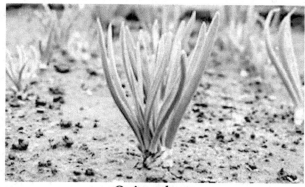

Onion plants
Image 8-77

Description: green grass-like leaves; pink or white flowers; onion bulb in ground

Onion medicine is often used to treat and prevent the common cold, flu, congestion, respiratory problems, cough, asthma, allergies, bacterial infections, cuts, wounds, angina, and body toxicity (heavy metals). Adding onions to your diet regularly may lower cholesterol, lower blood sugar levels, and support heart health. The antioxidant properties of onions may help prevent cancer. Its antibacterial and antifungal properties make it useful medicine in treating cuts, wounds, skin fungus, toothaches, preventing infections, and as an insect repellent. Onion acts as a natural anti-blood clotting agent. Onions are a rich source of quercetin, vitamins C, B6, B1, and K, biotin, chromium, calcium, dietary fiber, and folic acid. They are also a source of sulfur, which promotes healing and supports the liver.

I first became aware of onion medicine when my grandmother prepared an onion poultice on a deep wound I got as a child. It was one summer when my brothers and I stayed with her in Kaaawa, Hawaii in the early 1970's, and I cut my foot climbing up the famous "big rock" at Waimea Bay. That evening, my grandmother, Tutu, told me that if a piece of that volcanic rock or coral was in my foot, it could grow (how daunting). She said that the onion poultice would pull it out and draw out the infection, too. It worked! Today I have a foot without a rock or coral growth.

Preparation and application

Tea/tonic/decoction

Use 1/2 to 1 cup of raw, chopped or sliced onions to 1 cup of warm water. Cover and steep for 10 to 15 minutes and drink. For stronger brew or to make a decoction, increase the ratio of onions to water and after covering and steeping for 10 to 15 minutes, let sit for 30 to 60 minutes, then drink. Optional: add a few slices of fresh, raw ginger while steeping and sweeten with honey.

Onion cough syrup (coughs, congestion)

Slice one onion evenly. Place the base of the onion sliced-side up in a glass jar and pour honey over it. In the same way you would make a sandwhich, place an onion slice on top of the onion base with the honey in between, and pour more honey on top. Continue to layer the onion slices with honey to the top

Onion (continued)

of the jar. Optionally, other healing herbs can be added in the jar as the onions are being layered, such as garlic, mullein, peppermint or slippery elm bark. When finished, tightly close the top on the jar. Let mixture sit for 24 hours in a safe place on the counter or in a cabinet. The honey will pull out and absorb the onion medicine. Take a teaspoon of onion-medicated honey as needed to relieve cough, congestion, and throat irritation. You can leave the onions in the jar or remove after 2 days. Keep refrigerated.

Poultice

Onion poultices draw out infection and relieve inflammation. Chop the onion in small pieces and crush in a mortar and pestel bowl or something comparable. Take the onion paste and apply to the affected area; for example, a cut, wound, boil, on chest to relieve congestion, inflamed joints, behind the ear to treat ear infection. Cover with a flannel or wool cloth, wrap, or adhesive bandage depending on size of affected area.

Alternatively, to treat small cuts and bites, slice a piece of raw onion, crush slightly to release the medicine and then place it on the affected area. Cover with an adhesive bandage. Best to replace with a new piece of onion and cover every 3 hours, but at least twice daily. Clean affected area with cool water before replacing with fresh onion.

Soup or broth

Peel and slice 2 onions. Heat 2 tablespoons olive or coconut oil in a stock pot, then sauté the onions in the heated oil. Add 2 to 3 garlic cloves, making sure to crush the cloves to release the medicine. Sauté for 3 to 5 minutes. Add 2 cups of vegetable, chicken, beef and/or bone broth. Add vegetables and seasonings like salt, pepper, cayenne, or bay leaf. Bring to boil, then simmer for 20 to 30 minutes.

Tonic for colds, flu and infection

Put equal parts of onion, garlic, and ginger root in a mason jar so that these ingredients fill the jar to approximately 1 inch from the top. Add 1 teaspoon of cayenne pepper and 1 to 2 tablespoons of honey. Fill the jar with organic apple cider vinegar (ACV) and place in a cool, shaded place for 2 weeks. Shake vigorously at least twice daily. After 2 weeks, strain the mixture into another glass jar with an air-tight lid. Take 1 to 2 tablespoons a day for colds and as a preventive health tonic. For flu and infections, take 4 to 6 tablespoons daily and drink plenty of water.

Orange Weed

(skin rashes, sores, ringworms, poison oak/poison ivy)

Botanical name

Impatiens capensis

Also known as

jewelweed, orange jewelweed

Medicinal properties

antibacterial, antifungal, antiseptic, carminative

Health benefits

Used in African American healing traditions to treat a variety of skin conditions, body sores, ringworms, and itchy rashes like poison oak and ivy.

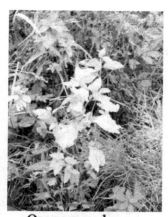

Orange weed
Image 8-78

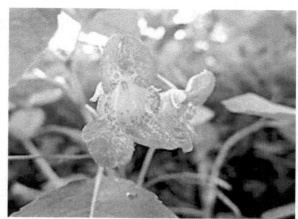

Orange weed flower
Image 8-78a

Description: green leaves; orange to yellowish-orange flowers, summer bloom

Preparation and application

Crush the leaves to release the medicine and rub on affected area several times a day.

Salve

Crush or bruise leaves to release the medicine, then make a salve, poultice, or bath from the leaves to treat the skin condition. Soak in bath, apply salve and apply poultice directly to the affected area.

Wash

Make a wash by crushing or bruising enough leaves to fill a pot. Place them in a pot of cool water, making sure the water covers the leaves about 1 inch over. Bring to a slow boil, remove from heat, and cover. Let cool and strain liquid into a clean glass container. Apply the wash/liquid on affected area several times a day.

Oysters

(aphrodisiac)

Medicinal properties

anti-inflammatory, antioxidant, supports male and female hormone balance, increases libido

Health benefits

Eating oysters has the reputation of being an aphrodisiac. This reputation may have come from the fact that they do contain two amino acids that raise levels of both sex hormones, testosterone and estrogen. Oysters also contain high amounts of zinc, which plays an important role in both male and female reproductive health. Oysters are a good source of protein and are also high in omega-3 fatty acids, potassium, magnesium, and vitamins A, B, C, D, and E.

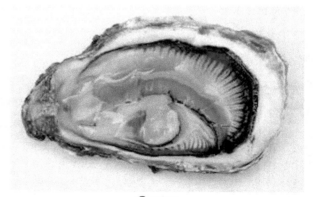

Oyster
Image 8-79

Description: gray-brown shell, light gray oyster meat

Eating oysters may help support good heart health, reduce inflammation, and protect against cell damage. However, oysters are also high in sodium, which is not good for health.

Preparation and application

Eat raw or steamed by themselves, garnish with lemon or hot sauce, or drop in a soup or stew.

Paregoric

(colic, fretfulness in babies, teething, pain, diarrhea, coughs)

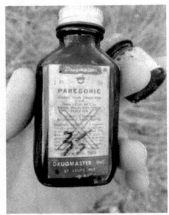

Paregoric bottle
Image 8-80

Also known as

paragat, paragor[162]

Medicinal properties

analgesic, antitussive, antidiarrheal

Health benefits

Paregoric is an elixir that was commonly used in the 18th, 19th and up to the mid 20th centuries to treat a number of ailments including pain, coughs, diarrhea, and colic, teething, and fretfulness in children. Paregoric is a mixture of powdered opium and camphor and may also include anise oil and honey. In the early 20th century, Paregoric became regulated and classified as an "Exempt Narcotic," still available at pharmacies without a prescription until 1970. Today, Paregoric is available in the United States only with a prescription and is often used to wean infants born from women addicted to opiates.

Preparation and application

Dosage was prescribed on bottle or by a physician.

Peach Tree Leaves

(fevers, colds, congestion, sore throat, "high sugar")

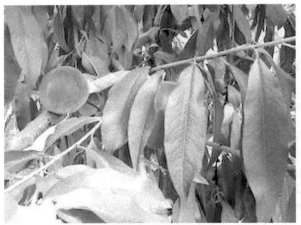

Peach tree leaves
Image 8-81

Description: green leaves; pink blossoms in early spring followed by large peaches

Botanical name

Prunus persica

Also known as

peach leaves

Medicinal properties

diaphoretic, mild diuretic, laxative, sedative

Health benefits

In African American healing traditions, peach tree leaf medicine was used to treat fevers, colds, congestion, sore throats, and—in combination with other medicines—to treat "high sugar." Peach tree leaf medicine may also have been useful in treating diarrhea and dysentery, chronic bronchitis, and stomach problems.

---

[162] These common names are spelled phonetically based on how they were pronounced during the interview with Ms. Chavis from North Carolina.

Preparation and application

Use 2 teaspoons dried leaf to 1 cup boiling water. Infuse for 20 minutes. Use as a gargle for sore throat or for chills, or drink 1/2 cup per hour. Use freely.

Peppergrass or Pergiegrass

(colds, flu, seasonal tonic)

Botanical name

Lepidium sativum

Medicinal properties

abortifacient, antiasthmatic, antibacterial, antitussive, aphrodisiac, bitter, cardiotonic, depurative, diuretic, emmenagogue, galactagogue, ophthalmic, stimulant, tonic, thermogenic

Health benefits

Peppergrass leaves are nutritious and detoxifying. Peppergrass tea was drunk to treat colds, flu, coughs, sinus congestion, asthma, kidney stones, poison ivy, arthritis pain, indigestion, flatulence, and intestinal worms. A poultice of the leaves was applied to the chest to treat croup. The bruised leaves were rubbed on the body to treat poison ivy rash and scurvy and to draw out blisters. A poultice made from seeds relieves joint pain and headaches.

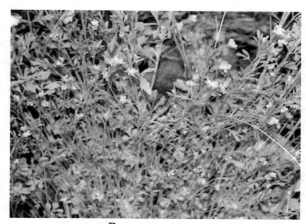

Peppergrass
Image 8-82

Description: bright green leaves with small white flowers June-July

Peppergrass leaf is rich with vitamins A, C, folate (vitamin B9), iron, and calcium, and is high in dietary fiber.

Preparation and application

Tea

Add 1 teaspoon of the dried leaves or 3 to 4 teaspoons of fresh chopped leaves to 1 cup of hot water. Cover and steep for 10 to 15 minutes. Drink 1 to 2 cups daily.

Poultice/Bruised leaves

Take fresh leaves and rub them together to bruise them and release the oils from the leaves. Rub bruised leaves onto affected area or make a poultice.

Pickash or Prickly Ash Bark/Tree

(teeth, cleaning, toothaches, healthy gums; the black gum, dogwood, and pickash or prickly ash trees are all commonly referred to as the toothbrush tree)

Botanical name

Zanthoxylum clava-herculis

Pickash or Prickly Ash Bark/Tree (continued)

Also known as

toothache tree, toothbrush tree

Medicinal properties

alterative, antiseptic, astringent, carminative, circulatory stimulant, diaphoretic, hepatic, sialogogue, general health tonic

Health benefits

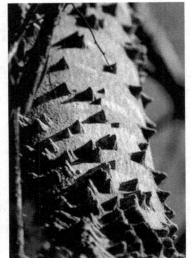

Pickash tree bark
Image 8-83

Prickly ash bark was used to treat a wide variety of problems in both Native American and African American healing traditions. The twig and bark were used for cleaning teeth and treating tooth and gum pain. Prickly ash bark works well at improving circulation for any specific targeted area in the body that is ailing. It worked well to decrease or eliminate toothache pain, tighten gums, and reduce inflammation caused by rheumatism and arthritis. Prickly ash bark may also help treat digestive problems, colic, and stomach cramps. A poultice or salve of prickly ash bark was used directly on the skin to treat open sores. Prickly ash bark medicine also stimulates the entire lymphatic system, and thus encourages elimination of toxins from the body.

Preparation and application

Prune small, live limbs and strip off the bark. Most potent after flowering.

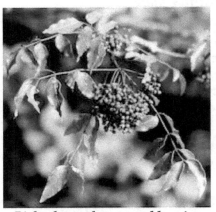

Pickash tree leaves and berries
Image 8-83a

Tea (decoction)

Best method to stimulate circulation, digestion and reduce inflammation.
* Add 2 teaspoons of the dried bark to 1 cup of hot water. Cover and let steep for 20 minutes. Drink 3 cups daily.
* If using fresh bark, use 1 teaspoon per 2 cups of water and bring to boil in a pot. Cover and let steep for 20 minutes, strain and put liquid in a jar. Drink 1 to 3 cups per day. As a digestive aid, drink before eating.

Description: dark green leaves; sharp prickles on stem and leaves; greenish yellow flowers; female flowers produce reddish-brown berries in summer; blooms in spring

For toothache, mouth sores, bleeding gums, or general health maintenance

Chew a small amount of the bark, moistening it with saliva, and then pack the mass around the painful tooth or other affected area to alleviate pain and begin the healing. The antiseptic and stimulant properties help to keep the mouth healthy.

Note: Recurring tooth pain and bleeding gums may be indicative of an underlying problem that may require the attention of a dental professional.

Salve (topical) for pain and inflammation

Method 1

Chop and grind the dried bark into a powder. Mix with a natural fat such as coconut oil, olive oil, or shea butter to make a salve.

Method 2

In a covered pot, simmer fresh cut bark in a natural fat for 30 minutes to extract the medicinal oil. Strain or remove the bark before it solidifies, then cool. Use the oil to rub on areas affected by pain and inflammation.

Tincture

* Use 1 part bark to 5 parts alcohol/water mixture using 80% grain alcohol and 20% purified water.
* Prepare in a mason jar and keep in a cool dark place for 30 to 45 days. Shake once daily for the first week then let sit until tincture is ready to strain.
* To separate the matter from the liquid, strain by pouring mixture into a sieve or into cheesecloth spread over a glass bowl. Store liquid in a blue or brown colored glass jar and close the top tight. Store in a cool, dry place.
* Take 10 to 20 drops before meals as a digestive aid.

To brush teeth and gums

Use the twigs or bark to scrub teeth and stimulate gums and as a floss.

To make a toothpowder

Chop and dry small pieces of the bark. Grind in a coffee grinder or food processor or use a pestle and mortar bowl to grind into a powder. Dip wet toothbrush in powder and proceed to brush teeth.

Pine Tree, Cone, Tar/Resin, Needles, Bark

(colds, congestion, coughs, virus, immune booster)

Botanical name

Pinus aphremphous

Also known as

abies, acer, Eastern pine, pitch pine, scotch pine, shortleaf pine, Virginia pine, white pine

Medicinal properties

antibacterial, anti-inflammatory, anti-tumor, antiviral, immune booster

Health benefits

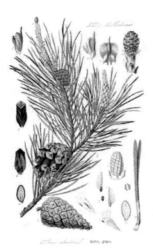

Pine is a potent medicine that was used alone or as an ingredient in other medicinal recipes. All parts of the tree were used in both Native American and African American healing traditions: pine tops or needles, pine tar, sap and resin, the seed cones, pine bark, twigs, and wood. Pine medicine was often used to treat a variety of ailments, including colds, chest and sinus congestion, coughs, respiratory ailments (using an external liniment plaster), hypertension, arthritis, rheumatism, bladder and kidney problems, eye health, skin conditions/rashes, fungal infections, abscesses, intestinal worms. It also promotes healthy brain functions. Pine tar and pine sap salve were applied externally to pull out splinters and glass, bring boils to a head, heal wounds, and more.

Note: In African American healing traditions, the term "pine tar" may have been used interchangeably with "pine sap." Pine tar is different from pine sap. Pine sap or resin naturally oozes from the tree. Pine tar is a sticky substance rendered from wood by burning it under pressure and with very little air.

Pine tree illustration
Image 8-84

Description: green needles; brown cones; reddish-brown bark

Pine Tree, Cone, Tar/Resin, Needles, Bark (continued)

Preparation and application

All parts of the pine tree were used as medicine. The needles, sap/pitch/resin, cone, wood, twigs, bark, and pine tar were all used individually to be made into a tea, cough syrup, extract, salve, or wash. Pine tar and sap (resin/rosin) were also used topically in the form of a linament plaster or salve. An extract is made from the pine cone or it is made into a tea or decoction, and often used with other herbs.

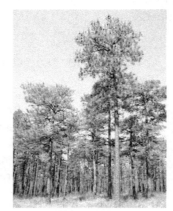

Pine trees
Image 8-84a

Pine cone tea

Pick 2 to 3 green pine cones that have resin in them (do not use the brown cones because they are dry and contain no resin). Put pine cones in 1 pint of boiling water and simmer for 10 minutes then let cool. Add lemon for added benefit and medicine. Strain, and add honey to taste.

Pine needle tea

Pick 1 cup of fresh pine needles, rinse with cold water, and chop. Add pine needles to 3 cups of boiling water, cover and low simmer for 20 minutes. Squeeze the juice from 1 lemon into the mixture and then add the remains of the squeezed lemon to the pot. Slow simmer another 20 minutes. Strain liquid into a glass mason jar. Drink 3 cups daily, adding honey to taste.

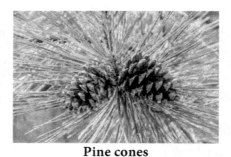

Pine cones
Image 8-84b

Description: green needles; brown cones; reddish-brown bark

To expel intestinal parasites, gather enough fresh pine needles to fill a pot or saucepan. Clean and rinse, then cover with clean, cool water, bring to a boil, cover the pot or saucepan and simmer for 20 to 30 minutes. Let cool and then strain into a glass jar. Drink 1 to 3 cups daily until better. Refrigerate between uses.

Pine twig tea or decoction

Make a strong tea or decoction from pine twigs to treat colds, congestion, achy joints, or rheumatism. Gather enough twigs to fill a small pot or saucepan. Rinse and cover with water. Cover the pot and bring to a slow boil. Let cool and strain. Drink 1 to 2 cups daily.

Pine sap/pitch tea or decoction

Heat the pine sap in a pot and add 1 cup of water per 1 to 2 tablespoons of pine sap. Cook slowly until all ingredients are blended. Can add other herbs, lemon and honey. Drink 1 cup 1 to 3 times daily.

Pine bark

Use the interior layer of the bark that contains resin and antioxidants in a tea or decoction with other herbs to treat cold, flu, coughs, and congestion and as an immune booster.

Pine cone

Pine cone medicine has been used as early as 500 AD. Pine cone medicine boosts the immune system and is said to have antiviral, anti-tumor, and antibacterial properties.

Pine needles

Pine needles contain medicine that helps loosen congestion, treat colds, ease rheumatism, and expel intestinal parasites. They are also a good source of vitamin C, which is essential for the immune system. A medicinal tea is usually made from the pine needles.

Pine sap/Resin/Pitch

Pine sap is a resin that has strong antibacterial properties. Pine sap medicine may effectively treat coughs, kill bacterial infections, improve breathing, and treat bronchitis. Pitch (pine sap resin) can be made into a poultice to "draw out" boils, splinters, and abscesses, and is used to treat rheumatism, broken bones, cuts, bruises, and inflammation.

A honey can be made from pine sap to treat colds, flu, cough, sore throat, congestion, and infection.[163]

Pine tar

A thick brown liquid derived from applying heat and pressure on pine wood in a closed container. Traditionally it has been used as an antiseptic to treat skin conditions such as eczema, psoriasis, dandruff, ringworm and other skin fungi, rashes from poison oak and ivy, bug bites, and to treat wounds on animals.

Pine wood

Add small pieces of pine wood (preferably containing resin) as an additional ingredient to your medicinal concoction of steeping tea or pot of medicinal herbs to treat colds and congestion.

Pine cone extract

The Japanese use pine cone extract to treat anything from the common cold to cancer, and they claim that drinking pine cone tea promotes longevity of life. Pine cone extract is purported to have immune boosting, antiviral, and anti-tumor properties.

Pine needle tonic (high in vitamin C)

To preserve all the vitamins found in fresh pine needles, fill a wide-mouthed jar with pine needles and pour room-temperature apple cider or white vinegar over them until they are completely covered. (Optional: Add 1 to 2 teaspoons of cane or brown sugar along with the vinegar.) Cover with an air-tight lid and soak for 6 weeks in a cool dark shelf or cabinet. Shake once a day for the first week. When ready, strain into a clean glass jar and use to make a tea or in salads.

Pine sap or resin cough and cold drops

To treat colds, flu, cough, sore throat, congestion, and infection: Simply slowly heat the sap in a pan and slowly add natural cane sugar and mix until the two blend together. If using honey instead of cane sugar, mix in after the pine sap has cooked and softened because of the heat. Optional: add lemon, mint, or other herbs to the mixture. Take a spoon and pour 1/4 teaspoon dollops of the liquid onto waxed paper and let cool. When dollops cool, they will look like cough drops. Take as needed.

Pine sap tincture

Collect pine sap from wounds in the trees, or scrape it off pine cones. Put sap in a mason jar, barely covering the sap with 80 proof or more grain alcohol. Close lid tightly. Place in a cool, dark place (can put jar in a brown paper bag, for example). Let sit for 6 to 8 weeks, shaking jar vigorously once daily. Use 5 to 10 drops 1 to 3 times daily when ready.

Salve/plaster liniment

Gather 2 cups of pine sap. Break up the hard chunks into small pieces so they can break down easier in the salve. Put pine sap in a pint-sized mason jar and fill the jar with olive oil or coconut oil. Put top on the jar and put jar in a pot of boiling water. Make sure boiling water does not come up more than the halfway point of the jar. Turn heat to a simmer and keep jar in pot until the pine sap chunks have dissolved. Strain the oil through a mesh to get out any bark or other particles. Add beeswax or shea butter for thickening. Store pine salve/oil in a glass jar and use on affected area for rheumatism, cuts, wounds, insect bites, boils, abscesses, infection, fungus and other conditions.

---

[163] See the "Preparation and application" section below for how to prepare pine sap honey.

Poke Sallat, Poke Berries, Poke Leaves, Poke Roots

(skin conditions, eczema, cancer, rheumatism, inflammation, wounds)

Poke may have gotten its name from an Algonquian word "pokan," which means any plant used to produce a red or yellow dye.

Botanical name

Phytolacca americana

Also known as

American nightshade, cancer jalap, cancer root, chui xu shang lu (Chinese medicine), coakum, garget, inkberry, pigeon berry, pocan bush, poke salad, pokeweed, red ink plant, redweed, scoke

Medicinal properties

alterative, antibiotic, anti-inflammatory, anti-cancer/anti-HIV, anticatarrhal, antifungal, antiparasitic, antirheumatic, antiviral, immuno-stimulant, mitogenic

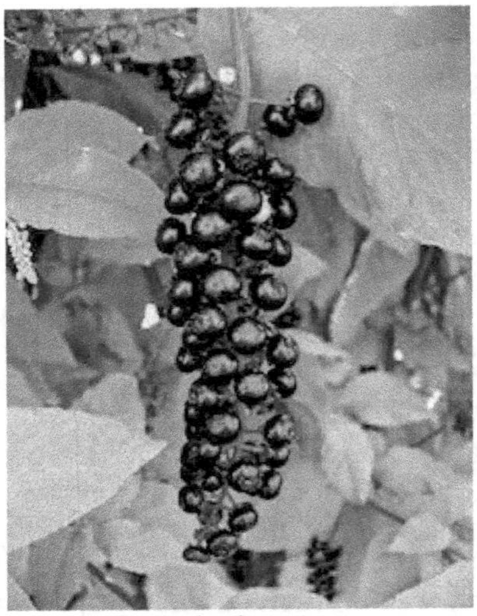

Health benefits

Poke berries
Image 8-85

Description: dark green leaves; magenta stem; white blooms from summer to fall; dark purple berries/fruit

Poke is a powerful plant! Poke medicine has been used for centuries in many healing traditions including Chinese, Ayurvedic, Native American, African American, and early American folk medicine, particularly in Appalachia.

I call poke the Jedi of the plant world (from the *Star Wars* movies). Why? Because it has a wide range of beneficial applications from use as food, medicine, ink, dye, paint, and most recently as a solar absorbent. And like the Jedi, poke has both a light side and a dark side. As a medicine, it is a potent and concentrated substance that, like the light side of "the Force," can effect a powerful healing. However, like the dark side of "the Force," if used incorrectly, poke can harm, even kill.

Traditional healers who worked with poke knew that using any part of the poke plant for medicine should be done with caution. Today, any attempt to use poke medicine should be done under the advice of a health care professional.

All parts of the poke plant—root, berry and leaves—were used as medicine that was made into teas, tinctures, poultices, or wine or taken directly, as is the case with the berries. Poke medicine was used to boost immunity as well as to treat a wide variety of ailments including skin conditions (eczema, psoriasis, impetigo, ringworm, and rashes), lymphatic congestion, internal infections, throat and mouth infections, fever, severe colds, rheumatism and arthritis, boils, cysts, mastitis, breast cancer, and other internal growths/tumors.

The leaves of the poke plant were commonly used as a food staple in the Southern United States. This dish was generally referred to as "poke sallat" or sometimes called "poor man's greens." However, there is a danger to such use. Poke leaves or sallat contain phytolaccatoxin and phytolaccigenin, both of which are poisonous to mammals. To make poke sallat greens safe and edible, the leaves were blanched twice in water, each time throwing the water off and thereby reducing the toxins within. Only after cooking a third time and seasoning like traditional Southern greens was the poke sallat dish ready to eat.

As an alternative, some people purposely used the toxins in the poke leaves to "clean themselves out" (that is, purge their intestinal system of toxins). They would only cook the poke sallat leaves once, so that some of the toxins remain in a reduced and tolerable amount. Eating the leftover toxins in the once-cooked leaves would give you stomach cramps, diarrhea, or possibly vomiting. The diarrhea and vomiting are part of the desired purging process.

Poke berries are by far the most versatile part of the poke plant. Pokeberry has been used as an effective medicine to treat rheumatism, arthritis, and skin conditions as well as other ailments. Again, there is some danger in improper use. The seed inside the berry is toxic. Fortunately, the seeds are very hard and difficult to crack, even with your teeth. Your body does not digest the seed, rather it comes out in your poop. People who use pokeberry medicine usually swallow the berry whole or remove the seed before ingesting. The other danger is with improper dosage. Taking too much poke medicine is poisonous and may give you diarrhea, vomiting, headache, or diziness. A general rule is to start with 1 dose or 1 berry a day and work up to no more than 3 doses or 3 berries while carefully monitoring to see that there are no side effects.

Pokeberries have other uses besides the medicinal. The deep sanguine color of the berry juice has been used as a dye, an ink, or made into a paint. Many American Civil War soldiers wrote their letters in pokeberry ink, and practicing wiccans often use pokeberry ink to write their spells. Native Americans also painted their horses with the pokeberry dye and rubbed their skin with the berry juice to repel mosquitoes in addition to using poke for its other medicinal benefits. It was Benjamin Lay, the outspoken abolitionist Quaker, who came up with one of the most creative uses for the pokeberry. He burst into a 1738 meeting of Philadelphia's Quaker leaders and slave owners and plunged a sword into a hollowed out Bible filled with blood-red pokeberry juice, which he then sprayed in the shocked faces of the slave-owners. From here on, pokeberry juice became a symbol of blood for the anti-slavery movement.

The root is the most potent part of the poke plant. It is where the medicines are most concentrated and should be used with great care. Poke root is also known as "cancer root" because the tincture and poultices have been used to treat cancer as well as many other ailments specifically listed below.

Today poke's healing capabilities are being used to help curb and "heal" our voracious appetite for fossil fuels. A coat of pokeberry dye is applied to fiber-based solar panels because it helps the panels absorb twice as much solar energy. That poke is some strong medicine!

Poke medicine and food are derived from three different portions of the poke plant: the leaves, the berries, and the root. Specific ailments that poke berry, root or leaf medicine were used to treat are listed below along with preparation and application methods.

Preparation and application

Poke medicine was used with caution. It was taken internally starting with very small doses and working up slowly to determine the body's tolerable dosage. One would wait 24 hours in between dosages to determine if there were any adverse side effects such as diarrhea, vomiting, or dizziness. If no side effects occurred, the dosage was increased by 1 increment, usually to a maximum of 3. If side effects were felt, the dosage was reduced to the previous, or ended entirely if side effects occurred after the smallest dosage.

Berries

Pokeberry juice, salves, and oils

Pokeberry juice, salves, and oils were used for topical skin conditions: eczema, psoriasis, acne, impetigo, infection, bites, rashes, ring-worm/fungus, boils, scabies, cuts, and other wounds. It was also used to treat and dissolve lumps, boils, breast abcesses bumps, growths, tumors, cysts, fungal infections, bedsores, breast cancer, chicken pox, melanoma, mastitis, measles, psoriasis, ringworm, shingles, and to reduce swollen lymph glands.

Pokeberry juice can be rubbed directly from the berry itself onto the affected area to relieve these conditions.

Alternatively, a salve or oil can be prepared to treat the above conditions.

Salves are a creamy, thick solution often made with a combination of melted beeswax, shea butter, and/or cocoa butter. A natural lighter oil (called the carrier oil) like olive or coconut isoften added to make the salve more malleable. Medicinal herbs or herb-infused oils are added to the salve mixture while it is melting and slow cooked for 2 to 4 hours in a crockpot. This infusion can also be achieved

Poke Sallat, Poke Berries, Poke Leaves, Poke Roots (continued)

by placing the herbs in a jar, covering with the carrier oil and then placing the jar in a sunny area for 2 or more weeks.

The process of slow cooking pulls the medicine out and concentrates it in the salve or oil solution.

The difference between salves and oils is not in their application, but in their consistency. Salves are thicker, oils are thinner, and the difference between the two is achieved by what one uses to "cut" the medicine: shea butter, beeswax, or cocoa butter are thicker and olive oil or coconic oil is thinner. The thinner oils are called carrier oils.

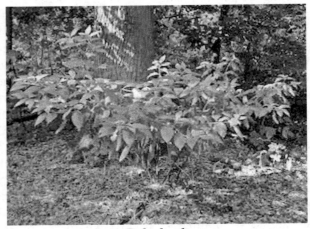

Poke bush

Image 8-85a

Description: dark green leaves; magenta stem

To prepare a pokeberry salve:

* In a bowl crush and strain the berries so there are no seeds left
* Melt shea butter, beeswax, or cocoa butter in a pot into a cream mixture
* Mix in an equal amount of the cream mixture into pokeberry juice; the pokeberry juice will further cream the mixture
* Pack in a jar; keep in refrigerator to prevent from spoiling
* Let sit for 24 hours, then use

To make the thinner pokeberry oil mixture, or something in-between, substitute the olive or coconut oil instead of shea butter, beeswax, or cocoa butter, and vary the amount of oil to the amount of pokeberry juice in order to achieve the desired consistency.

Once prepared, both salves and oils can be applied and rubbed onto the skin to treat affected areas.

Pokeberries swallowed whole

For treatment of skin conditions, cysts, swollen glands, abscesses, boils, arthritis, rheumatism, and joint pain, some people swallowed the berries whole, raw, or dried instead of making a tincture. They were careful not to chew the seeds, which are poisonous. The seeds are very hard, and if swallowed whole, they pass through the system intact and harmless.

To dry the berries, pick a bunch, rinse with cool water, spread out on a paper towel or brown paper bag, and leave them to air dry in an area that is sunny and warm/hot but is not humid. Humidity will cause the berries to mold. If you are drying outside, bring the berries inside during the night. Alternatively, you can spread the berries on a cookie sheet and dry in low oven heat, approximately 130 degrees for approximately 1 to 2 hours. Leave the oven door cracked when drying. When the berries have shriveled, remove them from the oven and allow them to cool. Whether air drying or oven drying, once the berries are dried, store in a glass jar, close the lid and keep in the refrigerator until used.

Swallow raw or dried berries whole, not biting into seed. Start with 1 per day working your way up to your tolerance level, but usually no more than 3 if taken regularly[164]. Wait 24 hours after each increase in dosage in order to notice any changes.

For arthritis, rheumatism and joint pain, some people take 1 to 3 berries a day for 7 days straight, depending on their tolerance level, then wait 1 to 2 weeks and start the treatment again.

Pokeberry tincture

Used for the treatment of skin conditions such as eczema, psoriasis, impetigo and fungal infections like ringworm. Also used to treat arthritis, rheumatism, fibromyalgia, inflammation, joint pain, and general body aches, colds, respiratory and throat infections, infected and swollen gums, ulcers, swollen lymph glands, breast cysts, and autoimmune diseases. Pokeberry medicine also acts as an immune

---

[164] One healer mentioned giving 9 pokeberries at one time once per year to treat impetigo.

builder and energy stimulant.

Combine equal amounts of fresh pokeberry juice (strained, without seeds) to 80+ proof alcohol in a mason jar. Make sure all the seeds have been taken out of the crushed berries. Cover in a bag and place in a cool, dry cupboard for 6 to 8 weeks. Make sure you shake vigorously at least 1 time daily.

Take 2 or more drops a day (depending on tolerance level). It was common for users to take the medicine up to 7 consecutive days and then take up to 7 days off, depending on how their body and the symptoms responded.

Pokeberry wine

For arthritis, rheumatism, fibromyalgia, inflammation, joint pain, and general body aches.

Recipe #1
* Gather 1 gallon of fresh, ripe berries
* Crush and strain over cheesecloth into a glass container, taking out all the seeds
* Add equal amount of red wine
* Add 1/2 cup or more of cane sugar or other natural sweetner to taste
* Stir well
* Cover and let sit in a cool, dark shelf for 6 to 8 weeks, shaking vigorously once daily
* Strain and bottle

Dosage: 1 to 3 tablespoons or a shot glass of fresh pokeberry wine for 3 to 7 days, depending on tolerance level. Then take 3 days off and begin again. Note: adding sweetner is optional.

Recipe #2
* Gather fresh, ripe berries only
* Crush and strain over cheesecloth, making sure all the seeds are out. Add equal amount of water, boil and strain
* Let cool and place in a glass fermentation jar
* To each quart of juice, add 1 to 2 cups or more of cane sugar to taste
* Cover and let ripen in a cool dark place for 6 months
* Strain and bottle

Dosage: 1 to 3 tablespoons or a shot glass of fresh pokeberry wine for 3 to 7 days, depending on tolerance level. Then take 3 days off and begin again.

Roots

Poke root poultice

Grated poke root was used as a poultice to treat inflammations and rashes.

Poke root salve or oil

Used to treat wounds, skin conditions (psoriasis, eczema, impetigo), acne, scabies, fungal infections, bedsores, chicken pox, measles, ringworm, shingles, boils, breast abscesses, mastitis, and cysts, and to reduce and dissolve growths, lumps, bumps, tumors, melanoma, breast cancer, clear lymphatic congestion, and treat swollen lymph glands.
* Grate and crush poke root so it is fine
* Melt beeswax, shea butter, coconut and/or olive oil in a pot so it is thick and creamy
* Mix equal amounts of grated poke root with the hot salve mixture and place in a jar

Use after 3 days, allowing time for the medicine to soak into the cream.

Poke root tincture

Poke root tincture was used for the treatment of arthritis, rheumatism, fibromyalgia, inflammation, joint pain, and general body aches. The tincture also treated sore throats, strep throat, tonsillitis, severe colds, respiratory infections, infected and swollen gums, ulcers, swollen lymph glands, lymphatic congestion, breast cysts, boils and other growths, skin conditions, and autoimmune diseases. It acted as an energy stimulant and immune builder.

Poke Sallat, Poke Berries, Poke Leaves, Poke Roots (continued)

Recipe # 1

Dig up the root in the fall, after the plant has died back in preparation for the winter. This is when the plant is the most medicinal and the least toxic. The next best time to dig the roots is in the early spring, when the leaves are just coming out.

* Wash the root, chop it into small pieces, fill a jar with the plant material, and then add enough 80+ proof alcohol to cover the roots.
* Secure the cover on the jar and place the jar in a paper bag. Store in a cool, dry cupboard and keep it there for 6 weeks. The paper bag and cupboard storage provide extra darkness, security, and isolation. Shake once daily for the first week, then once a week until tincture is ready to strain. Strain out the roots using cheesecloth.
* Take 1 drop then wait 24 hours. If no side effects, take another drop. Continue taking drops if you experience no side effects until you reach a 9-drop maximum. Take for as little as 3 days on, then 3 days off, or for 7 days on and up to 7 days off.

Recipe #2

Cut enough poke root slices so they are approximately 2 inches thick when stacked. Chop the slices in half and put in a quart of whiskey. Let stand for 7 days. Take 1 tablespoon 3 times daily for 7 days.

Wait 1 to 2 weeks and repeat.

Leaves

Poke sallat

Poke sallat was not intentionally eaten for any health reasons; usually it was eaten because poke was the only type of greens available. If not prepared correctly, eating the greens had the danger of purging the stomach because not all of the toxins were washed off during the preparation process. Some people mentioned that they ate poke greens to clean out their insides, however, this result was most often an unintentional side effect of carelessness.

To make poke sallat, pick a healthy bunch of the young tender leaves, wash. Place in a pot filled with water and boil for 2 minutes. Drain and rinse off with cold water. Put leaves back in a pot with water and bring to boil again. Drain and rinse with cold water. Cook again for the third time, as if you were cooking a pot of Southern-style greens, and season with garlic, onion, meat (optional), salt, peppers, and vinegar.

Note: People did not eat the leaves raw. They contain the toxins phytolaccatoxin and phytolaccigenin, which are poisonous to mammals and can give you stomach cramps and diarrhea. Each time you boil the leaves in water and throw the water away reduces the toxins.

Potato

(burns, arthritis, rheumatism, inflammation)

Botanical name

Solanum tuberosum

Also known as

ash (Irish) potato, spuds, taters

Medicinal properties

anti-inflammatory, antiscorbutic, detoxifying

Health benefits

Sliced or grated raw potato (with the skin left on) was sometimes used as a poultice to treat burns and to ease joint pain from arthritis and rheumatism. Potatoes are an anti-inflammatory food and are highly alkaline. Eaten baked, boiled, or raw, potatoes may help reduce an acidic body which contributes to arthritis, rheumatism, gout, and other chronic diseases. Potatoes are rich with vitamins A and C, potassium, calcium, and phosphorous. Many of the medicinal benefits of potatoes are in the skin.

Preparation and application

Burns

Apply sliced or grated raw potato directly on a burn. Leave the skin on the potato. Wrap with a guaze or cloth. Apply a fresh pack 2 to 3 times per day.

General health

Add potatoes to your diet, leaving the skin on. Do not cook longer than 20 minutes. Drink the broth from boiled potatoes. Today, many people juice raw potatoes and take 2 to 4 tablespoons daily.

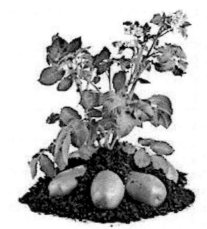

Potato plant
Image 8-86

Description: dark green leaves; white, pink or lavender flowering tops; pink to cream tubers

Rheumatism, arthritis, joint pain, de-acidification, and detoxification

Slice or grate a potato together with the skin and soak in a glass of distilled water overnight. Drink in the morning before meal.

Pot Licker (or Pot Liquor) from Cooked Greens

(nutrient rich immune booster)

Pot licker is the broth that's left after cooking a big pot of greens, which could be any variation of collard, mustard and/or turnips. African Americans have been drinking nutrient-dense pot licker for centuries. In fact, it is one of the reasons why African Americans endured and persevered through colonization and slavery.

The collard plant itself is very resilient and hardy; consequently, the greens can be tough. During slavery, African Americans cooked the greens down and season with fat back or ham hock. Most of the nutrition in the greens was cooked out and was then contained in the broth, the "liquor." The pot licker left from a pot of cooked collards contains the following nutrients: vitamins A, C, D, E, K, B-6, folate, niacin, riboflavin, and thiamin. It also contains the following minerals: potassium, magnesium, iron, calcium, phosphorus, sodium, and zinc.

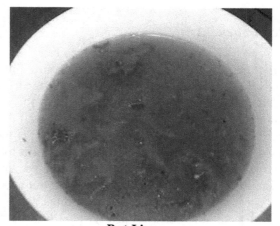

Pot Liquor
Image 8-87

Description: greenish-brown broth with residue of chopped collards and seasonings

Raw collard greens contain the most nutrients because heat is not being used to cook them. Below is a recipe for Kwahuumba's delicious raw collard green salad.

Pot Licker (or Pot Liquor) from Cooked Greens (continued)

Ingredients:

Collard greens – 1 bunch

Dino kale – 1 bunch

Swiss Chard – 1 bunch

(Optional: use any combination of greens listed above and add shredded carrots)

Olive oil

Seasoning: cayenne, sea salt, apple cider vinegar (ACV), chopped garlic, scallions/green onions, lemon or lime juice, sesame seeds.

Roll the greens up and slice them thin, put them in a big bowl or pot. Saturate the greens with olive oil, massaging the oil into the greens to soften them, for about 2 to 3 minutes. Add the seasonings, stir and massage together so all the ingredients are mixed well. Let sit together for at least 30 to 60 minutes before serving.

Prickly Pear

(scalp, hair and skin health, burns, cuts and insect bites)

Botanical name

Opuntia ficus-indica

Also known as

barbary fig, cactus fruit, cactus pear, nopal, nopales, indian fig, opuntia, paddle cactus, tuna (referring to the fruit)

Medicinal properties

anti-inflammatory, antioxidant, antiviral, astringent, antidiarrheal, digestive, emollient, immunostimulant, mucilagenous

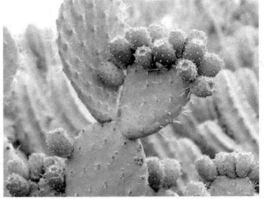

Prickly pear cactus fruit
Image 8-87a

Description: flat fleshy pads, pale green in color, with white cactus spines and red, purplish or yellow fruit

Health benefits

Prickly pear is a cactus that produces succulent fruits and pads (leaves) that are both edible and medicinal. Originating in Mexico and native to the western hemisphere, it has been used as food and for healing for centuries in many cultures around the world. Prickly pear is rich with vitamins, minerals, and other nutrients, such Vitamins C and B, magnesium, calcium, potassium, copper, iron, amino acids, saponins, and dietary fiber. It also includes antioxidants such as flavonoids, polyphenols, and betalains.

In African American healing tradition, prickly pear was primarily used as a topical medicine. The inside gel of the cactus pad was scooped out and used to maintain healthy scalp, hair, and skin. It was also applied to burns, cuts and insect bites.

Other medicinal uses of prickly pear include:

- a poultice made from the pulp inside the pad is applied to affected area to reduce inflammation and pain
- eating regularly may reduce internal inflammation, reduce cholesterol levels, lower blood pressure, regulate insulin levels, boost immunity and treat and prevent colds; the high fiber content helps treat constipation and gastrointestinal problems.

Prickly pear is a very common traditional food of Mexico and the southwest United States. The fruit can be eaten with or without the seeds, and can also be juiced. Jams and jellies can be made with the fruit. The pads (nopales) are eaten raw, dried, or cooked, and have a taste similar to okra. Cooking prickly pear is similar to cooking squash, so it does not need to cook long. Before eating or preparing in foods, it's important to peel off the skin and remove all the spines.

Preparation and application

Hair

Make a cream for your scalp and hair. Skin a prickly pear pad, making sure all the spines are removed. Chop into small pieces and place in a cast iron skillet along with Vaseline or a natural vegetable oil like coconut or olive. Slow cook until mixture turns green. Strain mixture through 2 to 3 layers of cheesecloth into a glass jar. Place in refrigerator to congeal and then use as needed on scalp (for dry scalp or dandruff) or on hair (to moisturize and strengthen).

Poultice/topical

Remove the meat from the pad, mash slightly, and place in cheesecloth. Apply to affected area to help reduce inflammation, pain, or to treat cuts, burns, or insect bites. Alternatively, gel can be applied directly to affected area without the use of cheesecloth.

Skin

To moisturize and soothe skin, apply gel from the pad directly to skin or mix into a natural vegetable oil like coconut or olive and then use.

Food

Pads: wear gloves when handling the pads. Peel the skin back with a knife and remove all the spines. Especially check for the small hard spines. Slice or dice the prickly pear and add to omelets, stews, casseroles or with other vegetables. Similar to squash, it does not need to cook long. Grill the entire pad in a slightly oiled pan with seasoning until soft and brownish in color.

Fruit: wear gloves and use a knife to harvest the tunas or fruit darker in color. Rinse and peel back the skin by making lengthwise cuts (similar to peeling mangoes), making sure all the spines are removed. Eat and enjoy with or without the seeds.

Pudge Grass/American Pennyroyal

(colds, cough, fever, skin conditions/rashes, eye problems)

Botanical name

Hedeoma pulegioides

Also known as

fleabane, mosquito plant, pennyroyal, pudding grass, pennyroyal, squaw mint, stinking balm, tickweed

Medicinal properties

abortifacient, antibacterial, antifungal, antioxidant, antiseptic, antiviral, aromatic, blood cleanser, digestive, emmenagogue, fever reducer

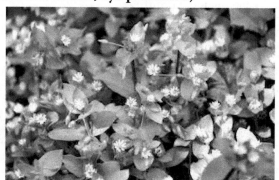

Pudge grass
Image 8-88

Description: medium-green leaves; white flowers with yellow stamens

Health benefits

I was unable to find a written reference for pudge grass (phonetically pronounced) in African American healing traditions. However, the name is very similar to pudding grass which is pennyroyal and grows widespread in North America. This herb was often used in some Native American healing traditions to alleviate similar ailments that pudge grass treats.

Pudge grass/pennyroyal tea was drunk as a digestive aid to relieve gas and bloating and to treat headaches, colds, coughs, congestion and fevers. It was used by women to bring on suppressed menstruation and abortion. The leaves were bruised to release the oil and rubbed on skin to alleviate rashes, insect bites, repel fleas and insects, treat acne and other skin problems. American pennyroyal oil is very toxic and should be ingested with caution and under the advice of a healthcare professional.

Pudge Grass/American Pennyroyal (continued)

Preparation and application

Tea

Use 1 to 2 teaspoons of dried pudgegrass/pennyroyal, or 3 to 4 teaspoons of fresh, to 1 cup of water, cover and steep for 10 to 15 minutes. Drink one cup daily for three days.

Poultice or topical medicine

Gather fresh pudge grass/pennyroyal and bruise or crush the leaves to release the oil and rub on affected skin area.

Wash

Gather fresh pudge grass/pennyroyal, place in a pot, and cover with water. Bring to boil, remove from heat, and cover. Once cooled, the medicated water can be applied to treat skin conditions. Store remaining liquid in a glass jar and refrigerate.

Pumpkin Seeds

(expels intestinal worms)

Botanical name

Curcubita maxima

Medicinal properties

anthelmintic, anti-inflammatory, emollient, diuretic, taeniacide, vermifuge

Health benefits

In African American healing traditions, a mixture of pumpkin seeds, Jerusalem weed, and molasses was used to expel intestinal worms and parasites. Pumpkin seeds are packed with protein and essential minerals, including magnesium, zinc, potassium, iron, mangagnese, phosphorous, amino acids, and vitamins A and C. Eating pumpkin seeds may also support a healthy prostate, liver and heart, prevent kidney stones, reduce post-menopausal symptoms, help prevent bed-wetting and ease arthritis.

Preparation and application

To expel intestinal worms, crush 2 tablespoons of pumpkin seeds and 1 tablespoon Jerusalem weed and mix with molasses so that it has the consistency of porridge. Eat first thing in the morning on an empty stomach. Drink plenty of water. Repeat if necessary.

Add pumpkin seeds to foods such as salads, cereal, deserts, muffins, and as a snack.

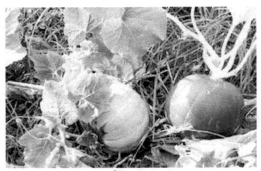

Pumpkins on vine
Image 8-89

Description: green leaves; green then orange fruit (pumpkin); yellow flowers

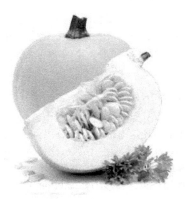

Pumpkin seeds
Image 8-89a

Description: pale orange-yellow seeds

Queen's Delight

(digestive disorders, blood cleanser, fertility)

Botanical name

Stillingia sylvatica

Also known as

cockup hat, marcory, queen's root, racine royale, raíz de la reina, silver leaf, yaw root

Medicinal properties

alterative, diaphoretic, diuretic, expectorant, sialagogue

Health benefits

Queen's Delight is used for its medicinal and hoodoo properties in Black folk medicine. As a "blood cleanser," it promotes sweating and the removal of toxins from the body through the skin. In spiritual hoodoo medicine, drinking the tea is said to help a person embody positive energy and to help women conceive.

Preparation and application

Tea, hot or cold infusion

Put 1 teaspoon of the dried root in a cup of boiled hot water, cover and steep 10 to 15 mintues for the tea and 30 minutes for the infusion. For cold infusion, cover and steep in cold water overnight and drink.

Tincture

Add 1 dropper full to a cup of warm water and drink.

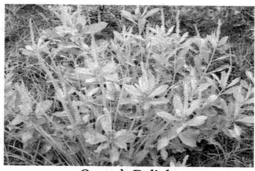

Queen's Delight
Image 8-90

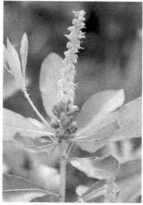

Queen's Delight fruit
Image 8-90a

Description: green leaves; yellow petal-less spike flowers; small capsule fruit, green to brown in color

Quinine Tree

(fever reducer, malaria treatment)

Botanical name

Cinchona rubra

Also known as

fever tree

Medicinal properties

analgesic, anesthetic, antiarrhythmic, antibacterial, antimalarial, antimicrobial, antiparasitic, antiprotozoal, antipyretic, antiseptic, antispasmodic, antiviral, appetite stimulant, astringent, bactericide, bitter, cytotoxic, febrifuge, fungicide, insecticide, nervine, stomachic, tonic for general health

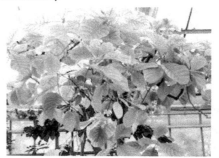

Quinine bush
Image 8-91

Description: brownish-gray bark; green leaves; white, pink or red flowers; green to yellow fruit containing seeds

<u>**Quinine Tree (continued)**</u>

Health benefits

There were two types of quinine medicine that were frequently used in African American, Native American, and early American folk healing traditions. One is the quinine from the cinchona tree indigenous to South America, and the other is "wild quinine," *Parthenium integrifolium*, native to eastern North America and common throughout Virginia and the Carolinas.

The name quinine comes from the indigenous word "quina," which means bark. Quinine medicine from the bark of the cinchona tree was often used to treat malaria, fever, colds, flu, pneumonia, diarrhea, dysentery, wound inflammation and pain. The cinchona trees were called "fever trees" because the bark is an effective fever reducer as well as a preventative against and cure for malaria.

Quinine medicine from the cinchona tree could not be produced in the United States, so it was imported first in the form of the bark to be made into medicine. Later, a derivative of the bark was made into a powder and pill, which was easier to import. Quinine was an effective and popular treatment during the Civil War to prevent malaria. Quinine was also used as a tonic to treat digestive disorders.

Preparation and application

Infusion

An infusion was made from cinchona bark by putting 1 teaspoon of the powdered bark in 1 cup of boiled water, covering and steeping for 30 minutes. This treatment was taken 3 times a day.

Pills were taken as prescribed on bottle or by doctor.

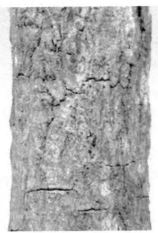

Quinine tree bark
Image 8-91a

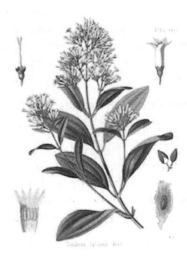

Quinine flower illustration
Image 8-91b

Description: brownish-gray bark; green leaves; white, pink or red flowers; green to yellow fruit containing seeds

Quinine "Wild"

(colds, fever, infection, immune booster, inflammation)

Botanical name

Parthenium integrifolium

Also known as

feverfew, prairie-dock, snakeroot

Medicinal properties

anti-inflammatory, bitter, detoxifier, febrifuge, immuno-stimulant, promotes wound healing

Health benefits

Wild quinine was used in Native American and African American healing traditions in the southeastern United States. The flower tops were effective in treating fevers; hence, that is how it earned the name "wild" quinine. The leaves were used whole or crushed and mashed to make a poultice to place on burns. Wild quinine root was brewed and drunk as a tea to treat colds, congestion, infections, inflammation, missed periods, to boost immunity, and to detoxify the blood. Wild quinine was also used to treat animals. It contains Vitamin A and zinc.

Preparation and application

Tea

Put 1 teaspoon of the dried tops or 1 teaspoon of the dried root in hot water, cover and steep for 10 to 15 minutes. Drink 1 to 3 times daily until fever breaks or ailment subsides.

Poultice

For burns, wash area first, mash or crush leaves into a paste and place on burned area, wrapping with a gauze to keep in place. Apply a fresh bandage daily. Alternatively, bruise whole leaf and place on burn, wrapping with a bandage. Change daily.

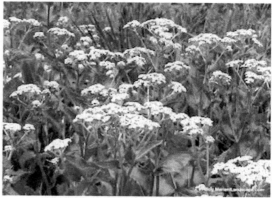

Wild quinine flowers in field
Image 8-92

Description: green leaves and stem; wooly white flower heads bloom spring to summer

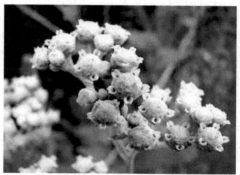

Wild quinine flowers close up
Image 8-92a

Description: green leaves and stem; wooly white flower heads bloom spring to summer

Rabbit Tobacco

(colds, congestion, flu)

Botanical name

Gnaphalium obtusifolium

Also known as

cat's foot, everlasting, Indian posy, Life-Everlasting, old field balsam, poverty weed, sweet balsam, sweet cudweed, sweet everlasting, white balsam

Medicinal properties

anti-inflammatory, antispasmodic, antiviral, diuretic, expectorant, sedative (mild)

Health benefits

Rabbit tobacco was a popular medicine and a tobacco substitute used by children in rural areas because of its mild sedative effects. Rabbit tobacco medicine was smoked for respiratory ailments or

Rabbit Tobacco (continued)

made into a healing and relaxing tea. Smoking the leaves was also good for sinusitis, head colds, and congestion. In hot teas, it was used to treat viral infections, sore throats, fevers, diarrhea, colds, congestion, flu, pneumonia, asthma, and coughs. Rabbit tobacco may also have diuretic and antispasmodic properties. Rabbit tobacco was often used in combination with other healing herbs in remedies to treat a variety of ailments.

Preparation and application

Tea

Pick the brown, silvery leaves, rinse, put in a pot, and cover with water. Use 1 to 2 teaspoons of rabbit tobacco leaves to 1 cup of water. Bring to boil and let sit for 15 to 30 minutes. Let cool and drain. You can squeeze the juice of 1/2 to 1 whole lemon into the tea while it is brewing and drop the lemon rind in the pot to stew along with the rabbit tobacco. Sweeten to taste. Drink 1 to 3 cups daily.

Poultice

Slowly warm 1 cup of the dried flower and leaves in talla or a natural vegetable oil (i.e., olive, castor, or other). Pack mixture on affected area and wrap with a wool or cotton cloth to hold in place for at least 1 hour or more.

Smoke

Use a pipe or make a cigarette from the dried leaves and flowers. Inhaling the smoke from the herb helps treat coughs, lung and chest congestion, and headaches. Pack rabbit tobacco leaves in a pipe and inhale the smoke deeply 2 times to bring up the phlegm, open sinuses, and clear lungs.

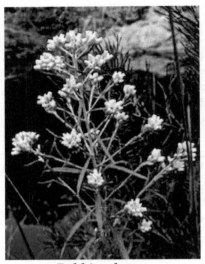

Rabbit tobacco
Image 8-93

Description: green to gray silvery leaves; lower leaves dried; white or pale yellow flower tops; looks gray when dry

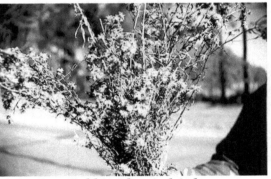

Rabbit tobacco dried
Image 8-93a

Description: green to gray silvery leaves; lower leaves dried; white or pale yellow flower tops; looks gray when dry

Rat Vein (aka Spotted Wintergreen)

(poison oak, poison ivy)

Botanical names

Chimaphila maculate or Chimaphila umbellata

Also known as

dragon's tongue, ground holly, pine tulip, rat tail, rheumatism root, rheumatism weed, striped pipsissewa

Medicinal properties

antiseptic, diuretic

Health benefits

Rat vein was used as an effective remedy for poison ivy and oak. Make a strong solution from the leaves and apply to affected area with a cotton ball or soak a compress in solution and apply. Drinking rat vein tea may also support kidney and liver health by helping the body eliminate excess fluids. This herb may also be effective in treating rheumatism, fever, sore throat, skin conditions, and general aches and pains.

Preparation and application

Tea

Put 1 teaspoon of dried or 2 teaspoons of fresh leaves in 1 cup of hot water, cover and steep for 10 to 15 minutes. Drink 1 to 3 cups daily.

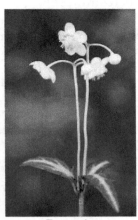

Rat vein

Image 8-94

Description: medium to dark green leaves with stripes; white to pink flowers June-August; red berries after flowering

Poultice

Gather rat vein leaves. Rinse and crush or bruise, then rub leaves directly on affected area. Let some leaves remain on affected area and wrap with a cloth or bandage. Alternatively, place leaves in cloth and bundle up, douse with hot water and, when cool, place on affected area.

Wash

Gather rat vein leaves, rinse with cool water, and let them dry. Place in pot and cover with water about 1 inch above leaves. Bring to boil and remove from heat. Let cool. Apply to affected area with cotton or soaked compress with leaves wrapped inside.

Red Shank

(blood cleanser)

Botanical name

Ceanothus americanus

Also known as

New Jersey tea, red root, wild mountain snowbell

Medicinal properties

anti-inflammatory, antimicrobial, antiseptic, antispasmodic, astringent, cathartic/laxative, expectorant, nervine/relaxant

Health benefits

Red shank was used as a blood cleanser and blood strengthener in African American healing traditions. An infusion of the root was drunk as a tea to strengthen and cleanse the blood and lymphatic system. In general, it boosted the immune system.

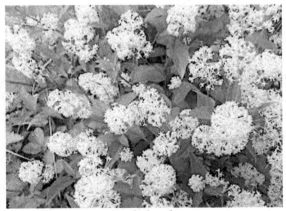

Red shank

Image 8-95

Description: dark green leaves, gray and hairy underside; white flowers in late spring

<u>**Red Shank (continued)**</u>

Preparation and application

Tea – hot or cold infusion

The bark is the part of the plant that is used. Harvest in the Spring after the last frost. Chip the root from an exposed area or dig down into the soil to expose the root. Make a tea by adding 1 teaspoon of dried or fresh root to 2 cups of water. Drink 1 cup daily. For hot tea, cover and steep 10 to 15 minutes. For cold infusion, cover and steep overnight in cold water.

Sage Bush

(stimulant, colds, flu, congestion, digestion, skin irritations, spiritual cleansing)

Botanical name

Salvia officinalis

Also known as

sage

Medicinal properties

antibiotic, antifungal, anti-inflammatory, antimalarial, antimicrobial, antioxidant, antirheumatic, antiseptic, antispasmodic, anxiolytic, bitter, bile stimulant, carminative, diuretic, digestive, expels worms, expectorant, induces perspiration, menstrual regulator, uterine stimulant

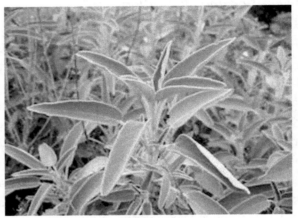

Sage bush
Image 8-96

Description: gray-green leaves; lavender-blue flowers in late spring

Health benefits

Sage medicine has been used for its many medicinal properties and benefits, both physical and spiritual. Sage tea was often drunk in the morning to prevent and treat colds, as well as an energy stimulant to boost memory. It also has diuretic, and expectorant properties.

Sage medicine used topically provided antibacterial, antifungal, and antiseptic effects for sores and other skin conditions. Drinking sage tea was also effective in treating fevers, headaches, and digestive disorders. It was used as a gargle to relieve sore throat.

Sage tea is rich with antioxidants that help prevent the damaging effects of free radicals and protect the body from the metabolism of unhealthy foods and environmental toxins like smoke and pesticides. Antioxidants work to prevent free radicals from attacking the cell tissues, preventing the signs of early aging and the risk of conditions like cancer and heart disease.

Preparation and application

Tea

Put 2 teaspoons of fresh or 1 teaspoon of dried sage leaves in 1 cup of moderately hot water (if the water is too hot it will vaporize the essential medicine). Cover with a ceramic or glass top and steep for 10 to 15 minutes. Drink 1 to 2 cups or use as a gargle for sore throats. If desired, sweeten to taste and add other herbs like peppermint or ginger while steeping.

Spiritual cleansing and for ceremonies

Burning dried sage has been used to greet, cleanse and heal the energy around a person or space. Take a dry leaf or bundle of sage leaves and light with a match, blow the fire out, and fan the smoke around the body or throughout the area to be cleansed. Use a non-plastic container to catch the ashes that may drop. Burning sage results in an aromatic scent that freshens, cleans, and kills germs.

Wash

Place sage leaves in a pot, cover with water, place cover on pot, and bring to a slow boil. Remove from heat and let cool. Strain into a glass container and use as a wash on affected areas. Can also use as a gargle.

Sardines & Oil

(mumps, arthritis/rheumatism and associated inflammation and pain)

Medicinal properties

anti-inflammatory, nutritive

Health benefits

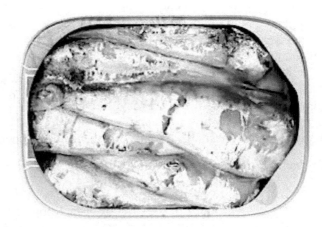

Sardines and oil in can
Image 8-97

The oil from sardines was used to treat and cure mumps and to relieve pain and inflammation from arthritis and rheumatism. The sardine oil was rubbed on the body of the infected person and the sardines were eaten. Sardines are considered a superfood because they are rich with essential nutrients, including omega-3 fatty acids, protein, calcium, niacin, copper, vitamins B12, B2, and D, selenium, choline, and phosphorous. Eating sardines sup ports heart health and healthy bones and is an energy and immune booster. The omega-3's in sardines may reduce inflammation.

Description: light gray-brown in color with yellowish oil

Preparation and application

Diet

Add sardines to your diet as a snack with crackers or in salads, 1 to 2 times per week.

Salves and ointments

Use sardine oil alone or mix with tallow, vegetable oil, or a healing salve, cream or ointment. Apply to affected area.

Sarsaparilla Root

(winter tonic for colds, fever, blood cleanser, rheumatism, gout)

Botanical name

Smilax pumila

Also known as

Honduran sarsaparilla, Jamaican sarsaparilla, zarzaparilla

Medicinal properties

antifungal, antibacterial, anti-inflammatory, alterative, carminative, diaphoretic, testosterone (libido) enhancer, tonic for general health

<u>Sarsaparilla Root (continued)</u>

Health benefits

Sarsaparilla root is a vine-like plant that grows in the southern hemisphere of the Americas. In African American healing traditions, a tea made from the sarsaparilla roots was drunk as a blood cleanser, to treat colds, and as a health tonic. Topically it was used to treat ringworm, itching, and other skin conditions like psoriasis, eczema, and acne. Sarsaparilla root medicine detoxifies and strengthens the body, tones the nervous system, and may regulate hormones.

Sarsaparilla root tea has also been used to treat rheumatism, arthritis, gout, fevers, urinary tract infections, and syphilis. The medicine has been used internally and externally simultaneously to treat boils, abscesses, and leprosy. Sarsaparilla is nutrient-rich with amino acids, vitamins A, B-complex, C, and D, and also the minerals iron, manganese, magnesium, sodium, silicon, sulfur, copper, zinc, and iodine.

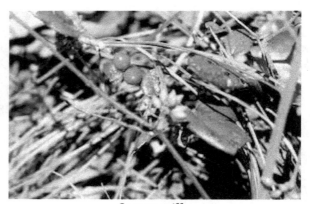

Sarsaparilla
Image 8-98

Description: dark green leaves; whitish-yellow flowers; small red fruits

Preparation and application

Tea

Put 1 to 2 teaspoons of the dried root in 1 cup of hot water, cover and steep for 10 to 15 minutes. Strain the root out and drink the tea warm. Drink 1 to 2 times a day.

Poultice

Chop and mash the root and apply mixture to affected area. Wrap with a gauze or bandage. Change daily.

Sarsaparilla "Wild"

(rheumatism, skin conditions, sores, detox, colds, digestion)

Botanical name

Aralia nudicaulis

Also known as

false sarsaparilla, small spikenard

Medicinal properties

alterative, diaphoretic, diuretic, pectoral, stimulant

Health benefits

Wild sarsaparilla is a small, flowering plant that grows throughout the United States from Canada to the Carolinas. When the people I interviewed spoke of using sarsaparilla medicine, they may have actually meant wild sarsaparilla and not the sarsaparilla native to South America. The root of the wild sarsaparilla plant was also used to treat some of the same

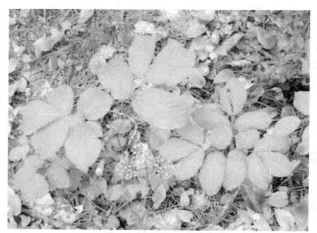

Sarsaparilla (wild)
Image 8-99

Description: light green to dark red-purplish leaves; greenish white flowers bloom spring to summer; purplish black fruit-berries after flowering; brown-gray bark

ailments as the South American plant—colds, rheumatism, ringworm, stomach problems—as well as being used for detox and as a substitute for making root beer. Wild sarsaparilla root was also used topically to treat ulcers, swellings, burns, and wounds. A strong elixir was made from the root to make a cough syrup. A root beer-like beverage was made from the root stock.

Preparation and application

Tea

Put 1 to 2 teaspoons of fresh or dried root in 1 cup of hot water, cover and steep for 10 to 15 minutes. Sweeten to taste. Drink 1 to 2 cups daily.

Beverage

Slow boil the root in a pot until the water is reddish-brown. Let cool. Sweeten and add other flavors if desired during cooling phase.

Poultice

Chop and pound the root so it is like mush. Apply to affected area and wrap with a bandage or gauze.

Sassafras

(colds, health tonic, blood cleanser, wounds, skin conditions, fevers)

Botanical name

Sassafras albidum

Also known as

ague tree, cinnamonwood, saloip, saxifrax, sassafrax, sassafract, smelling-stick

Medicinal properties

alterative, anodyne, antiseptic, aromatic, carminative, diaphoretic, diuretic, stimulant, vasodilator

Health benefits

Sassafras was commonly used as a treatment for colds where it was often combined with other herbs in a remedy, as well as a seasonal health tonic during winter and spring.

The leaves were made into a tea or a poultice that was applied to relieve inflammation or to treat skin conditions, wounds, and sores. But it is the root that contains the medicine: safrole, an essential oil. Dig up the roots at the end of October or November, when the leaves start falling. Clean the root and let dry. According to Mrs. Ruth Patterson, *"Make sure the roots are red and not white. The white will run ya blind."* Others say there is no difference.

Sassafras medicine has been used to treat a variety of ailments, including rheumatism, arthritis, gout, inflammation, scurvy, fevers, digestive problems, liver and kidney ailments, head lice, and as a blood purifier.

A tea and the beverage root beer was made from the root bark.

Sassafras was and still is used in cooking and food preparation. In the South the roots were boiled, then combined with molasses, and allowed to ferment into the first root beer. The Choctaw Indians used a paste of dried sassafras leaves to thicken and flavor their soups and stews. The filé in gumbo is made from ground sassafras root and is a derivative of the Choctaw stew.

An important warning note about sassafras and safrole

Sassafras has been used in traditional medicine for centuries. People understood that a dosage could either be healing or toxic. They were sensible about ingesting sassafras and didn't use it as long-term medicine.

Sassafras (continued)

This was because the active ingredient in sassafras is safrole. While safrole is a compound found in many plants, including ginger, cinnamon, mace, nutmeg, rosemary, dill, black tea, tamarind and witch hazel, it is also known to have harmful effects if ingested over a period of time in large and concentrated quantities. In the 1960s the FDA banned the use of sassafras and safrole as food or medicine because research from a study at that time found that when laboratory rats were fed large amounts of sassafras for an extended period of time, the rats developed cancer. That ban focused on instances where safrole was present in a food or flavoring in large or concentrated dosages. However, in its 2014 13th Report on Carcinogens, the U.S. Department of Health and Human Services found that "safrole may be ingested in edible spices, including sassafras [etc., all of which] contain naturally occurring safrole at low levels. For this reason filé (commonly used in preparing gumbo) containing sassafras is still sold and used in the United States without any restrictions.

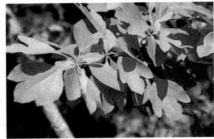

Sassafras leaves
Image 8-100

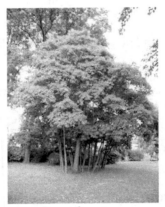

Sassafras tree
Image 8-100a

Preparation and application

Leaf tea

The ratio is 1 to 2 teaspoons of leaves to 1 cup of water. Place leaves in a pot, cover with hot water, cover and let steep for 10 to 15 minutes. Strain and drink. Sweeten to taste.

Root tea

The ratio is 1 teaspoon of dried root to 1 cup of water. Place root in a pot and add cold water, bring to a boil, remove from heat, cover and let steep 10 to 15 minutes. Strain and drink 1 to 3 cups daily. Sweeten to taste. Add other herbs or lemon as desired.

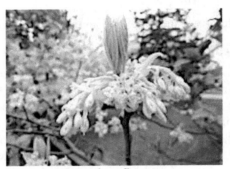

Sassafras flowers
Image 8-100b

Poultice using root

Cut, chop, and mash the root. Cover with just enough apple cider vinegar (ACV) or water to soak into the root. Continuing mixing. Put in a gauze and apply to affected area.

Description: bright green leaves turn yellow, purple and red during fall; greenish-yellow flowers appear in springtime; blue-black berries on pollinated female trees

Poultice using leaves

Bruise and/or crush leaves and rub directly on affected area. Alternatively, mash and mix with ACV or a natural vegetable oil and apply to affected area. Wrap with a gauze or wool cloth.

Wash

Make a strong solution by filling a pot halfway with leaves and/or root and covering with cold water. Bring to boil, remove from heat, cover and let steep for 20 to 30 minutes. Strain and use on affected areas for wounds, skin conditions, cuts, and rashes. Keep remaining liquid in a glass jar in the refrigerator for later use.

A note about the origins and medicinal properties of gumbo, and a recipe

I grew up watching my grandmother and mother make filé gumbo. That was the only gumbo I knew until my early twenties. Our family would eat filé gumbo two to three times a year usually on the holidays: Christmas, Easter, and Thanksgiving.

My grandmother's gumbo was better than any gumbo I have ever tasted in my entire life, whether made by all the other grandmothers of the world or made and served in a restaurant.

Maw-Maw, my grandmother, Eveline Prayo-Bernard, would send to New Orleans for her filé and Louisiana hot sausage. If a family member or friend had a plentiful crop of hot peppers from which they made their very own Louisiana-style hot sauce, Maw-Maw would get that, too. The basic ingredients were all back-home Southern. There was nothing comparable or acceptable as a substitute up North.

Making Maw-Maw's gumbo was an all-day affair. It was slow-cooked in a big stockpot, which we always called the gumbo pot even when it was used for other dishes. The fresh ingredients were strategically added, one by one, each in its own particular time, so that the flavor would not be cooked out or the texture of the gumbo turned too mushy. Nothing that had been previously-frozen was used, and we didn't know anything about such a thing as farm-raised seafood. The shrimp, oysters, and crab were tender, not rubbery, and had a sweet aftertaste that melted in your mouth. They were wild-caught, fresh from an ocean that had not yet been too polluted to eat from.

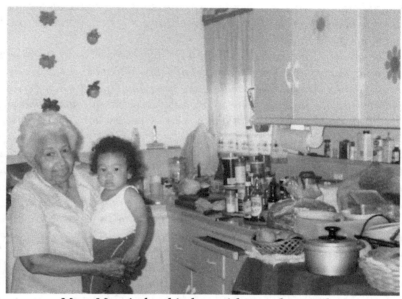

Maw-Maw in her kitchen with grandson Milon
Image 8-100c

My grandmother, who was all of 4 feet 11 inches tall, barely tall enough to reach the stove or counter without aid, used a step-stool to get to all the needed utensils and ingredients and to reach the top of the gumbo pot. Maw-Maw was very deliberate and precise in her cooking, never using measurement tools. She was the gumbo scientist.

Maw-Maw's gumbo was always slammin' good. Similar to how soup is sometimes the first course in a multi-course restaurant meal, Maw-Maw's gumbo was served first at family meals in special gumbo bowls. A scoop of white rice would be put in the bowl, then the gumbo, rich with crab, shrimp, oysters, Louisiana hot sausage, chicken wings, ham, and all the fixings, would be added. After that it was get-down time.

The crab parts that had a lot of meat and were steeped in the gumbo juice were my favorite. I'd break the shell in the right place at the top to reveal the meat, then suck it out with such delight, the juice dribbling between my fingers and down my chin to my napkin or bib.

Sometimes, Maw-Maw would make hog's head cheese as well. This was almost as involved as making the gumbo, but in a different way. She would carry a bucket on the bus through North Oakland downtown to Housewives Market, buy a whole hogs head at the fresh meat counter, and bring it back home in the bucket on the bus. Maw-Maw would put the whole hog's head in the big gumbo pot, fill it with water, and slow-cook it until the meat could be pulled out with her fingers. She'd strain out all the gel-like innards from the brain cavity, chop the meat into the smallest pieces possible, then drop it into a pot mixed with onion, garlic, celery, bay leaf, peppers, basil, salt, cayenne, other herbs and spices, and an all-purpose creole seasoning. Taking about four cups of the liquid that remained from straining out the brain innards, she would slow-cook the mixture for about 20 minutes. When it was finished

A note about the origins and medicinal properties of gumbo (continued)

cooking, she would pour it into a casserole pan to be chilled in the refrigerator until it would gel.

Maw-Maw's hog's head cheese was served with saltine crackers along with the gumbo. I would put a slice on a cracker, dip that in the gumbo juice, and put it straight into my mouth. All the flavors and textures slowly tantalized my tastebuds. I'd repeat that as much as I could get away with.

When I was growing up, I thought that filé gumbo, the type of gumbo Maw-Maw made, was the only authentic gumbo that existed. Filé is made from dried and ground sasafrass leaves. It gave the gumbo its earthy taste and texture. Maw-Maw always added the filé at the end, both while the gumbo was cooking and just after it was finished, using the seasoning for thickening and flavoring.

I later learned from family members that our grandmother actually often made okra gumbo, rather than filé gumbo, when she lived in New Orleans. She made either one or the other, but never combined them together. Both the filé and the okra are thickening agents, adding both to a gumbo at the same time made it too thick.

For my grandmother, deciding on the type of gumbo to make was more a seasonal matter than a seasoning matter. Okra is a summer/fall crop. When okra was available for harvest during the summer or fall months, Maw-Maw would make okra gumbo, but when okra was out of season, she'd make her gumbo with filé instead. This is probably how many gumbo-making people in old traditional New Orleans decided which type of gumbo they would make. It was a practical decision laden only with the bias of availability.

Gumbo, particularly okra gumbo, is often associated with its African origins, as the Bantu word for okra is ki ngombo. Besides using okra as the thickening agent, Africans used it to give the gumbo its distinct flavor.

In reality, however, gumbo is both of African and Choctaw origin.

One holiday when the family was eating gumbo, my Uncle Alvin Poyadue shared with everyone that the filé gumbo we eat has Native American roots, specifically from the Choctaw. His father was Mississippi Choctaw and some family relations refer to themselves as Creole-Choctaw. The Mississippi Choctaw first used filé as a seasoning, often in stews. Even the word "gumbo" may have been derived from the Choctaw word, kombo, meaning for filé.

Both the okra and filé (ground sasafrass leaves) have medicinal properties. Filé powder is purported to detoxify the body, regulate blood pressure, and alleviate arthritis, rheumatism, bronchitis, gastrointestinal problems, and skin eruptions. Okra's mucilage (the slimy stuff) acts as a laxative and lubricant of the intestinal tract. It is high in dietary fiber and is effective against diarrhea and constipation.

As I got older, I learned that there were other types of gumbo besides filé or okra. Texas style gumbo uses tomato sauce as a base, something I'd never seen in filé or okra gumbo until recently at my sister-in-law's house, where she uses all three! And what was called the "poor man's gumbo" had chicken and sausage instead of the usual seafood medley.

Michele Lee

Maw-Maw's (Eveline Prayo-Bernard's) filé gumbo recipe
perfected for over 100 years
(feeds 20 people)

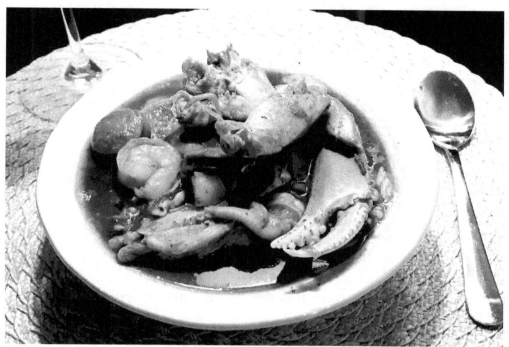

Seafood filé gumbo
Image 8-100d

Ingredients:
    4 to 5 pounds of shrimp
    6 to 8 pounds of chicken drumettes
    4 packages of hot sausage
    Ham chopped (optional)
    3 to 4 jars of oysters
    3 to 4 crabs
    2 onions chopped
    1 garlic bulb chopped
    1 bunch of celery chopped
    1/2 to 1 package of crab boil and/or chicken stock and/or vegetable stock
    Filé
    Flour
    Oil
Seasonings: salt, cayenne, bay leaf, garlic powder, creole/cajun seasoning[165]

1. Season drummettes (flour optional) and sauté in oil. Only brown the meat; don't cook all the way. Take out, put aside, and save the oil.
2. Sauté sliced hot sausage in oil and put aside. Only quick sauté if sausage is already cooked. (Do this to flavor the oil and brown the sausage.) Save the oil sausage was sautéd in.
3. If using ham, chop and sauté ham, put meat and sauté oil to side to use later.
    Note: Meats will finish cooking in the pot with the roux.
4. Shell the shrimp and put aside. Boil the meatless shells in water and save the water for the stock.
5. Chop the celery, onion, and garlic. Sauté in oil and put aside.

---

[165] For okra gumbo, see instructions below substituting okra for filé in the ingredients and the recipe

Maw-Maw's Filé Gumbo Recipe (continued)

6. Take the seasonings and the oil used from sautéing the meats and put in bottom of gumbo pot. Gradually heat up. Gradually add 1/2 cup of flour to make the roux[166]. Stir up so flour is mixed in well with no lumps. Cook until brown. Mix in celery, onion, and garlic.
7. Add meats or, alternatively, wait to add meats after #9.
8. Gradually pour in shrimp stock, oyster stock, and any other stock you choose to use, all the time stirring the mixture and checking thickness.
9. Add water along with crab boil and/or chicken stock and/or vegetable stock to fill half the pot.
10. Starting with 1 to 2 tablespoons, slowly add in the filè. Stop when the mixture reaches the desired taste and thickness.
11. Season to taste with salt, cayenne, and creole and/or cajun seasoning.
12. Add crab and continue to slow boil.
13. Add oysters and shrimp last.
14. Turn off fire. Cover and let seafood cook in the heat of the stew.

Alternative: If making okra gumbo, add 2 cups of sliced okra at #9 above instead of the filé. Adding okra and filé will make the gumbo too thick.

Saw Palmetto

(prostate health, urinary tract disorders, insect bites, infection, digestion aid)

Botanical name

Serenoa repens

Also known as

dwarf palmetto, pan palm, sabal

Medicinal properties

anti-inflammatory, antiseptic, aphrodisiac, diuretic, expectorant, sedative

Health benefits

Saw palmetto is native to the Southern United States coastal regions, and has been used as medicine for hundreds of years. It flourishes in Florida and was especially important to the Seminole Nation and surrounding Native tribes who used it for food, medicine, and for making utilitarian objects such as brooms, baskets, and rope. The powder from dried, ground palmetto berries was used to make nutritious flour or a tonic to treat stomach, digestion, respiratory, and urinary tract disorders or to increase milk in nursing mothers. The inner bark of the trunk was made into a poultice to treat snakebites, insect bites, skin ulcers, and infection. Saw palmetto medicine is popularly known today for its support of prostate health, treating bladder and testicular inflammation, and urinary tract disorders.

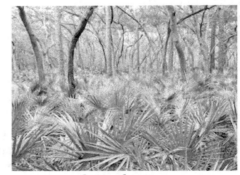

Saw palmettos
Image 8-101

Description: green palm leaves; thorny stems; white flowers; yellow berries turn brownish black when ripe

---

[166] Pronounced "roo." A roux is comprised of flour and a small amount of various liquids to make a thickener for soups and sauses and a thickener base for gumbo.

Preparation and application

Tea

Put 1 tablespoon of dried and crushed berries or 2 tablespoons of fresh berries in 1 cup of hot water, cover and steep for 10 to 15 minutes. Strain and drink. Can sweeten to taste if desired.

Berry tonic/infusion

Use 1 tablespoon of dried and crushed berries or 2 tablespoons of fresh berries to 1 cup of cold water. Place berries and water in a pot, bring to boil, cover, and simmer for 30 minutes. Remove from heat and let sit overnight. Strain liquid into a clean glass container and drink 2 to 3 cups per day for ailment.

Poultice

Scrape out the inner bark of a saw palmetto trunk and mash. Apply to affected area directly and wrap or put in a gauze poultice and apply. Change 1 to 2 times daily.

Senna

(constipation, laxative)

Botanical name

Senna hebecarpa

Also known as

American senna, locust plant, wild senna

Medicinal properties

cathartic, diuretic, laxative, purgative, stimulant, vermifuge

Health benefits

Senna was used as a laxative to help treat constipation and as a purgative to get rid of intestinal worms. It was also given at the onset of colds. A tea was made with other herbs such as mint or lemons to help lessen the purgative effect of the medicine.

Preparation and application

Tea

Hot

Put 1 teaspoon of dried leaves in 1 cup of hot water, cover and steep for 10 to 15 minutes. Drink right before bedtime.

Cold

Use 1/2 to 1 teaspoon fresh leaves per 1 cup of cold water. Let sit 24 hours and drink the next day. Adding ginger to senna tea helps to aid digestion and counteract any negative purging effects.

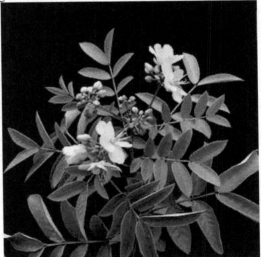

Senna
Image 8-102

Description: dull green leaves; yellow to orange flowers bloom July-August

Important: Stop using after 5 days or immediately after you have purged, whichever comes first.

Sheep Shallots Tea

(measles, whooping cough)

Also known as

manure tea, nanny tea

Medicinal properties

Not known at the present time

Health benefits

In African American healing traditions, sheep manure was made into a tea and sweetened to treat measles and whooping cough. Sheep shallots tea is nutrient rich with a high potassium and nitrogen level and digestive enzymes. In early 17th century England, manure tea was drunk to treat a variety of ailments, specifically for measles, smallpox, whooping cough, and jaundice.

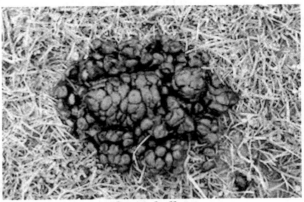

Sheep shallots
Image 8-103

Description: varies between brown, brownish-black, and ink-black in color

Preparation and application

1 cup of sheep manure was scooped up and put in a white cloth free from dye. Other ingredients were added such as lemon, peppermint tea, candy, sugar or honey, to sweeten and mask the taste. It was placed in a small pot and covered with fresh water, then brought to a boil and simmered, still covered, for 30 to 40 minutes. The mixture was cooled, then strained. A big, warm cup was drunk up to 3 times per day, one of those times being right before bedtime.

Snakeweed

(colds, cuts, insect bites, snake bites)

Botanical name

Gutierrezia sarothrae

Also known as

broom snakeroot, broom snakeweed, rabbit weed, snake root, turpentine weed

Medicinal properties

anodyne, antispasmodic, astringent, bitter, diaphoretic, diuretic, emetic, fumigent, nervine, stimulant

Health benefits

Snakeweed grows wild in Texas and other parts of the western United States and Mexico. In African American healing traditions, snakeweed medicine was mostly used to treat colds, snake bites, insect bites, wounds, and cuts. The medicine was made into a poultice or tea.

Snakeweed medicine has also been used in Native American healing traditions to treat numerous other ailments including respiratory problems, whooping cough, colds, fever, vertigo, diarrhea, bruises, bites (snake and insect), wounds, headaches, stomach ache, rheumatism, and more. The roots, leaves, and flowers were used and made into a tea for internal healing or poultice for topical healing.

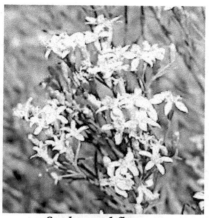

Snakeweed flowers
Image 8-104

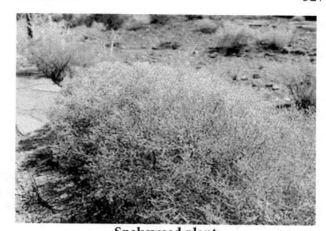

Snakeweed plant
Image 8-104a

Description: green to brown stems; clusters of yellow flowers bloom July-September

Preparation and application

Tea

Leaf and flower
Use 1 teaspoon of dried leaves and flowers, or 2 teaspoons of fresh leaves and flowers, to 1 cup of hot water. Cover and steep for 10 to 15 minutes.

Root
The Dine (Navajo) made a strong tonic of the root to treat stomach aches, colds, fever, and painful urination.

Poultice

Crush the leaves and make a paste or grind or chew the stem and apply directly to affected area to treat stings, cuts, bites, wounds, rheumatism, and skin conditions.

Snuff (aka Gooferdust or Goofadust)

(bee stings, insect bites, cuts, wounds, infection, boils)

Also known as

graveyard dirt

Medicinal properties

antibiotic, antiseptic, disinfectant, promotes wound healing, insecticide, stimulant

Health benefits

Snuff is fine-ground tobacco. It is used similarly to chewing tobacco by grabbing a "pinch" of the powder (referred to as "dipping snuff") and placing it in the bottom part of your inside lip or the back side of your mouth. The user holds it in place until the saliva build-up and then spits it out into a "snuff can" specifically used for "spitting snuff."

Snuff was used similarly to tobacco as a topical medicine to treat bee stings, cuts, wounds, sores, boils, to relieve pain, and stop infection.

Snuff (aka Gooferdust or Goofadust) (continued)

Spiritual properties

Gooferdust (also known as goofadust) comes from the Kikongo word "kufwa," which means "todie." Some Southerners say gooferdust is the same as snuff and others say it is synonomous with graveyard dirt, which is dirt actually removed from a grave. Gooferdust is used in hoodoo medicine as a powder to cast a spell that can cause harm, trouble, or even to kill. Sometimes gooferdust is used in love spells to coerce the target to "love me." Gooferdust can refer to any powder (not just snuff), to cast a spell using ingredients such as ash, dried manure, herbs, spices, ground insects, powdered sulfur, salt, or blacksmith anvil dust.

Southerners also used the term "Gooferdust" euphemistically to mean "poison" and in a very broad sense to include spells and physical illness, as being poisoned by dipping snuff.

Preparation and application

For bee stings, insect bites, open wounds and sores, moisten snuff powder so it is the consistency of a paste and apply to affected area. Moisten with water, apple cider vinegar (ACV), or a natural vegetable oil such as castor, olive or aloe vera gel. Wrap with a bandage. Repeat 2 to 3 times a day as necessary until area is healed.

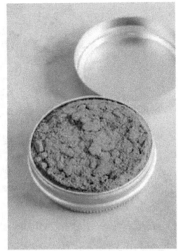

Snuff
Image 8-105

Description: light brown to brown powder

Spanish Moss, Tree Moss

(fever reducer, diabetes, skin conditions)

Botanical name

Tillandsia usneoides

Also known as

Florida moss, grandfather's whiskers, graybeard, old man's beard

Medicinal properties

analgesic, antibacterial, antipyretic (reduces fever)

Health benefits

Spanish moss tea was used in African American healing traditions to treat "high sugar" or diabetes (it may regulate glucose levels), reduce fevers, and was packed on as a poultice to treat skin rashes. Native Americans in the South and Southeast also used Spanish moss to make textile products, clothing, bedding, padding, diapers, home insulation, and more. African Americans and the European colonizers also adopted these uses. Spanish moss is not a traditional moss but a plant known as an angiosperm that hangs from big oak and cypress trees in the sunny, warm, and humid climate of the Southeastern United States.

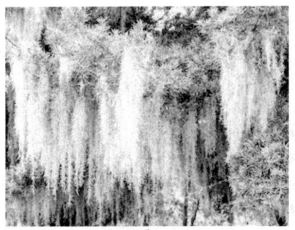

Spanish moss
Image 8-106

Description: a plant that grows from hanging on tree branches; grayish-green in color with tiny flowers; habitation for thousands of insects

Preparation and application

Tea

Wash a bunch of Spanish moss in cool water. Using a small pot, place enough to cover the bottom. Cover moss with water and slowly bring to a boil. Remove from heat, cover and let steep for 10 to 15 minutes. Drink 3 cups daily to treat ailments. Pour remaining liquid in a clean glass container for later use. Store in refrigerator.

Poultice or salve for skin conditions

Wash a bunch of Spanish moss in cool water, and let dry. Take the dried moss, grind it into a powder, and apply to affected area that has first been cleaned. Cover with gauze or bandage. Can also mix with a natural vegetable oil to make a cream. Apply to affected area 2 to 3 times daily until ailment is gone.

Spider Web

(stitching for cuts, suture, wound healer)

Also known as

spider silk

Medicinal properties

antimicrobial, regenerative

Health benefits

Spider webs have been used for centuries as an effective suture, bandage, or dressing for deep wounds and cuts. It was the material of choice to treat deep cuts and wounds when access to a doctor was not possible and stitches were needed. Spider webs are a natural fiber that may help fight infection, stop bleeding, and promote wound healing by supporting the regrowth of skin, tissues, and nerves in wounds.

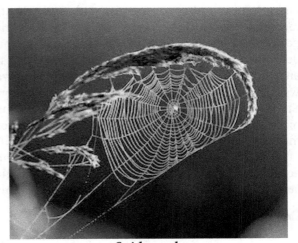

Spider web
Image 8-107

Description: delicate silk strands, transparent and silver-like in color

Preparation and application

Use fresh or abandoned spider webs to stitch and patch deep cuts and wounds and to stop bleeding. Clean out the wound with cool water and pack with spider webs as well as another healing herb such as aloe vera or comfrey. Spread web across the wound onto the skin on either side. Wrap with bandage. Change bandage and medicines daily or every 2 days for fresh injuries. As wound heals, you can leave on longer than 2 days at a time. (See also Anon Forrest's story on the healing power of spider webs and aloe vera under *Aloe vera and spider webs* page 174.)

Stinging Nettles

(allergies, general health tonic)

Botanical name

Urtica dioica

Also known as

nettles

Medicinal properties

anti-inflammatory, antiseptic, expectorant, diuretic, haemostatic

Health benefits

Children remember running through a patch of stinging nettles and getting stung by the plant's stinging hairs. In African American healing, stinging nettles tea was traditionally prepared to alleviate colds and allergies and as a general health tonic. Nettles medicine may also reduce swelling, treat arthritis, gout, increase lactation in humans and animals, decrease hemorrhaging (nose bleeds, heavy menses) and more. A poultice using stinging nettles powder was used to treat wounds, cuts, insect bites and burns. Stinging nettles is nutrient-rich with calcium, magnesium, iron, potassium, phosphorous, manganese, silica, iodine, silicon, sodium, sulfur, vitamins C and B complex, beta-carotene, amino acids, chlorophyll, and is high in protein. Stinging nettles tea may also help treat gout, diarrhea, worms and stomach problems.

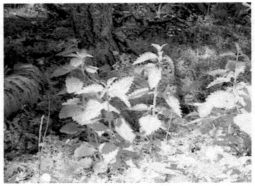

Stinging nettles
Image 8-108

Description: green leaves that have sharp stinging hairs; fuzzy white flowers

Preparation and application

Tea

Boil or steam fresh nettles for 5 to 15 minutes until tender. The leaves can be prepared to eat immediately, or frozen to eat later. The water used to boil can be drunk as tea.

Poultice

Grind dried stinging nettles leaves into a powder. Mix with a little water, aloe gel, or a natural vegetable oil. Apply to affected area and wrap with a bandage. Change 1 to 2 times daily until healed.

Sulfur

(wound healing, infection, health tonic)

Medicinal properties

antibacterial, anti-inflammatory, antimicrobial, antiseptic

Health benefits

Sulfur is an essential component in all living cells that is important for forming connective tissue and responsible for healthy skin, hair, and nails. Sulfur is also necessary for a healthy respiratory system, boosts energy and reduces fatigue, reduces inflammation, detoxifies the body, and allows for better absorption of food and nutrients. It is naturally found in eggs, onion, garlic, cabbage, brussel sprouts, broccoli, collards, kale, raw milk, fresh fruits, meats, and seafood.

The sulfur referred to here is the nutritional organic form of sulfur[167] and not the chemical sulfur oxide. Organic sulfur is a naturally occurring vital nutrient and an important mineral found primarily in muscular tissue, skin, and bones of our bodies.

A salve of sulfur and molasses was used in African American healing traditions as a topical medicine to heal wounds. It was also ingested as a health tonic. Water containing high amounts of sulfur usually smelled like rotten eggs, but was sometimes sipped as a health tonic.

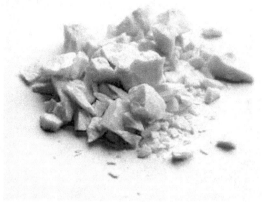

Sulfur
Image 8-109

Description: pale-yellowish color mineral

Preparation and application

Mix 1 tablespoon of molasses with organic sulfur powder and apply to affected area.

Organic sulfur powder or crystals (commonly known today as MSM, or methylsulphonylmethane) can be purchased from a natural medicine or health food store. MSM sulfur is an organic compound found in the tissues of all animals and plants. It is an essential nutrient necessary for proper health. MSM sulfur supports the connective tissues of ligaments, muscles, and tendons and is necessary for cell oxygenation and detoxification. MSM sulfur should be differentiated from sulfur, the chemical element also known as sulphur or sulfur oxide and which can be processed into sulfuric acid, which is *not* necessary or beneficial for proper health, but is actually toxic and poisonous to the human body.

Sweet Gum Tree—Bark and Fruit/Balls

(burns, colds, flu, cough, ringworm, sores)

Botanical name

Liquidambar styraciflua

Medicinal properties

anti-inflammatory, antiseptic, antiviral, astringent, carminative, diuretic, expectorant, parasiticide, stimulant, vulnerary

Health benefits

Medicine in the sweet gum tree is found in the resin, bark, and the fruit/balls. The resin is secreted from the tree bark and trunk and has been used externally to help heal wounds, ringworm, skin sores, boils, and other skin conditions. A tea was made from the resin or a small piece can be sucked on to treat colds, sore throat, coughs, and chest congestion. The bark has been used to make a tea to treat diarrhea.

Preparation and application

Sweet gum fruit/balls for burns, ringworm, sores

Gather sweet gum fruit/balls and crush them to break them into small pieces. Put them in a saucepan or skillet and cook them on medium heat until they turn to ashes. Take fresh cream from the top of cow's milk and mix the cream in with the ashes until it is smooth and completely blended together. Put the salve in a glass jar with an air-tight lid. Apply to affected area several times a day, washing the area with warm water and soap each time before application. Store in a cool, dry place for future use.

---

[167] aka MSM sulfur

Sweet Gum Tree—Bark and Fruit/Balls (continued)

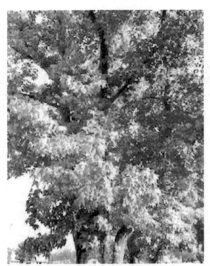

Sweet gum tree
Image 8-110

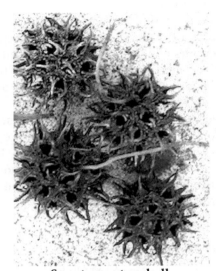

Sweet gum tree balls
Image 8-110a

Description: glossy green leaves that turn yellow, orange, purple and red in fall; yellow-green flowers in April and May that give way to dark brown gum balls

Sweet gum bark to treat diarrhea

Put 1 teaspoon of the bark in 1 cup of hot water, cover and steep for 20 minutes. Drink 1 cup daily until symptoms relieved.

Sweet gum resin for colds, coughs, chest congestion, sore throat

To collect the resin, slap the tree with a stick to release the resin if it is not easily seen. Break off 1 or more pieces of the resin as needed. Suck on a piece throughout the day as you would a lozenge. Alternatively, drop 1 teaspoon of the resin in a cup of hot water, let dissolve, and drink 2 to 3 cups daily.

Sweet gum resin salve for external use

Gather the resin as indicated above and soften by warming in a pot. You may need to add a natural vegetable oil or tallow to make creamy. Mix well and let cool. Apply to affected area 2 to 4 times daily.

Tallow

(chest congestion, colds, skin irritations, moisturizer)

Also known as

talla, tallah

Medicinal properties

antioxidant, anti-inflammatory

Health benefits

In the rural South, tallow was made by scraping the fat off of what was cooked from cow, sheep, or bison. The fat was used to make medicines, body creams, cooking grease, soaps, candles, and as an ingredient in the tanning of hides. It was also used as a base ingredient to make salves to treat chest congestion and colds. Topically, tallow is soothing and may help treat skin irritations like eczema, acne, and dryness. Nutritionally, tallow is an excellent source of niacin, vitamins B6, B12, K2, selenium, iron, phosphorus, potassium, and riboflavin.

Preparation and application

Making Tallow

Put pieces of beef or lamb into a pan, add a little water, cover, and cook on a low setting stirring occasionally. Remove from heat when you have mostly clear liquid and meat is cooked. Strain liquid into a glass jar using a metal strainer lined with paper towel, cheesecloth, or coffee filter. Refrigerate. When liquid is cool, the fat will be a thick layer that has risen to the top. Scrape off fat and reheat when ready to use. Keep jar of unused tallow refrigerated.

Another option is to put pan with meat and liquid in refrigerator once it has cooled and let fat rise to top in a thick layer, then scrape off when ready to use.

For oven cooking, place meat in the pan, add a little water (and spices), cover with foil or a top, and cook until liquid fat is clear and meat is cooked. Strain, same as above or let cool first in pan, then refrigerate and scrape layer of fat off once it has risen to the top.

To use as medicine, heat fat slowly in a small pot or sauce pan and use as a salve in a compress or as a poultice.

Compress

Soak warm, melted tallow on a flannel cloth and put on the chest to relieve congestion.

Poultice

Put tallow in a bandage and place on your chest.

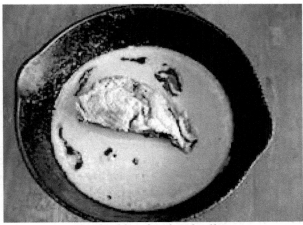

Cooked beef in beef tallow
Image 8-111

Description: Cooked beef surrounded by solidified fat grease (tallow) in black cast iron skillet

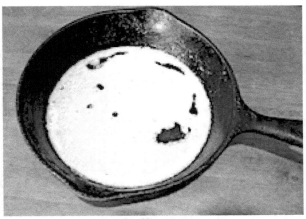

Beef tallow in pan
Image 8-111a

Description: White grease residue (tallow) from cooked beef solidified in a black cast iron black skillet

Three Sixes Cold Preparation (666)

Medicinal properties

analgesic, antibacterial, antifungal, antispasmodic, bitter digestive, febrifuge, nervine,

Health benefits

666 Cold Preparation (Three Sixes) has been used as a cold and flu remedy for over 100 years. The original formula had a high concentration of the active ingredient quinine. It also contained magnesium sulfate (Epsom salt) and alcohol. It was taken to relieve fevers due to colds, flu, coughs, nasal congestion, headache, constipation, malaria, and body aches and pains. Due to its quinine content, some say it saved the lives of countless people during the malaria epidemic that accompanied the building of the Panama Canal (circa 1881-1914).

666 got its name from the prescription pad number on which the patent holder, Tharp Spencer Roberts (Roberts Remedies #666) wrote a formula to treat a rural preacher with a severe case of

Three Sixes Cold Preparation (666) (continued)

malaria and the formula saved his life. Because Roberts wrote the prescription formula as "Roberts Remedies #666," the formula came to be requested as "Number 666," which eventually evolved into referring to the medicine as simply "666."

The original formula of 666 Cold Preparation has since been discontinued. Today it is artificially red in color and the active ingredients are acetaminophen, dextromethorphan and phenylephrine. There are also a host of inactive ingredients that range from FD&C Red #40, polyethylene glycol and sucrose, to name a few.

Original dosage

Taken as directed on the bottle. For example: Adults: 1 tablespoon taken with a full glass of water, every 4 hours, no more than 3 times daily; children (12 and under): 1 teaspoon with a full glass of water, every 3 hours no more than 3 times daily.

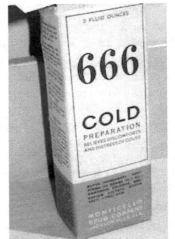

Three Sixes Cold Preparation
Image 8-112

Thyme or Tinthyme Tea

(circulation, cough, congestion, insect repellent)

Botanical name

Thymus vulgaris

Also known as

wild thyme

Medicinal properties

analgesic, antibacterial, anticancer, antifungal antioxidant, antiperspirant, antispasmodic, antiseptic, antitussive, antiviral, aromatic depurative, digestive, expectorant, insect repellent, nervine, vermifuge, warming (improves circulation)

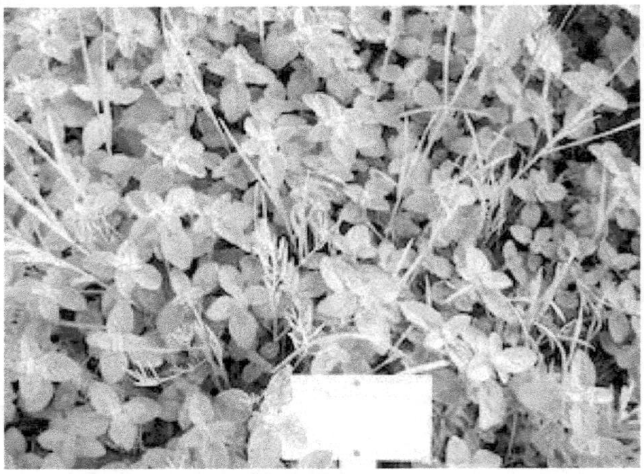

Tinthyme/Thyme
Image 8-113

Description: green leaves; white to lilac flowers

Health benefits

Thyme or Tinthyme tea was most often used for its expectorant and antiseptic properties to treat coughs, colds, flu, sore throats, and chest and sinus congestion. Thymol and carvacrol, the medicinal antiseptic components in thyme, also made it effective in treating cuts, wounds, and in preventing infection. Thyme medicine has also been used to reduce headaches, calm upset stomach, and bring down fever.

Preparation and application

Tea

Add 1 tablespoon of fresh thyme, or 1/2 tablespoon of dried, chopped thyme, to 1 cup of hot water. Cover and let steep for 10 to 15 minutes. Add lemon and sweeten to taste. Drink 2 to 3 cups daily.

Gargle

Make a strong solution by putting 1 to 2 tablespoons of thyme in 1 cup of hot water and covering and steeping for 30 minutes. Strain and let cool. Store remaining liquid in glass jar and refrigerate for future use.

Poultice/topical

Gather thyme leaves, put in a bowl, and pour just enough hot water over them to cover. Mash the leaves to release the medicine, until they are mixed well with the water. Let cool and apply to affected area. Wrap mixture with a cloth to hold in place.

Titiweed, Tetterwort

(see "Coon Root" this chapter)

Tobacco

(bee stings, insect bites, earaches, skin irritations)

Botanical name

Nicotiana tabacum

Medicinal properties

antiseptic, antispasmodic, cathartic, depressant, diaphoretic, diuretic, emetic, expectorant, narcotic, nauseant, sedative, sternutatory

Health benefits

Tobacco has been the go-to remedy in African American healing traditions for bee stings, insect bites, snake bites, earaches, skin wounds, and other skin irritations. Externally, the nicotine in tobacco acts as an antiseptic. Small doses of tobacco taken internally may have also treated constipation, expelled intestinal worms, and alleviated ulcers. Tobacco is native to the Americas and has been used as medicine and in ceremonies among the indigenous people of both the Americas and Africa for centuries.

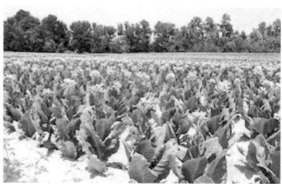

Tobacco field
Image 8-114

Description: green leaves; white flower clusters

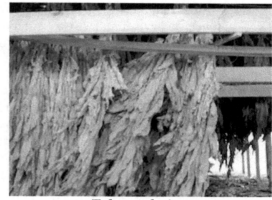

Tobacco drying
Image 8-114a

Description: ochre-colored dry tobacco leaves

Preparation and application

Poultice to treat bee stings and insect bites

Traditionally, someone chewing tobacco would pull a little from their mouth and apply to the bee sting or bite. Essentially, the medicine would be tobacco mixed with saliva as it was chewed. Alternatively, the dried tobacco leaf was chopped and ground up using a pestle or grinder, getting it as close to a powder consistency. Water or aloe vera gel was added to make a paste. It was wrapped with a bandage that was changed 1 to 2 times daily until condition improved.

Tobacco (continued)

Poultice to treat snake bites, skin wounds and irritations

Use whole tobacco leaves or chop and mix with another healing agent like aloe vera or vinegar.[168] Bind whole leaf or chopped mixture to affected area and wrap with a bandage. Change bandage 2 to 3 times a day.

Tobacco smoke to treat ear infections and nasal congestion

Put dried tobacco in a pipe or roll it in cigarette papers. Light it and pull on the pipe or cigarette to draw smoke into your mouth, but do not inhale. Using both hands, cup them around the area you want to blow the smoke into, so you can direct the smoke. Blow onto the affected area. Do this 2 to 3 times a day until relief.

Toothbrush Tree

(see "Black Gum Tree," "Dogwood," and "Pickash or Prickley Ash Bark/Tree" this chapter; these are all trees that are sometimes commonly referred to as the toothbrush tree)

Turmeric

(anti-inflammatory)

Botanical name

Curcuma longa

Also known as

turmeric root, Indian saffron

Medicinal properties

antiangiogenic, antiasthmatic, antibacterial, anti-cancer, anticataract, anticatarrh, anticolitic, antichron's, antieczemic, antihalitosic, anti-inflammatory, antimetastatic, antimutagenic, antioxidant, antiseptic, detoxicant, fungicide, hepatotonic, metal chelator

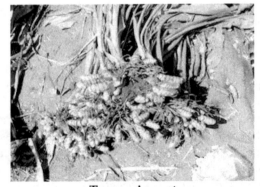

Turmeric root
Image 8-115

Description: green leaves; yellowish-orange underground tubers (turmeric root); white, green or reddish-purple flowers in August

Health benefits

Turmeric root is a powerful medicine that has been used in Ayurvedic medicine for centuries and has recently become popular in the United States. It is used to relieve general inflammation and pain in the whole body, including the digestive tract and the reproductive system and for arthritis-related ailments. It may also detoxify the liver, protect against cancer, and used topically, may treat skin conditions and speed wound healing. Turmeric root medicine can be used whole or as a spice and made into a tea or poultice or added to food and smoothies. Turmeric is high in vitamins C and E, and contains curcumin, which is a powerful anti-inflammatory and antioxidant.

---

[168] Apple cider vinegar has more medicinal properties than white vinegar, and would be the preferred type. However, white vinegar can be used if ACV is not available.

Traditional use

This herb was not used in early traditional African American healing practices. However, it is a popular herb used today and is benefical for those seeking natural remedies to treat inflammation, arthritis, and similar ailments.

Preparation and application

Add turmeric spice to add a deep yellow color and the medicinal benefits when cooking rice, vegetables, meats, stews, and your favorite recipes.

Alternatively, make a decoction using the root powder or slices of the fresh root to drink as a tea. Add 1 teaspoon of turmeric per 1 cup of hot water, simmer low for 20 minutes, then drink. Sweeten with honey, add ginger slices, or use milk (almond, rice, soy, cow) instead of water.

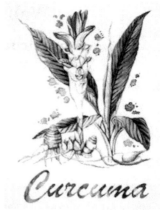

Turmeric plant
Image 8-115a

Description: green leaves; yellowish-orange underground tubers (turmeric root); white, green or reddish-purple flowers in August

Turpentine

(snake bites, congestion, colds, intestinal parasites, health tonic)

Also known as

gum turpentine, pure gum turpentine oil

Medicinal properties

antibacterial, anti-inflammatory

Health benefits

Small doses of 100% pure gum turpentine oil was used as a preventive health tonic and a cure-all that treated a variety of ailments, including intestinal parasites, wounds, cuts, constipation, colds, chest congestion, lung problems, snake bites, arthritis, rheumatism, and muscle and joint pain. Pure gum turpentine oil is made from the distillation of pine tree resin or sap. That differentiates it from the industrial version of turpentine, mineral turpentine, which comes from petroleum. 100% pure gum turpentine medicine was used in small doses, and with caution.

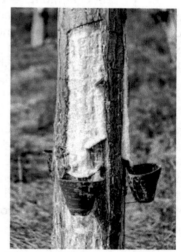

Turpentine harvested from tree
Image 8-116

Description: harvesting cream-colored pine resin from pine tree for processing into turpentine

Preventive health tonic and for coughs and colds

During the fall and winter season, a few drops (3 to 7) of turpentine oil were added to 1 teaspoonful of sugar, taken once a day for 3 days, and then stopped. This remedy was also taken at the first onset of cold or flu.

Topically for chest congestion, arthritis, joint pain

Mix a few drops in a natural oil base (olive, tallow, castor, or vegetable). Rub on affected area twice daily to reduce inflammation and relieve pain.

Walnut Tree, Walnut Hull

(ringworm, skin fungus, intestinal worms, skin irritations)

Botanical name

Juglans nigla

Also known as

black walnut

Medicinal properties

alterative, anti-inflammatory, antiparasitic, astringent, immune booster, laxative, sudorific

Health benefits

The inside of the green walnut husk was used to treat ringworm and other skin conditions like psoriasis, eczema, and ulcers. The unripe walnut husk, shell, and peel have astringent and antiparasitic properties. A medicinal wash made from walnut hull, bark, and leaves was applied to treat a variety of skin conditions. Drinking a tea made from the bark and leaves kills and expels intestinal worms, promotes sweating, and is an effective laxative. Placing a piece of the green husk into a hollow tooth eased the pain. Using an infusion as a gargle relieved sore and inflamed throats and mouth.

Walnuts are very nutritious. They are high in protein, B vitamins, and minerals. Walnuts are also a rich source of omega-3s and two other essential fatty acids: linolenic acid and alpha-linoleic acid. Linolenic acid reduces cholesterol, inflammation, prevents blood clot formation, supports nerve tissue formation, and produces antibodies to fight disease.

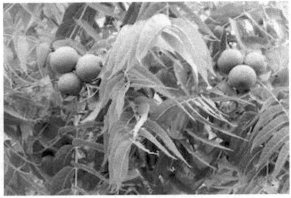

Walnuts on tree

Image 8-117

Description: green hulled walnuts growing on tree

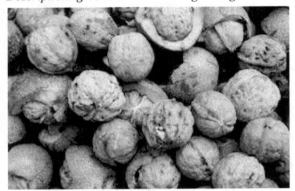

Walnuts

Image 8-117a

Description: light green hulls with tan walnuts

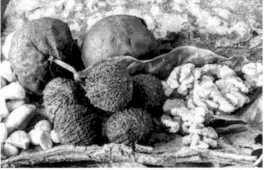

Walnut hulls

Image 8-117b

Description: blackened husks and walnuts

Preparation and application

Decoction for internal use

Add 1 oz. of dried bark or leaves to 1 pint of hot water. Bring to boil slowly, cover and let cool. Strain and drink 1 cup, 3 times per day to expel worms. Can be used as a wash.

Gargle

Follow directions to prepare a wash. Gargle with the mixture. Can add honey to sweeten.

Infusion for internal use

Add 1 oz. of dried bark or leaves to 1 pint of boiling water. Let stand for 6 hours, then strain. Drink 3 times a day. This solution can also be used as an external wash.

Poultice for ringworms, fungus and skin conditions

Separate the green husk from the walnut and apply the meaty inside of the husk to the affected area several times a day.

Wash

In a pot of water (enough to cover the top of the husks), bring to boil 3 to 5 green husks. Let cool. Pour liquid into a mason jar and use a cotton ball to apply the medicine to affected area at least 3 times a day until healed.

Watermelon, Watermelon Rind

(moisturizer, detoxifier, hydration)

Botanical name

Citrullus lanatus

Also known as

melon

Medicinal properties

antifebrific, anti-inflammatory, antioxidant, antiscle-rotic, choleretic action, demulcent, diuretic, emollient/moisturizer, febrifuge, purgative, vermifuge, lowers blood pressure

Health benefits

Originating in Africa and brought to America by enslaved Africans, watermelon was cultivated in North America as early as the 16th century. Eating watermelon on any hot and humid day in the South prevented dehydration. Eating and drinking watermelon also detoxifies the body. Watermelon rind was rubbed on the face to cleanse and moisturize the skin. The rind contains vitamins B6 and C, and eating it or making a tea from the rind may boost the immune system. Pickled watermelon rind is a common dish in the South, and the rind may also be prepared in preserves and relishes. Watermelon is nutrient rich with potassium, magnesium, calcium, fiber, protein, vitamins C, A, and B6, niacin, thiamin, carotenoids, and phytonutrients.

Preparation and application

Rub watermelon rind directly onto the face and skin. The rind can also be boiled and taken as a tea. Eat watermelon or make a juice to detox the body and benefit from the nutrients.

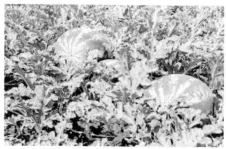

Watermelons in field
Image 8-118

Description: green leaves; pale green flowers; smooth green fruit with white striping; white inner rind with sweet edible juicy flesh that is red, pink or yellow

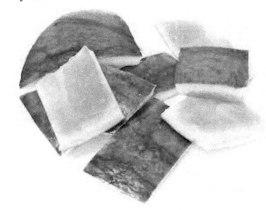

Watermelon rind
Image 8-118a

Description: green leaves; pale green flowers; smooth green fruit with white striping; white inner rind with sweet edible juicy flesh that is red, pink or yellow

Wormwood

(colds, flu, bronchitis, digestion, detoxifier, fever, intestinal worms)

Botanical names

Artemisia absinthium or Artemisia vulgaris

Also known as

absinth, ajenjo, common wormwood, green ginger, old woman

Medicinal properties

antiparasitic, antiseptic, antispasmodic, aromatic, carminative, cholagogue, detoxifier, febrifuge, immunity booster, stimulant, stomachic, tonic

Health benefits

Wormwood is a bitter herb that was used to treat coughs, colds, flu, bronchitis, and fever, and to aid digestion and detoxify the body. It is also known for its ability to expel parasites and worms from the body. Applied externally as a compress or poultice, wormwood supports the healing of insect bites, bruises, and other skin conditions. Wormwood medicine has also been used to treat jaundice, regulate women's periods, and ease constipation.

Preparation and application

Tea

Put 1 teaspoon of dried leaves and stems in 1 cup of boiled water, cover and steep for 10 to 15 minutes. Add a sweetener and lemon to improve taste. Drink wormwood tea at least 20 to 30 minutes before a meal to benefit from its medicinal properties. Drink 1 to 3 cups daily for 1 week, rest for 1 week, then resume.

Compress

Soak a clean cloth in a wormwood infusion of leaves and stems. Strain mixture into a large glass bowl or pot. Put cloth in liquid and leave in for 30 minutes. Wring out cloth, spread open, and put leaves and stem in the center. Wrap up

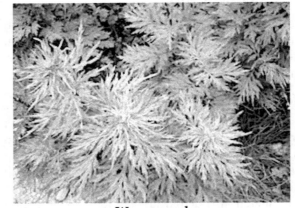

Wormwood
Image 8-119

Description: gray-green stems; silvery green leaves with silky white hairs; yellowish-gray flower heads

with cloth into a bundle. Re-soak the bundle in the liquid and apply to affected area. Alternatively, simply soak cloth in liquid for 3 to 5 minutes, wring slightly, and apply as a wrap or bundle with leaves to affected area. Can also rub liquid directly onto affected area.

Yellow Root

(winter and spring tonic, colds, headaches)

Botanical name

Xanthorhiza simplicissima

Also known as

eye balm, goldenseal, ground raspberry, Indian paint, jaundice root, poor man's ginseng

Medicinal properties

antibacterial, antifungal, antibiotic, antiparasitic, anti-inflammatory, astringent, bitter, immuno-stimulant, laxative

Health benefits

Yellow root is a bitter that when drunk as a tea boosts immunity and was known as a cure-all treatment for a wide range of ailments such as: colds, flu, congestion, sore throat, sinus infections, mouth sores, bladder problems, earache, uterine fibroids, gum disease, and PMS. It was also helpful as a digestive aid. Yellow root was also used in combination with other herbs to make a tea to treat high blood pressure and diabetes. Yellow root medicine is also a liver stimulant.

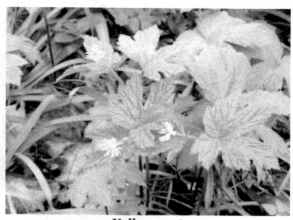

Yellow root
Image 8-120

Description: green leaves; yellowish green-greenish white flowers with white stamens; blooms in spring

Warning: Taking yellow root may stimulate uterine contractions, and should be avoided if pregnant.

Preparation and application

Make a tea using the standard tea preparation (put 1 teaspoon dried root in 1 cup of water, cover and steep for 10 to 15 minutes) or use the traditional decoction below.

Traditional Decoction

* Clean the root. Let it dry by hanging or use it immediately.
* Chop the stems and root and put enough in a mason jar so it is 1/4 full.
* Pour lukewarm water into the jar over the mixture, filling the jar. Let the yellow root sit until the medicine is released out and water turns yellow. Sip on the mixture daily directly out of the jar or drink 1 to 3 cups a day. You can refrigerate it or leave out at room temperature for later use.

Chapter 9 - Working The Powers: Conjurin'
And Hoodoo Remedies

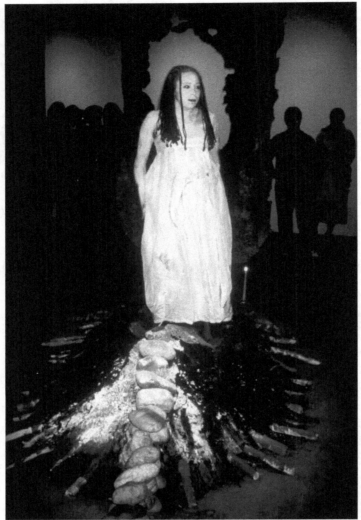

Transformation of Spiderwoman
Image 9-1

Getting A Spell Off Of Someone

"Her mind jus kep' comin', and in, I say, 'bout thirty minutes, she was back to normal jus' like she always was. After she got better, we took her to another root doctor to get the spell off. The woman tol' her, "Whoever done dis, dey got yo mother's hair. I don' know how or where she live, but look under da north corner down under the pillar, dig down dere and find dat hair, and take it and throw it in da runnin' water. Make sure da water runnin' and not no standin' water and get dat hair and throw it." We found dat hair, got it and put it in paper and threw it in this creek over yonder. It wasn't but a few days befo' my step daddy was gone. He was tryin' to git rid of my mama so he could go be wit dis other woman. He did'n say nuthin' but he knew that we knew what wuz goin on. People down heah use root doctors to do devilment. It ain't bad as it used to be years ago. People was bad 'bout dem root workers. I don't hear tell of it too much now."

Luther Stelly Smith, Mr. Red, North Carolina

Frizzy hen to find, scratch up, and dispel conjure or a spell that was put on you

"Now they got guinea hen in Africa which is a bird that is eaten and there's a lot of folklore and stuff about the guinea hen down South. They call that a frizzy hen. It was a special thing if you had a frizzy hen. Now, frizzy hen was a magical thing, actually. You let a frizzy hen move in the yard to scratch up conjure. If someone pays somebody to throw something at you[169], then you let a frizzy hen loose in the yard and the frizzy hen would find it and undo it. That's right! I knew people who kept a frizzy hen on a leash at the front door. Now where did that come from? It was a tradition that came from Africa where conjure was done around foot tracks for protection against evil and to undo roots or a spell. Cleaning, sweeping, or washing areas of foot travel with herbs, or minerals (like salt) would restore balance and luck. The frizzy hen is able to scratch up conjure and dispel it."
Luisah Teish

To ward off evil and for protection

For protection, to ward off evil and establish your territory:
*   Use red brick powder or dust

*   Scrub the steps down in this for security and to ward off evil, establish your territory (today people paint their steps red).
*   Scrub your steps down with urine on the first Friday of every month, early in the morning
*   Put red brick powder in your pocket for protection

To prevent someone from returning to your house:
"If somebody came to your house and you didn't want them to come back anymore, when they leave get the broom, sweep them out, take the broom and hang it up behind the door upside down and they never come back. That's right, and throw some salt after them."
  Eveline Elizabeth Prayo-Bernard

Efun/Cascarilla to hold in the good and repel the bad

Efun is powdered snail shell and lime chalk that comes from Nigeria. You can put Efun in a bath or directly on your body. Efun is a medicine that holds the goodness in and repels anything that conflicts with that. Cascarilla is the United States counterpart to Efun and used for the same purpose. It is made of powdered egg whites and eggshell.

Gooferdust (also known as graveyard dirt)

This material is used if you need protection. Carry it in your medicine bag, or put in the corners of your home and around your home outside or under your porch. Can use either actual dirt from the graveyard or snuff. (In North Carolina, snuff is also called gooferdust because of its harmful effect on the body.)

Gooferdust can also be used to harm or injure a person, which I do not recommend, as energy always comes back around to its originator (what Southerners speak of as "what comes around goes around" or the concept of "karma").

---

[169] Meaning, to put a spell on you.

High John the Conqueror Root

(see also under "Good Luck" below)

Put some root in a medicine bag and carry on your person. Wear High John the Conqueror oil.

Freezer conjures

Use to protect yourself and prevent someone from harming you, talking bad about you (i.e., spreading gossip and lies), or to stop negative actions toward you.

Freezer conjures have been used successfully by many people using lemon, cow tongue, or a written conjure on paper. The freezer conjure "freezes" the offenders actions and sends the negativity back to its source of origin.

Lemon freezer conjure

Write the name of the offender or offenders on a piece of natural fiber paper. You can also write the desired outcome. The name and/or outcome can be written in pencil or in some natural berry ink like pokeberry. Be careful not to write something that will harm the offender as conjures which are energy can come back to you.

After completing the writing, fold the paper up small. Cut the lemon so it opens up, but do not cut in half. Sprinkle alum powder and vinegar in the lemon and in the conjure, then place the written conjure in the lemon. Use sewing needles to close the lemon where you cut it. Wrap the lemon in aluminum foil with the shiny side down and place in the back corner of your freezer or in the bottom freezer drawer in the corner. Place a wooden board over it. Only use this drawer for your conjures. Alternatively, you can place the lemon conjure in a small mason jar, close the lid tight, and place in paper bag. Put the conjure jar in a small dark corner that is hidden from your normal activity.

Cow tongue freezer conjure

Write the conjure paper following the instructions for the lemon vessel, above. Take a cows tongue and slice it lengthwise. Add the alum and vinegar to both the tongue and the conjure. Place the written conjure inside the opened tongue. Sew up the tongue with 9 sewing needles and then wrap the sewed-up tongue in aluminum foil with the shiny side down. If desired, you can then place the conjure in a brown paper bag. Place the conjure in your freezer conjure drawer as described in the lemon freezer conjure above, making sure the wooden board covers the conjure from the rest of the items in your freezer.

Paper freeezer conjure

Write the offender's name three times in pencil or natural berry ink in the middle of the paper (parchment, brown paper bag or natural fiber). Write the desired outcome and/or what you want to happen around the name. Sprinkle with alum powder and saturate in vinegar. Squeezing lemon juice on the conjure is optional. Fold the paper as small as possible. Wrap in aluminum foil with the shiny side down and place in your freezer.

Getting Rid Of Malintent, Absorbing Negativity, Purification

Bay Leaves

Take a branch from a tree with bay leaves on it, hang it from the ceiling or over a doorway. The negativity rises and the bay leaves will absorb it. The leaves will absorb the negativity until they are dry. When the leaves are all drawn up and dried out, burn to dispel and transform the energy.

To get the same effect, you can also take bay leaves off the stem and line them up around the window sill openings and hang them on the ceiling.

Efun/Cascarilla to hold in the good and repel the bad

Gather a bundle of white sage, wrap it in string, and let it dry. Light the wrapped sage and burn, directing the smoke to cleanse or smudge your house, your body, another person, or whatever you want to heal. Smudge your house weekly, or smudge yourself prior to participating in ceremonies and prayer.

Sage/Smudge

Efun is powdered snail shell and lime chalk that comes from Nigeria. You can put Efun in a bath or directly on your body. Efun is a medicine that holds the goodness in and repels anything that conflicts with that. Cascarilla is the United States counterpart to Efun and used for the same purpose. It is made of powdered egg whites and eggshell.

Other ways to get rid of something bad

To get rid of a bad thought, memory, an illness, a growth, or anything that is not healthy for you in your life, take a cloth or a fruit and rub it on your body. While you are doing this, hold the affirmation that you are releasing or transferring this entire bad thing into the article you are rubbing your body with. Then, go bury the article in some soil that is barren. Leave it there, because nothing grows there. It will dissipate and disappear.

To Command A Situation

High John the Conqueror Root

(see under "Good Luck" below)

Calamus Root

Calamus root is used for control and domination of a situation or person. This could be a love spell or controlling someone's decisions and actions to your benefit. Calamus root chips can be burned (like dry sage or on charcoal) in an area before the person you want it to affect enters, or while you are meditating on the situation you wish to affect. Calamus root can be put in the corners of the home of the person you want to affect or an area they frequent. Alternatively, you can make a conjure bag in order to dominate the situation along with your desired outcome written on a piece of paper in pencil.

To Help A New Idea Or Venture Grow, To Reinforce An Attribute, Or To Give Something Positive Energy For Growth

Take a cloth or a fruit and rub it on your body, thinking about your intent while you do so. Go bury the object in fertile soil. If we need something to grow then we use fertile soil. Say a prayer for this to manifest and exactly what your intent is.

Obi Kola for success and to strengthen the power of what you say to be successful

"Obi Kola is a nut from Nigeria that is used to make the words that come out of our mouths stronger. It is a medicine that is used with the Orishas Oya or Chango and/or given as food or nutrition. The divine infinite Orisha we call Chango is specifically associated with success. And, the power of our word helps us to achieve success. If given an Obi Kola nut, you can just chew or nibble on it like you would a licorice stick."
Amani Ajaniku, Priestess Ochunike

Power of Intent, Prayers to E-QUE-CO

"If I need to ask for something, I will do more than what I ordinarily do. One of the things I do is prayers to E-que-co (pronounced "A kay co"). I did this one of the times I went to Puerto Rico. E-que-co is a little guy, his mouth is wide open and it's big enough to put a cigar in it. So if something happens that you've been praying for, you give him a cigar and it's really cool. I love my little E-que-co because he looks like my dad's people. And my dad's people used to keep cigars and beer lying around all over the house. Every Tuesday and Friday, I talk to E-que-co. You put a candle around him and I say, where's my studio, you been slackin off a little bit here. Then every once in a while you hold up a cigar and say, "See this, wouldn't you like to have this." You have to learn how to have fun with this stuff too. So E-que-co's message came back and said it's about my intent and the law of attraction, what you're bringing and what you're not bringing. It's an island thing, it's an African thing, it's a Caribbean thing as well as a New Orleans thing. E-que-co is special; it's a minor entity that is spirit-based for a particular intention or thing that you are asking for. [E-que-co and spirits] are merely messengers anyway, pure energy."
Anita Poree

Good Luck

Bee Shame

Herb of unknown origin. It is possibly bergamot mint, which is used to bring good luck, attract love, and reverse a bad situation. Carry the herb in your medicine bag, make a wash and rub on your body, put in your bath and soak, or use the essential oil.

Devil's Shoestring

Brings luck and protection. Use the root to "trip up the devil," to reverse the energy and stop bad luck or negativity coming toward you. Also good for success in gambling, getting a job, or for other personal goals that bring you balance and positivity.

Carry or bundle the roots in your medicine bag or hang in your home on your altar, doorway, or window sill. Alternatively, you can bury the roots in your yard near your porch.

High John the Conqueror

The origins of High John The Conqueror as an individual, before the name became associated with a medicinal plant, evolved in the days of the African slave trade and the enslavement of African people in America. Surrounding High John are many stories, legends, and songs—some of the latter by blues musicians Muddy Waters and Willie Dixon—which represent his ability to conquer any situation. Some of the stories describe the "actual" High John as an African prince, possibly of Senegalese or Congolese origin, who was captured and put into slavery and who never became subservient to his "masters," but was able to outwit and outsmart them through cunning and nerve. High John is a shapeshifter, time traveller, a trickster in the mold of Bre'r Rabbit or the orishas Eshu and Ellegua. When High John the man was supposed to have departed this earthly plane, he is said in the stories to have left his powers in the root of the Ipomoea Jalapa plant so that those powers could be accessed at any time by those with the knowledge and faith to invoke his spirit. This High John the Conqueror root, as it is commonly called, is used for protection, good luck in love and money, to command any situation and for success in court cases.

Court cases and legal conflicts

Carry the root on your person or in your medicine/mojo bag to bring good luck, especially in court cases and legal conflicts. In a legal situation, for example, use a pencil to put the name of the case and all the participants and your desired outcome on a piece of paper. Place the paper in the medicine bag along with the root to carry around with you.

Chew the root before your court case and spit the juice on the floor or in front of the court house prior to the case beginning. Dress candles in High John the Conqueror oil and burn for 7 days.

To attract the opposite sex

Wear the oil to bring good luck and to attract the opposite sex. Wrap your desired affection's hair or personal item around the root.

Calamus Root

Also used for good luck in the southern Black rootworking and conjuring tradition. For good luck, put a few pieces of the root in your pocket, medicine bag or in the corners of your house.

Queen's Delight tea

Used to bring positive energy into your life. One cup of this tea was often drunk daily by women who wanted good luck in getting pregnant.

Finding Water With A Stick, Water Divining

1. Survey the area and observe the direction the tree tops are leaning. They should all be leaning toward the water source.
2. Find a branch from a fruit-bearing tree about 3 to 4 feet in length. Break it off the tree, then say a prayer and give thanks. Take any fruit off if it is heavy enough to influence the flexibility of the branch, otherwise leave on.
3. Bend the branch into an arc and hold out in front of your waist.
4. Relax your body and say a prayer to the divine energy that asks to release yourself from your ego and allows you to become a vessel to find water. Realize that energy finds energy and you and water have the same molecules and energy source.
5. Let the branch lead you in the direction of the water. You will be pulled in many directions: left, right, north, south, east, west, 180 degrees, 360 degrees. When the branch points down and you feel the water under the ground, then stop.

Finding Water With A Stick, Water Divining (continued)

6. Pop the top of the arced branch on the spot and let it bounce up and down until it stops. It could bounce 20 to 80 times or more. Make sure you count the number of times it bounces up and down. This is the number of feet you need to drill down in order to reach clear water.
7. Give thanks and praise to the divine energy and drink water.

To Help You Decide, Indecision

Peony seeds

"Get a string of Peony seeds with a hole bore in em and strung. It's a red seed with a black dot on it. Now we may look at it and see a pretty seed that you can plant and will grow a flower, but there is folklore that talks about how when the Creator was giving everything it's property, Creator asked the Peony, 'What color do you wanna be?'

"And the Peony said, 'I wanna be a black seed.' And it changed it's mind and said, "Oh no, I wanna be a red seed." And so Creator made it black and then threw red paint on it and most of it is red and only the tip of it is black. So, it's not just the flower that you grow, it's a seed that you give to somebody when they're suffering from indecision."
Luisah Teish

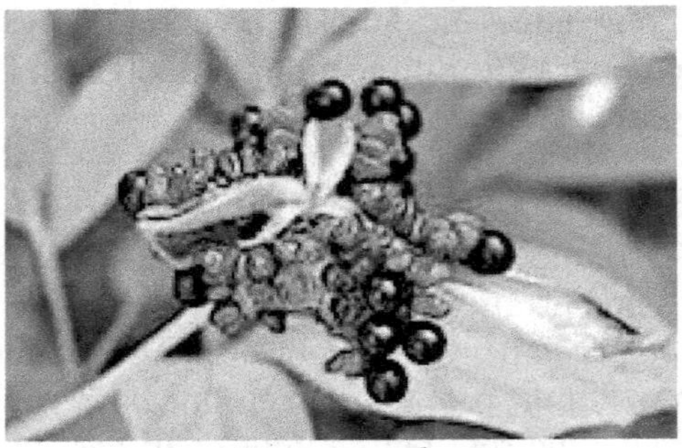

Peony seeds
Image 9-2

brownish-red seeds bursting out of dull brown or beige pod, green leaves

Raw egg

Use this conjure technique when you want to know if a decision you make will be fruitful. Do this at night before you go to bed:

1. Take a raw egg in the shell and cleanse it with water. Hold it in the palm of your hands, pray and share your thoughts about your dilemma. Ask if you take a certain direction, if there will be growth.
2. Get a glass and fill it with water. Crack the egg into the water. Place it in a sacred place like on your altar, near an ancestor picture, near your Bible, or near or on something else sacred and safe. Let it sit overnight. When you awake the next morning, if the egg whites are spread across the water in the glass like a web or netting, your decision will grow and be fruitful. If there are no egg white strings throughout the water and the yolk sits at the bottom of the glass, your decision will not be fruitful for you.

Asking For Divine Help And Support Through Spiritual Consultation

Talking to your Ancestor (Egun)

Take a stick and pound it three times and call the name of your ancestor three times. For example "Mama Edmonia, wake up. Mama Edmonia, wake up. Mama Edmonia, wake up. This is your daughter Michele Elizabeth." In Ifá, Lucumi, Voudoun, and other religions from the African Diaspora, when a person wants to talk to their ancestor, an Egun (ancestor) stick is pounded on the ground while calling out to the ancestor three times, "wake up, hear me, hear me, hear me."

Diloggun Divination

Diloggun divination is an ancient and sacred system of divination, foretelling the future and giving advice and guidance that has its roots in West Africa. Diloggun is used in many of the African-based spiritual beliefs throughout the African Diaspora, such as Santería, Candomble, and Lucumi. It includes a complex ritual used only by priests and priestesses in the religion that involves the casting of 16 cowrie shells.

First, the shells are prayed over and bonded to a ceremony that makes them sacred and gives them the ability to "talk" when they are cast. The cowries are no longer cowries and are referred to as Diloggun, the oracle of of Odu (the Great Spirit, God, Cosmic Energy). The priest or priestess is able to interpret or read the pattern of the cast Diloggun

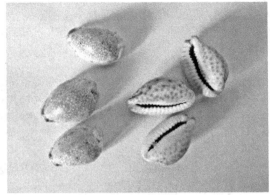

Cowrie shells
Image 9-3

Description: smooth cream-colored shells with ochre spots

that contains the advice, message, answer, or remedy for the practitioner or client. The process is similar to the ancient Chinese divination, the I-Ching.

"The Odu is very similar to a parable from the Bible or ancient wisdom from an Asian saying. It's usually applicable to what's going on with that person. The magic comes in when the problem is stated and the recipe is given to restore the balance. When that advice is followed, the balance is restored in that person. That's the defining moment. You have free will to accept the advice or not. If the advice is to make a cake with special ingredients then you put it together, bake it, and you have your cake. You have your medicine and it works! It's really beautiful. I've witnessed this time and time again. Lucumi is as old as time."
Imani Ajaniku

Moyuba Prayers to honor ancestors and call for support

Used to honor ancestors connected by blood or ancestors who may be in our spiritual lineage but not connected by blood. These can be living elders, priests, medicine men and women, or healers—anyone who has walked the road of truth all over. Start the Moyuba by calling out the ancestor's name. By using your hands, body and voice, it is another way for us to call on the four directions and get that unseen but felt support that we look for in our prayers. The Moyuba taps into the collective energy and uplifts our ancestors who also give us support in our lives.

Talking the fire out of someone

"God the father, God the son, take fire and put frost in." When someone's skin has been burned, say this three times and blow your breath on the area that has been burned—"on the fire"—and then place your hands over the area, palms down, and yank your hands back like you are pulling the fire out. Pause for a couple of minutes, then repeat.

Cycles

"To everything there is a season and a time and purpose under heaven." Ecclesiastes 3:1

"The timing for everything is important. Also, there are songs that go with that medicine and special

Cycles (continued)

times that you prepare it and take it. You have a relationship to the herb that ranges from what phase of the moon you planted in to what kind of offerings you make to the earth before you plant it . . . and, what kind of prayers you do before you harvest it, what the process is for preparing it, when you take it, and the folklore that embodies it. The relationship gives you the whole thing. You're not a lone somebody somewhere swallowing a pill made out of something you don't know nothing about."
Anita Poree

Energies and cycles of the moon, planets, and sun affect the outcome of your intent, affirmation, and goals. They also affect the natural movement of our physical world, whether intentional or not. The alignment of the moon, earth, and sun create the highest and lowest tides at the full moon and the new moon.

Timing and Cycles

* Cut your hair on a new moon so it grows healthy, long and fast
* Cut your hair on good Friday for healthy hair
* Never pierce your ear on a full moon because the ears will bubble up or keloid (raise a scar because of growth tissue)
* Start a new direction, project, venture, new idea at the new moon
* Plant above-ground crops between the new moon and the full moon
* Plant below-ground and root crops from the end of the full moon to the new moon
* The elders advised during thunder and lightning storms to turn off all the lights, be quiet and still so the lightening energy does not strike you. They felt that like energy finds like energy.
* East fruit and vegetables when they are harvested in their natural season.

Moon phases to achieve maximum effect of your conjures, affirmations, and intentions

* **New Moon:** new beginnings, new projects, new ideas, and new manifestations. This is when the first sliver of the moon is visible.
* **Waxing Moon:** growth and nurturing of new ideas, projects, and undertakings. This period lasts for about two weeks when the moon is getting larger in the sky, evolving toward the full moon.
* **Full Moon:** transformation, heightened psychic ability, and conjures for peace, love, fertility, and power. The moon has reached its zenith and forms a perfect sphere in the sky.
* **Waning Moon:** conjures to reverse, release bad habits, and end relationships; good for reflection and divination. The moon is decreasing in size, evolving toward the dark moon, and lasts about two weeks.
* **Dark Moon:** conjures to silence and stop your enemies, curses, and retributions. The moon is hidden behind the earth and sun and is not visible in the sky.

Days of the week to achieve maximum effect of your conjures, affirmations, and intentions

* **Sunday:** career, wealth, success, achievement
* **Monday:** intuition, spiritualism, dreams
* **Tuesday:** power, putting enemies in check
* **Wednesday:** healing, wisdom, communication, business
* **Thursday:** luck, happiness, growth
* **Friday:** love, relationships
* **Saturday:** spiritual and physical protection, metamorphosis, change

APPENDIX

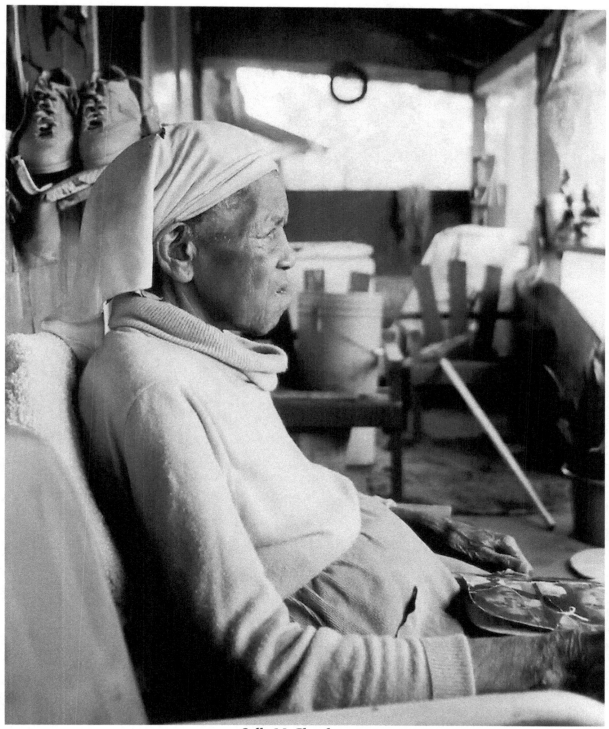

Sally McCloud
Image A-1

INDEX OF IMAGES

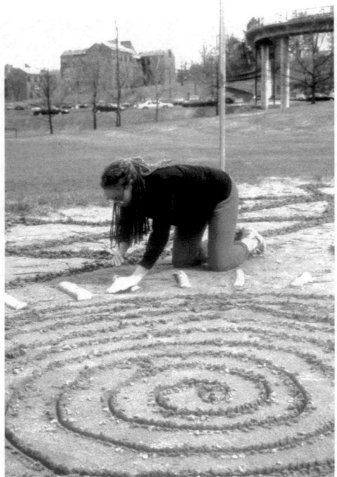

Michele E. Lee creating earthwork, "Volley Marks"
Image A-2

PART I HEALING NARRATIVES

Valena Noble

Image 1-24   *Ms. Valena Noble.* Image credit: Michele E. Lee

Etta Minor-Williams

Image 1-25   *Ms. Etta Minor-Williams.* Image credit: Michele E. Lee

Chapter 2 - Strong Medicine

Strong Medicine

Image 2-1   *Black Native American Pow Wow.* Don Littlecloud Davenport (RIP) & Bonita Roxie Aleja Sizemore, September 9-10, 2010 - First Black Native Pow Wow, Hayward, California hosted by the BNAA (Black Native American Association of Oakland, California. Image credit: Chantal Viellard / Copyright images2marquephotography (France)

Hattie Hazel Pegues-Clark

Image 2-2   *Ms. Hattie Hazel Pegues-Clark.* Image credit: Image provided by Hattie Hazel Pegues-Clark

Ola B. Hunter-Woods

Image 2-3   *Ms. Ola B. Hunter-Woods.* Image credit: Michele E. Lee
Image 2-4   *Ms. Hunter-Woods with one of her quilts in progress.* Image credit: Michele E. Lee
Image 2-5   *Refrigerated goods from Ms. Hunter-Woods' garden.* Image credit: Michele E. Lee

Ramona Big Eagle

Image 2-6   *Ramona Moore Big Eagle.* Image credit: Image provided by Ramona Moore Big Eagle (photographer unknown)

Beyond The African American

Image 2-7   *Native American Sacred Objects.* Image credit: David McKay

Ms. Chavis

Image 2-8   *Lumbee River, North Carolina.* Image credit: By Dincher (Own work) [Public domain], via Wikimedia Commons

Ms. Jacobs

Image 2-9   *Ms. Jacobs.* Image credit: Michele E. Lee

Chapter 3 - Spirit Work

Chapter 4 - Coming Full Circle

Breaking Halal

Image 4-5   *Eveline Prayo-Bernard, Luisah Teish, and Bonita Sizemore gathering at Yacine Bell's home in Oakland, CA to share medicine stories over lunch.* Image credit: Michele E. Lee

Image 4-6   *Black eyed-peas and cow peas.* Image credit: By Bubba73 (Jud McCranie) (Own work) [CC BY-SA 4.0 (http://creativecommons.org/licenses/by-sa/4.0)], via Wikimedia Commons

Image 4-7   *Luisah Teish.* Image credit: Asual Aswad

Image 4-8   *Eveline Prayo-Bernard.* Image credit: photographer unknown, image provided by James Allen Gordon, III

Image 4-9   *Bonita Sizemore.* Image credit: Courtesy One Sky Productions

Image 4-10   *Wooden image of Eshu from Nigeria.* Image credit: This file comes from Wellcome Images, a website operated by Wellcome Trust, a global charitable foundation based in the United Kingdom. [CC BY 4.0 (http://creativecommons.org/licenses/by/4.0)], via Wikimedia Commons

Image 4-11   *Bre'r Rabbit and the Tar-Baby.* Image credit: By Edward W. Kemble (1861–1933) (The Tar-Baby, by Joel Chandler Harris) [Public domain], via Wikimedia CommonsSee page for author

Image 4-12   *Peony flowers.* Image credit: By H. Zell (Own work) [GFDL (http://www.gnu.org/copyleft/fdl.html) or CC BY-SA 3.0 (http://creativecommons.org/licenses/by-sa/3.0)], via Wikimedia Commons

Image 4-13   *Peony seeds.* Image credit: By H. Zell (Own work) [GFDL (http://www.gnu.org/copyleft/fdl.html) or CC BY-SA 3.0 (http://creativecommons.org/licenses/by-sa/3.0)], via Wikimedia Commons

Image 4-14   *Yacine Bell.* Image credit: Jennah Bell

Imani Ajaniku

Image 4-15   *Imani Ajaniku in her Oakland, CA botanica.* Image credit: Asual Aswad

Image 4-16   *Imani Ajaniku's parents.* Image credit: provided by family

Image 4-17   *Imani Ajaniku in her altar room.* Image credit: Asual Aswad

Image 4-18   *Medicinal and ceremonial plants in Imani Ajaniku's garden.* Image credit: Asual Aswad

Image 4-19   *Obi kola nuts used in a divination tray.* Image credit: By Toluaye [Public domain], via Wikimedia Commons

Image 4-20   *Efun and Cascarilla.* Image credit: Michele E. Lee

Image 4-21   *Nkisi from Zaire (Congo).* Image credit: Photographer unknown [Public domain], via Wikimedia Commons, {PD-1923}

Image 4-22   *New Orleans Voodoo Dolls.* Image credit: By Mysticvoodoo Created by artist Denise Alvarado. (Own work) [CC BY-SA 3.0 (http://creativecommons.org/licenses/by-sa/3.0) or GFDL (http://www.gnu.org/copyleft/fdl.html)], via Wikimedia Commons

PART II - THE AILMENTS AND THEIR REMEDIES AND THE MEDICINES

Image II-1   Mr. Pete Smith with lion's tongue and rabbit tobacco. Image credit: Michele E. Lee

Chapter 8 - The Medicines

Image 8-16   *Blue cohosh.* Image credit: By H. Zell. (Own work) [GFDL (http://www.gnu.org/copyleft/fdl.html) or CC BY-SA

Image 8-17   *Boneset.* Image credit: SB Johnny, GFDL, Creative Commons 3.0 [GFDL (http://www.gnu.org/copyleft/fdl.html) or CC-BY-SA-3.0 (http://creativecommons.org/licenses/by-sa/3.0/), via Wikimedia Commons]

Image 8-18   *Buttongrass (weed).* Image credit: By Robert H. Mohlenbrock hosted by the USDA-NRCS 2015. The PLANTS Database / USDA SCS. 1989. *Midwest wetland flora: Field office illustrated guide to plant species.* Midwest National Technical Center, Lincoln.

Image 8-19   *Buttonwillow bush.* Image credit: By User:BotBln (Own work: User:BotBln) [GFDL (http://www.gnu.org/copyleft/fdl.html) or CC BY-SA 3.0 (http://creativecommons.org/licenses/by-sa/3.0)], via Wikimedia Commons

Image 8-19a   *Buttonwillow bush (detail).* Image credit: dugwy39/Shutterstock

Image 8-20   *Buzzard weed.* Image credit: By Marcia Stefani. [(Porophyllum ruderale Uploaded by berichard) [CC BY 2.0 (http://creativecommons.org/licenses/by/2.0)], via Wikimedia Commons]

Image 8-21   *Calmus plant.* Image credit: By J.F. Gaffard, Autoreille, France, 2004. [GFDL (http://www.gnu.org/copyleft/fdl.html), CC-BY-SA-3.0 (http://creativecommons.org/licenses/by-sa/3.0/) or CC BY-SA 1.0 (http://creativecommons.org/licenses/by-sa/1.0)], via Wikimedia Commons.

Image 8-21a   *Calamus plant flowering.* Shutterstock Image ID: 286571405, copyright jiki2

Image 8-21b   *Calmus root.* Image credit: By Krzysztof Ziarnek, Kenraiz (Own work) [CC BY-SA 3.0 (http://creativecommons.org/licenses/by-sa/3.0)], via Wikimedia Commons

Image 8-22   *Camphor tree.* Image credit By Abu Shawka. (Own work) [Public domain], via Wikimedia Commons

Image 8-22a   *Camphor plant.* Image credit: Franz Eugen Köhler. Franz Eugen Köhler's Medicinal Plants was published in 1887 in Germany. : *Kohler's medicinal plants – 1887*, public domain

Image 8-23   *Cascara tree bark.* Image credit: Jesse Taylor (Own work) [CC BY-SA 3.0 (http://creativecommons.org/licenses/by-sa/3.0)], via Wikimedia Commons [Note: the photographer is a different individual than the editor of this book.]

Image 8-23a   *Cascara leaves.* Image credit: Jesse Taylor (Own work) [CC BY-SA 3.0 (http://creativecommons.org/licenses/by-sa/3.0)], via Wikimedia Commons [Note: the photographer is a different individual than the editor of this book.]

Image 8-24   *Castor oil plant.* Image credit: By Alvesgaspar. (Own work) [CC BY-SA 3.0 (http://creativecommons.org/licenses/by-sa/3.0) or GFDL (http://www.gnu.org/copyleft/fdl.html)], via Wikimedia Commons. Public domain

Image 8-25   *Catnip.* Image credit: By Forest & Kim Starr. [CC BY 3.0 (http://creativecommons.org/licenses/by/3.0)], via Wikimedia Commons. Public domain

Image 8-25a   *Catnip (Illustration).* Image credit: By Johann Georg Sturm. Illustrated and painted by Jacob Strum. Public domain, via Wikimedia Commons. In public domain because copyright has expired {PD-1923}.

Image 8-26   *Cayenne.* Image credit: ChameleonsEye/Shutterstock

Image 8-27   *Cedar leaves.* Image credit: Solomiya Trlovska/Shutterstock

Image 8-27a   *Cedar leaves with seeds.* Image credit: Photogal/Shutterstock

Image 8-27b   *Cedar tree.* Image credit: YANGCHAO/Shutterstock

Image 8-39   *Cow chip.* Image credit: adirekjob/Shutterstock

Image 8-40   *Dandelion root.* Image credit: Brzostowska/Shutterstock

Image 8-41   *Devil's shoestring flowering plant.* Image credit: Debu55y/Shutterstock

Image 8-41a   *Devil's shoestring root.* Image credit: Michele E. Lee.

Image 8-42   *Dogwood flowers.* Image credit: By Robert H. Mohlenbrock @ USDA-NRCS PLANTS Database / USDA NRCS. 1995. Public domain. Northeast wetland flora: Field office guide to plant species. Northeast National Technical Center, Chester, PA. [Public domain], via Wikimedia Commons

Image 8-42a   *Dogwood tree.* Image credit: Steven Russell Smith Photos/Shutterstock

Image 8-43   *Ear wax.* Image credit: By Freak1972 aka Ulf Hundeiker. https://commons.wikimedia.org/wiki/File%3AOhrenSchmalzBrocken.jpg. (At home, selfmade) [Attribution], via Wikimedia Commons

Image 8-44   *Elderberry.* Image credit: SASIMOTO/Shutterstock

Image 8-45   *Epsom salt.* Image credit: Siriluck Ardsamatchai/Shutterstock

Image 8-46   *Eucalyptus leaves.* Image credit: Pat Hastings/Shutterstock

Image 8-46a   *Eucalyptus tree.* Image credit: Jakkrit Orrasri/Shutterstock

Image 8-47   *Figs.* Image credit: nbnserge/Shutterstock

Image 8-47a   *Fig tree.* Image credit: Natalie Barth/Shutterstock

Image 8-48   *Flax plant.* Image credit: Manfred Ruckszio/Shutterstock

Image 8-48a   *Flax seeds.* Image credit: MaraZe/Shutterstock Image ID: 25675793, copyright.

Image 8-49   *Garlic.* Image credit: Julie Clopper/Shutterstock

Image 8-50   *Ginger root.* Image credit: Rigamondis/Shutterstock

Image 8-50a   *Ginger plant flowering top.* Image credit: Rigamondis/Shutterstock

Image 8-51   *Goldenrod.* Image credit: SeDmi/Shutterstock

Image 8-52   *Hawthorn berry.* Image credit: muratart/Shutterstock

Image 8-53   *Heart leaves.* Image credit: Anna Grigorjeva/Shutterstock

Image 8-54   *High John the Conquerer.* Image credit: image credit: List of Koehler images, public domain {PD-1923} (454x597 pixels)

Image 8-55   *Hog hoof.* Image credit: Andrjuss/Shutterstock

Image 8-56   *Hog maws.* Image credit: Taurus 15/Shutterstock

Image 8-57   *Honey comb.* Image credit: Africa Studio/Shutterstock

Image 8-58   *Horehound.* Image credit: Chad Zuber/Shutterstock

Image 8-59   *Horny goat weed.* Image credit: By Maja Dumat. (Flickr: Elfenblume (Epimedium x versicolor)) [CC BY 2.0 (http://creativecommons.org/licenses/by/2.0)], via Wikimedia Commons

Image 8-60   *Horse milking.* Image credit: By Firespeaker (Own work) [CC BY-SA 3.0 (http://creativecommons.org/licenses/by-sa/3.0) or GFDL (http://www.gnu.org/copyleft/fdl.html)], via Wikimedia Commons

Image 8-60a   *Horse milk.* Image credit: By A.Savin (Wikimedia Commons · WikiPhotoSpace) (Own work) [FAL or CC BY-SA 3.0 (http://creativecommons.org/licenses/by-sa/3.0)], via Wikimedia Commons

Image 8-61   *Horsemint.* Image credit: By Sydenham Teak Edwards (1768-1819, {PD-1923}. [Public domain], via Wikimedia Commons https://commons.wikimedia.org/wiki/Commons:Copyright_tags#United_States

Image 8-62   *Huckleberry.* Image credit: Sergei Gorin/Shutterstock

Image 8-83a   *Pickash tree leaves and berries.* Image credit: This image or file is a work of a United States Department of Agriculture employee, taken or made as part of that person's official duties. As a work of the U.S. federal government, the image is in the public domain.

Image 8-84   *Pine tree illustration.* Image credit: By Prof. Dr. Otto Wilhelm Thomé [Public domain], via Wikimedia Commons, This work is in the Public Domain, (include the following tag) -- {PD-US}} – published in the US before 1923 and public domain in the US.

Image 8-84a   *Pine trees.* Image credit: By Chris M (Longleaf Pine) [CC BY 2.0 (http://creativecommons.org/licenses/by/2.0)], via Wikimedia Commons

Image 8-84b   *Pine cones.* Image credit: Gavin Budd/Shutterstock

Image 8-85   *Poke berries.* Image credit: By H. Zell (Own work) [GFDL (http://www.gnu.org/copyleft/fdl.html) or CC BY-SA 3.0 (http://creativecommons.org/licenses/by-sa/3.0)], via Wikimedia Commons

Image 8-85a   *Poke bush.* Image credit: By H. Zell (Own work) [GFDL (http://www.gnu.org/copyleft/fdl.html) or CC BY-SA 3.0 (http://creativecommons.org/licenses/by-sa/3.0)], via Wikimedia Commons

Image 8-86   *Potato plant.* Image credit: Madlen/Shutterstock

Image 8-87   *Pot Liquor.* Image credit: Michele E. Lee.

Image 8-87a   *Prickly pear cactus fruit.* By Tomás Castelazo (Own work) [CC BY-SA 2.5 (http://creativecommons.org/licenses/by-sa/2.5)], via Wikimedia Commons

Image 8-88   *Pudge Grass.* By Lazaregagnidze (Own work) [CC BY-SA 4.0 (http://creativecommons.org/licenses/by-sa/4.0)], via Wikimedia Commons

Image 8-89   *Pumpkins on vine.* Image credit: Evgenili Trushkova/Shutterstock

Image 8-89a   *Pumpkin seeds.* Christian Jung/ Shutterstock

Image 8-90   *Queen's Delight.* Image credit: By Craig N. Huegel, PhD.

Image 8-90a   *Queen's Delight fruit.* Image credit: Michel E. Lee

Image 8-91   *Quinine bush.* Image credit: By James Steakley (Own work) [CC BY-SA 3.0 (http://creativecommons.org/licenses/by-sa/3.0)], via Wikimedia Commons

Image 8-91a   *Quinine tree bark.* Image credit: By H. Zell (Own work) [GFDL (http://www.gnu.org/copyleft/fdl.html) or CC BY-SA 3.0 (http://creativecommons.org/licenses/by-sa/3.0)], via Wikimedia Commons

Image 8-91b   *Quinine flower illustration.* Image credit: By Franz Eugen Köhler, Köhler's Medizinal-Pflanzen (List of Koehler Images) [Public domain], via Wikimedia Commons – use this tag: {{PD-1923}} – published before 1923 and public domain in the US.

Image 8-92   *Wild quinine flowers in field.* Image credit: Mariani Landscape, Lake Bluff Illinois (Image taken taken in the native garden display at the Chicago Botanic Garden, summer, 2015.)

Image 8-92a   *Wild quinine flowers close up.* Image credit: By Adamantios. (Own work) [CC BY-SA 3.0 (http://creativecommons.org/licenses/by-sa/3.0) or GFDL (http://www.gnu.org/copyleft/fdl.html)], via Wikimedia Commons

Image 8-93   *Rabbit tobacco.* Image credit: By Fritzflohrreynolds. (Own work) [CC BY-SA 3.0 (http://creativecommons.org/licenses/by-sa/3.0)], via Wikimedia Commons

Image 8-93a   *Rabbit tobacco dried.* Image credit: Michele E. Lee.

Image 8-114   *Tobacco field.* Image credit: Kevinbercaw, Tobacco field, Rolesville, NC Date 4 July 2011 [CC BY-SA 3.0 (http://creativecommons.org/licenses/by-sa/3.0)], via Wikimedia Commons

Image 8-114a   *Tobacco drying.* Image credit: By Angelsharum (Own work) [CC BY-SA 3.0 (http://creativecommons.org/licenses/by-sa/3.0)], via Wikimedia Commons

Image 8-115   *Turmeric root.* Image credit: By Thamizhpparithi Maari. (Own work) [CC BY-SA 3.0 (http://creativecommons.org/licenses/by-sa/3.0)], via Wikimedia Commons

Image 8-115a   *Turmeric plant.* Image credit: Yudina Anna/Shutterstock

Image 8-116   *Turpentine harvested from tree.* Image credit: Discovod/Shutterstock

Image 8-117   *Walnuts on tree.* Image credit: public domain

Image 8-117a   *Walnuts.* Image credit: Xidong Luo/Shutterstock

Image 8-117b   *Walnut hulls.* Image credit: John A. Anderson/Shutterstock

Image 8-118   *Watermelons in field.* Image credit: ppi09/Shutterstock

Image 8-118a   *Watermelon rind.* Image credit: Natthapenpis Jindatham/Shutterstock

Image 8-119   *Wormwood.* Image credit: Rita Erfurt. [GFDL (http://www.gnu.org/copyleft/fdl.html), CC-BY-SA-3.0 (http://creativecommons.org/licenses/by-sa/3.0/) or CC BY-SA 2.5-2.0-1.0 (http://creativecommons.org/licenses/by-sa/2.5-2.0-1.0)], via Wikimedia Commons

Image 8-120   *Yellow root.* Image credit: By James Steakley. (Own work) [CC BY-SA 3.0 (http://creativecommons.org/licenses/by-sa/3.0) or GFDL (http://www.gnu.org/copyleft/fdl.html)], via Wikimedia Commons

Chapter 9 - Working The Powers

Image 9-1   *Transformation of Spiderwoman.* 1992. Installation and performance at the Santa Monica Museum, LAX Biennial. Produced and performed by Michele E. Lee. Image Credit: Beverly Lee

Image 9-2   *Peony seeds.* Image credit: Secundum naturam (Own work) [Public domain], via Wikimedia Commons

Image 9-3   *Cowrie shells.* Image credit: Sodabottle (Own work) [CC BY-SA 3.0 (http://creativecommons.org/licenses/by-sa/3.0)], via Wikimedia Commons

Appendix

Image A-1   *Ms. Sally McCloud.* Image credit: Michele E. Lee

Image A-2   *Michele E. Lee creating earthwork, "Volley Marks"* 1993 New York Image credit: image provided by Michele E. Lee

GLOSSARY OF CULTURAL TERMS

Ashé, Aché, Axé, or Asé   The term used in the West African religion Ifá and its branches that refers to the life force which runs through all things, living and inanimate. Ashé is the power to make things happen. Also used as an affirmation in greetings and prayers, as well as a concept about spiritual growth. Similar to how Christians use "Amen."

Bembé   A bembé is a party for the Orishas (African natural powers equivalent to saints or "Gods" that represent manifestions of nature). During a bembé, drummers play specific rhythms to call the Orishas who are praised and saluted, and who join the party through mounting or "possessing" one of the priests or priestesses in attendance.

Botanica   A retail store that sells folk medicine, herbs/roots, religious candles, statuary, amulets, oils, incense, and other products for spiritual practice or as alternative medicine. The name *botánica* is Spanish and translates as "botany" or "plant" store. Many practitioners of Ifá, Santería, Candomble, and other African-syncretized religions buy their spiritual products from a botanica.

Cooter   A word of West African origin from the area of the Bambara people which refers to turtle. It has been used as early as the 1700s in the southeastern United States from the Carolinas to Florida to refer to turtles or tortoises. The term "cooter" is used in the Seminole Nation and as an endearing term in other Native American Nations.

Cowrie shell   Used in Diloggun divination by the preist or priestess.

Diloggun   A divination that originated in the Yoruba religion of West Africa and is also used in Santería, Candomble, and other African-derived spiritual beliefs that rooted in the Americas during the trade of Africans to the Western Hemisphere. A priest or priestess prepares and blesses 16 cowrie shells and throws them out on a mat. The pattern that the shells form is interpreted by the priest or priestess and serves as advice for the client coming to seek help.

Efun/Cascarilla   A spiritual chalk from West Africa made of ground snail shell and limestone. Efun is used extensively in Orisha, Ifá, Lucumi, Santería, and Candomble rituals for cleansing, sanctification, and protection as well as for certain sacred writings and drawings. Cascarilla (powdered egg shell and egg whites) is used as a substitute due to Efun's limited availability in the United States and the Caribbean.

Egun   Among the Yoruba people, Egun means the collective representation of the ancestors.

Epele   Pieces of coconut shell on a chain used for Ifá divination.

Goofadust or Gooferdust

Gooferdust is a word used in the Southern United States to refer to a powder or dust that is used in conjuring and hoodoo work to trick, stop, or harm an enemy or predicament. In the Carolinas, some people call snuff "gooferdust." In New Orleans, gooferdust was also called graveyard dirt. The origin of the word "goofer" comes from the Kikongo word kufwa, which means "to die."

Gullah

The Gullah people are African Americans who have lived in and developed the coastal plain and Sea Islands region of the Carolinas, Georgia, and Florida since the 1700s. They are descendants of enslaved Africans who were from the rice-growing regions of West Africa centered primarily in Sierra Leone. The Gullah people and their language are also called Geechee. The term "Gullah" is possibly derived from the word "Angola," and "Geeche" is perhaps related to the Ogeechee River near Savannah, Georgia. The Gullah are known for preserving more of their African linguistic and cultural heritage than any other African American community in the United States. Gullah language also contains Native American and English words.

Hoodoo

An American term originating in the 19th century or earlier that refers to African American folkloric practices in spirituality and medicine and also with admixtures of Native American and European medical knowledge and folklore.

Ifá

A religion that originated in West Africa among the Yoruba people of present-day Nigeria and Benin as a form of traditional African spirituality and medicine. Some report Ifá to be 40,000 years old.

Juju

A word of West African origin, derived from the French joujou (toy) that refers to the supernatural power ascribed to an object or fetish. It can also refer to the use of such objects.

Lucumi (Lukumi)

A religious system originated by Yorubans who were captured in Africa and enslaved and brought to the island of Cuba. Lucumi survived by being syncretized or infused within Catholicism.

Madrina

Spanish word for godmother. The priestess or priest who initiates new practitioners into Santería and then becomes the Madrina (Godmother) or Padrino (Godfather) of the new initiate, guiding them in the faith.

Nkisi

Literally means sacred medicine and/or elevated spirit and is used to empower a variety of objects used in the spiritual and religious practice of many throughout the Congo Basin in Central Africa. Nkisi can represent a community agreement or contract, protection, or have other meanings to aid in the harmony of human life.

Obi

Coconut or Kola nut divination system used as an oracle in Ifá and its many branches (Santería, Candomble, etc.).

Odu

The primal sacred energies accessed in Ifá divination; the oracle; the message.

Olatunji Village
A traditional Yoruban village in Beaufort County, South Carolina, established in the early 1970s.

Olodumare
The supreme being, i.e., God, in the Ifá religion of the Yoruba people, primarily of Nigeria in West Africa.

Orisha
(also spelled Orisa or Orixa)
A spirit or deity that reflects one of the manifestations of Olodumare (God) in Ifá, the Yoruba religion brought to the Western Hemisphere by enslaved Africans. Orishas rule over forces of nature and the endeavors of humanity. Orishas embody attributes from that particular aspect of nature they rule over. For example, Ogun is the Orisha or god of iron, weapons, and tools and is considered a great warrior and protector of his people. Yemaya represents the ocean and seas and all that inhabit and are connected to that energy. Specific dance movements, songs, and colors are associated with each Orisha and are part of an intricate weaving of prayer and praise-calling for the Orishas to bless, counsel, and cleanse the initiated members.

Padrino
Spanish word for godfather. The priest or priestess who initiates new practitioners into Santería and then becomes the Padrino or Madrina (Godmother) of the new initiate, guiding him or her in the faith.

Santería
A branch of Ifá which is the traditional religion of the Yoruba people of Nigeria, West Africa. Enslaved Yorubans brought their religion with them across the Atlantic. Forbidden to practice and forced to baptize as Roman Catholic, they creatively fused and concealed their beliefs within Catholicism by choosing a Catholic saint and associating the saint to one of the Orishas of their traditional practice. As a result, Saint Barbara became Changó, the god of thunder; Saint Peter became Ogún, the god of politics, fire, and war; Our Lady of Mercy, the Virgin Mary, became Obatalá, the creator; Our Lady of Regla became Yemayá , master of seas; St Lazarus became Babalú Ayé, patron of the sick; and Olorún, the father of and wisest of all gods, was covered with the cloak of Jesus Christ.

Vodun, Vodou, Voodoo
A religious practice that originated from enslaved West Africans of the Fon and Ewe tribes from Dahomey in what is now present-day Benin. Vodun took root in Haiti and New Orleans, the infusion of traditional African beliefs with Catholicism that came to be called by the name Voodoo. Vodun means the power; that who is invisible, the creator of all things. Vodun practitioners believe in an Omnipresent Creator and the Loa or Orishas who act as intermediaries (like the saints in Catholicism) between the creator and the human world. The misconception that Vodun is associated with zombies or Satanism has been spread by Hollywood.

Voodoo dolls   Used as a focusing power object to help enrich the lives of its practitioners in the area of prosperity, love, health, protection, and other positive influences. The practice of sticking pins in objects has history in many traditional cultures, but not necessarily for evil. Its exact origins may have come from the Nkisi in Central Africa. Hollywood stereotypes helped perpetuate this practice as an evil method used to curse an individual.

Yoruba   Predominantly found in Nigeria, the Yoruba are one of the largest ethnic groups of West Africa. Many historians and anthropologists confirm that Yorubaland—Southwest Nigeria, Benin and Togo—has existed for several millennia. Their traditional religious practice is called Ifá. Enslaved Africans practicing Ifá brought this spiritual practice with them to the Western Hemisphere and infused or syncretized it with Catholic rituals. Today, versions of Ifá exist in Puerto Rico (Santería), Cuba (Santería and Lucumi,) Brazil (Candomble and Macumba) and Trinidad (Chango).

GLOSSARY OF MEDICINAL PROPERTIES

Abortifacient	induces abortion
Adaptogen	a classification of herbs that strengthens your body's response to stress and supports the health of your adrenal system
Allicin	compound in garlic that is antimicrobial and antiviral
Alterative	induces change to aid detoxification and restore healthy functions
Analgesic	relieves pain
Anesthetic	induces temporary loss of sensation
Anodyne	relieves or soothes pain
Anthelmintic	expels or destroys parasites
Antiandrogen	blocks androgen hormone
Antiangiogenic	reduces growth of new blood vessels which helps to stop or inhibit tumor growth
Antianxiety	reduces experience of and symptoms of anxiety
Antiasthmatic	prevents and reduces asthma symptoms
Antibacterial	kills or inhibits growth of bacteria
Anti-cancer	helps prevent cancer
Anticataract	helps prevent cataracts and promotes healthy eye function
Anticatarrhal	helps to reduce excess mucous
Anticholinergic	blockade of acetylcholine receptors resulting in the inhibition of parasympathetic nerve impulses; commonly used in the treatment of vomiting or diaharrhea
Anticholinesterase	used in the treatment of dementia and to improve alertness by slowing the breakdown of the neurotransmitter acetylcholine
Anticolitic	reduces and prevents colon inflammation, colic
Anticonvulsive/ Anticonvulsant	preventing or arresting seizures
Antiedemic	reduces and prevents edema (swelling and fluid retention)
Antieczemic	prevents and treats eczema

Antiemetic	treats and prevents nausea and vomiting (such as experienced in sea sickness)
Antiflatulent	prevents gas, flatulence
Antigingivitic	prevents gingivitis, gum disease
Antihalitosic	prevents bad breath
Antihistamine/ Antihistaminic	counteracts the effets of histamine (substance responsible for many allergies)
Anti-inflammatory	reduces swelling
Antimetastatic	prevents cancer growth and spread
Antimicrobial	kills bacteria, fungus and parasites
Antimutagenic	reduces mutation
Antineoplastic	inhibits or prevents the growth and spread of tumors or malignant cells
Antioxidant	acts as scavenger to clean up the free radicals of metabolism and other environmental toxins like smoke and pesticides in the body; antioxidants work to prevent free radicals from attacking the cell tissues and prevent the signs of early aging and the risk of conditions like cancer and heart disease
Antiparasitic	substance used to treat parasites
Antiperiodontic	helps to prevent gum disease
Antiplaque	reduces organisms that create plaque buildup
Antipyretic	helps to reduce fevers
Antirheumatic	alleviates or prevents rheumatism (inflammation, swelling, and pain in the joints or muscles)
Antiseborrheic	preventing or relieving seborrhea, a red, itchy rash with white scales which is called dandruff when on the scalp
Antiscorbutic	preventing or treating scurvy
Antiseptic	prevents infections by killing or inhibiting growth of micro-organisms and other harmful agents
Antispasmodic	prevents or eases spasms or cramps
Antithrombotic	reduces formation of blood clots
Antitussive	a substance that alleviates or suppresses coughing

Antiviral	kills viruses
Anxiolytic	anti-anxiety, anti-panic, mild tranquilizer
Aperient	relieves constipation
Aphrodisiac	increases sexual desire
Aquaretic	promotes loss of body water without losing electrolytes
Aromatic	having fragrance
Astringent	a substance or preparation that draws together or constricts body tissues and is effective in stopping the flow of blood or other secretions; can be used internally for diarrhea, sore throats, and peptic ulcers; can be used externally for cuts, insect bites, stretch marks, scars, etc.
Bile stimulant	stimulates the release of bile from the liver or gallbladder, which aids digestion
Bitter	cleanses blood stream, stimulates bile flow, astringent, laxative, appetite stimulant, regulates insulin secretion
Cardiotonic	tones and strengthens the heart
Carminative	anti-gas, rich in volatile oils, stimulates the peristalsis of digestive system and relaxes stomach, supporting digestion and helping against gas in digestive tract
Cathartic	helps to reduce emotional tension
Cholagogue	stimulates bile flow
Cicatrizing	promotes wound healing
Cytotonic	changing the morphology of a cell
Demulcent	rich in mucilage, soothes and protects irritated or inflamed internal tissue
Depurative	helps to cleanse waste products and toxins from the body
Detoxifier/ Detoxifying	aids the removal of a toxin
Diaphoretic	reduces fevers
Digestive	supports healthy digestion
Diuretic	increases urination and reduces fluid retention, aids kidneys

Emetic	induces vomiting
Emmenagogue	stimulates and normalizes menstrual flow, can also indicate any substance used as a tonic for the female reproductive system
Emollient	softens, soothes, and protects skin (works externally similar to how demulcents work internally)
Expectorant	brings up mucus and other material from the lungs, bronchi, and trachea; promotes drainage and lubricates the irritated respiratory tract
Febrifuge	helps the body to reduce fevers
Fungicide	inhibits or kills fungi or fungus spores
Galactogogue	promotes lactation as in breastfeeding
Germicide	kills germs or micro-organisms
Hepatotonic	supports gastrointestinal health
Hyperemic	increases blood flow to an area of the body
Hypertensive	lowers blood pressure
Immunostimulant	stimulates the immune system
Laxative	stimulates bowel movements
Lymph nodes	small ball-shaped organs of the immune system found throughout the body that act as filters or traps for foreign particles harmful to the body; they are important in proper functioning of the immune system
Metal chelator	removes heavy metals from the body
Mitogenic	breaks up chromosomes
Mucilaginous	containing mucilage, a thick, gluey substance
Nervine	tones and strengthens nervous system
Nutritive	high nutritional value, nourishing
Ophthalmic	relating to the eye, healthy eye support
Pectoral	general strengthening and healing effect on the respiratory system
Pesticide	a substance that attracts, reduces, and often kills pests
Proliferant	cell proliferant; promotes rapid cell growth
Purgative	promotes bowel elimination

Respiratory stimulant	promotes increased respiratory rate
Rubefacient	an herb that brings blood rapidly to a certain area, causing the skin to turn red
Sedative	relaxes, calms
Sialogogue	stimulates the secretion of saliva
Sternutatory	causes sneezing
Stimulant	provides an energy boost; makes you alert
Stomachic	stimulates and aids gastric digestion
Styptic/ antihemorrhagic	reduces or stops external bleeding
Sudorific	causes or increases sweat
Thermogenic	increases heat in the body, affecting metabolism rates
Tonic	strengthens and enlivens either specific organs or the whole body
Topical	on the surface, i.e., the skin
Toxins	poisonous substance produced by living cells or organisms
Vasodilator	widens blood vessels and reduces hypertension
Vermifuge	an anthelmintic medicine used to expel worms
Vulnerary	external aid to wounds and cuts

BIBLIOGRAPHY

It would be impossible to recreate a complete list of the many scholarly and lay materials that made up the research that were essential to the writing *Working The Roots: Over 400 Years of Traditional African American Healing*. Below is a list of the most important of those books and materials.

Print Sources

Foster, Steven and Duke, James, A. (1999). <u>A Field Guide to Medicinal Plants and Herbs: Of Eastern and Central North America Second Edition.</u> Houghton Mifflin Company, Boston, New York

Foster, Steven A. and Johnson, Rebecca L. (2006) <u>Desk Reference to Nature's Medicine.</u> National Geographic Society

Garrett, J.T. (2003). <u>The Cherokee Herbal.</u> Bear & Company. Rochester, Vermont

Mitchell, Faith. (1999). <u>Hoodoo Medicine.</u> Summerhouse Press. Columbia, South Carolina

Mitchem, Stephanie, Y. (2007). <u>African American Folk Healing.</u> New York University Press. New York, New York

Pinkney, Roger (2002). <u>Blue Roots.</u> Llewellyn Publication, St. Paul, Minnesota

Teish, Luisah (1988). <u>Jambalaya: The Natural Woman's Book of Personal Charms and Practical Rituals.</u> Harper Collins Publishers. New York, New York

Tenney, Louise. (1994). <u>Health Handbook.</u> Woodland Books. Pleasant Grove, Utah

Yronwode, Catherine (2002). <u>Hoodoo Herb and Root Magic,</u> The Lucky Mojo Curio Company, Forestville, CA

Online Sources

Annies remedies - herbs for self healing: Annies remedy A-Z medicinal herb chart. (n.d.). *Annie's Remedy website.* Retrieved 2012-2015 from http://www.anniesremedy.com/

Grieve, M., edited by Leyel, Hilda. Plant & Herb Index. Botanical.com: A Modern Herbal. (n.d.). *Botanical.com website.* Retrieved 2012-2015 from http://botanical.com/botanical/mgmh/comindx.html

Herbs In Alphabetical Order. Herbs2000: A practical guide for nutritional and traditional healthcare website. (n.d.). *Herbs2000 website.* Retrieved 2012-2015 from http://www.herbs2000.com/

Herbs: Alphabetical directory of herbs. (n.d.). *Medicinal Herb Info website, Lynn DeVries.* Retrieved 2012-2015 from http://medicinalherbinfo.org/herbs/Herb-index.html

Herbs: Organicfacts. (n.d.) *Organicfacts.net website,* Organic Information Services Pvt Ltd. Retrieved 2013-2015 from https://www.organicfacts.net/

CPSIA information can be obtained
at www.ICGtesting.com
Printed in the USA
LVHW010027040721
691856LV00004B/16